Cancer of the
UTERUS

Cancer of the
UTERUS

edited by

GEORGE COUKOS, M.D., PH.D

Assistant Professor, Department of Obstetrics and Gynecology
Division of Gynecologic Oncology
Hospital of the University of Pennsylvania
and
Director, Gynecologic Malignancy Research Program
Abramson Family Cancer Research Institute
Philadelphia, Pennsylvania, U.S.A.

STEPHEN C. RUBIN, M.D.

Chief of the Division of Gynecologic Oncology
and
The Franklin Payne Professor of Obstetrics and Gynecology
University of Pennsylvania
Philadelphia, Pennsylvania, U.S.A.

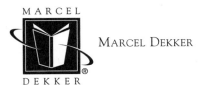

MARCEL DEKKER

NEW YORK

Library of Congress Cataloging-in-Publication Data
A catalog record for this book is available from the Library of Congress.

ISBN: 0-8247-5415-8

Marcel Dekker, 270 Madison Avenue, New York, NY 10016

Distribution Center
Marcel Dekker, Cimarron Road, Monticello, New York 12701, U.S.A.

To Alessandra, Dimitri and Alex
G.C.

To Anne, Mike and Ellie
S.C.R.

Preface

Cancers of the uterine corpus represent the most common gynecologic malignancies, with an estimated yearly incidence of 40,000 new cases in the United States, which is among the highest worldwide. A substantial increase in uterine cancers may be seen in the near future as a result of the epidemic of obesity and diabetes in the Western world. These statistics create a pressing need to understand the molecular basis of uterine cancers, improve their prevention and optimize their therapy.

We are extremely excited and humbled by the opportunity to invite a group of distinguished scientists and clinicians to discuss systematically the important basic, translational and clinical advances made in this field and review the many controversies still surrounding the management of uterine cancers. Dr. Goodfellow and colleagues discuss the current understanding of the molecular events underlying endometrial cancer and the identification of two distinct molecular phenotypes of endometrial cancer. Dr. Bandera reviews the role of the environmental and genetic factors modulating the risk of uterine cancer and discusses the counseling of women at risk for uterine cancer based on molecular epidemiology data. The molecular characterization of uterine cancers has unveiled novel targets for molecular therapy. Dr. Coukos and colleagues discuss these in relation to current compounds emerging from the industry pipeline. Understanding endometrial cancer and uterine sarcomas at the molecular level forces a rethinking of their pathologic classification, as it will be discussed by Drs. Kurman and colleagues and Dr.

Kempson, respectively. Although the role of steroid hormones in the pathogenesis of endometrial neoplasia is well established, the significance of steroid receptors as prognostic or disease classification biomarkers guiding therapy remains controversial and is discussed by Dr. Leslie and colleagues. Finally, Dr. Barakat reviews the effects of tamoxifen and other selective estrogen receptor modulators on the uterus and the management of patients receiving these drugs.

Important controversies remain in the clinical management of uterine cancers. Dr. Cooper and colleagues review the work up and management of abnormal uterine bleeding, while Dr. Randall and Bowman argue the case of conservative management of early endometrial cancer and its precursor lesions. Dr. Chu reviews the prognostic factors affecting outcome in patients with early stage endometrial cancer and discusses the rationale for surgical staging and different surgical approaches to define the optimal surgical management of early endometrial cancer. The public demand for minimally invasive surgical approaches has created a pressing need to define the value of laparoscopic approaches to uterine cancer surgery. Dr. Walker and colleagues review these issues in detail and present outcome evidence from recent studies.

Although high survival rates are attainable in early stage endometrial cancer, approximately 20% of newly diagnosed patients will have regional or distant spread of disease. Dr. Bristow and colleagues discuss the rationale and outcomes relevant to primary cytoreductive surgery for patients with stage III and IV disease. In addition, they review the recent literature addressing the surgical management of uterine papillary serous carcinoma, making the case that this histotype warrants aggressive management even in early stage.

One of the most controversial topics in the field of gynecologic oncology is the postoperative management of patients with endometrial cancer and uterine sarcomas. Dr. Grisby reviews radiation therapy recommendations for patients who are surgically staged and for those who have incomplete surgical staging, based on the results of existing prospective randomized studies or retrospective studies. He also describes the use of irradiation alone for medically inoperable patients and provide the techniques for both external irradiation and high dose rate brachytherapy.

The restored life expectancy of patients with early stage uterine cancer poses important questions on the safety of estrogen replacement therapy in this population. Dr. Runowicz and colleagues review the risks and benefits of estrogen replacement therapy in endometrial cancer survivors.

Recurrence is not uncommon in patients presenting initially with high risk early stage or advanced disease. There is a recognized role for surgery in carefully selected patients. Dr. Penalver and colleagues review the indications, technique, outcome, and complications of exenterative surgery for recurrent endometrial cancer in previously irradiated patients, and discuss palliative surgery approaches. In addition, Dr. Lu and colleagues discuss the medical management of recurrent endometrial cancer, reviewing the evidence on chemotherapy and hormonal therapy. Finally, Dr. Harris and colleagues review the postoperative radiation treatment of advanced and recurrent endometrial carcinoma, discuss palliative radiation therapy, and discuss the role of high dose radiation in this setting.

Uterine sarcomas represent a challenging group of tumors owing to their rarity and heterogeneity. Dr. Sutton and colleagues review the management of mixed müllerian mesodermal tumors, endometrial stromal sarcoma and leiomyosarcoma. They discuss the role of staging for apparently early disease and that of debulking for advanced sarcomas. They also discuss adjuvant therapies for early stage disease and the management of advanced disease.

We are grateful to all colleagues, friends, and authors for their time, wisdom, and technical expertise. We hope that this monograph will fill an important gap in the field of translational and clinical gynecologic oncology and provides the reader useful information for the management of these tumors.

George Coukos
Stephen C. Rubin

Acknowledgments

The editors gratefully acknowledge Jerry and Lucille Francesco and the St. Martha Foundation for their generous support of our translational research program in gynecologic cancers. We would also like to acknowledge Carmen Lord, our editorial assistant, for her tireless efforts on behalf of this text.

Contents

Preface . . . . *v*
Acknowledgments . . . . *ix*

1. Molecular Genetics of Uterine Malignancies *1*
Paul J. Goodfellow
Introduction *1*
Genetic and Environmental Factors *3*
Summary *17*
References *19*

2. Endometrial Cancer in the Hereditary
   Nonpolyposis Colorectal Cancer Syndrome *35*
Christina A. Bandera
Introduction *35*
Clinical and Pathologic Features of
      HNPCC-Related Cancers *36*
Genetic Basis of HNPCC *39*
Identifying the HNPCC Syndrome *40*
Counseling Regarding Screening and Prevention *44*
Conclusion *47*
References *48*

3. Steroid Hormone Receptors in the Normal
   Endometrium and in Endometrial Cancer *53*
Kimberly K. Leslie, Suzy Davies, Meenakshi Singh,
and Harriet O. Smith
Introduction: Endometrial Cancer and the Link to
      Steroid Hormones and Steroid Receptors *53*

Hormone Receptors in the Normal Endometrium *54*
Hormonal Effects and Hormone Receptors in
    Endometrial Cancer *56*
Ligand Binding Assays and Immunohistochemistry
    to Determine Steroid Receptor Status *58*
Cross-Talk and Expression in Endometrial Glands
    and Stroma *61*
Genomic Effects of SRs *62*
Receptor Isoforms *63*
Non-Genomic Effects of Steroid Hormones Through
    Membrane and Cytosolic Receptors *67*
References *68*

**4. The Effects of Tamoxifen on
    the Endometrium** **79**
Richard R. Barakat
Introduction *79*
Endometrial Carcinoma *80*
Histology of Tamoxifen-Associated
    Uterine Cancer *82*
The Role of Screening *86*
References *90*

**5. Pathology of Endometrial Hyperplasia
    and Carcinoma** **93**
*Brigitte M. Ronnett, Jeffrey D. Seidman, Richard J. Zaino,
Lora Hedrick Ellenson, and Robert J. Kurman*
Classification *93*
Precursors of Endometrial Carcinoma *96*
Endometrioid Carcinoma *108*
Serous Carcinoma *124*
Clear Cell Carcinoma *131*
Mixed Types of Carcinoma *133*
Malignant Mesodermal Mixed Tumor
    (MMMT)/Carcinosarcoma *134*
Undifferentiated Carcinoma *136*
Molecular Genetics of Endometrial Cancer *136*
References *142*

6. Pathology of Uterine Sarcomas *149*
Michael R. Hendrickson, Teri A. Longacre,
and Richard L. Kempson
Classification of Uterine Mesenchymal, Mixed
    Mesenchymal, and Epithelial Neoplasms *149*
Endometrial Stromal Sarcoma (ESS) *150*
Uterine Neoplasms with Sex Cord-like Elements *158*
Leiomyosarcoma *162*
Undifferentiated ESS *170*
Miscellaneous Pure Sarcomas *171*
Mixed Müllerian Neoplasms *171*
Adenosarcoma *172*
Carcinosarcoma *176*
References *180*

**7. Clinical Evaluation of Abnormal
    Uterine Bleeding** *195*
Jay M. Cooper and Barbara J. Stegmann
Definition *195*
History and Physical Examination *196*
Etiology *197*
Diagnosis *206*
References *223*

**8. Conservative Treatment of Endometrial
    Hyperplasia and Early Endometrial Cancer** .. *229*
Genesis Bowen and Thomas Randall
Introduction *229*
Clinical Characteristics *230*
Progestin Therapy *232*
Anticipation of Treatment Failure *237*
Treatment Regimens *240*
References *242*

**9. The Surgical Management of Early
    Endometrial Cancer** *245*
Christina S. Chu
Introduction *245*

Staging *246*
Prognostic Factors *248*
Surgical Approaches *260*
Conclusions *263*
References *264*

**10. The Role of Laparoscopy in the Management
     of Endometrial Cancer 275**
Joan L. Walker and Robert S. Mannel
Demand for Laparoscopic Surgery *275*
Surgical Techniques for Laparoscopic Treatment of
     Endometrial Cancer *280*
Current Treatment Algorithms Utilizing Laparoscopy
     in EC *284*
Surgical Candidate Selection *284*
Training *288*
Potential Benefits of Laparoscopic Surgery *289*
Complications of Laparoscopy *291*
References *297*

**11. The Role of Primary Surgery in Advanced
     Endometrial Cancer 305**
Robert E. Bristow and F.J. Montz
Introduction *305*
Theoretical Basis for Cytoreductive Surgery *306*
Stage III Endometrial Cancer *307*
Stage IV Endometrial Cancer *312*
Uterine Papillary Serous Carcinoma/
     Cancer (UPSC) *317*
Conclusion *320*
References *320*

**12.   Surgical Management of Recurrent
     Endometrial Cancer 327**
Nicholas Lambrou, Luis Mendez, and Manuel Penalver
Introduction *327*
Pelvic Exenteration *329*
Palliation *337*
References *338*

13. Radiation Treatment for Early Stage Endometrial Cancer and Uterine Sarcoma *343*
Perry W. Grigsby
Introduction *343*
Endometrial Cancer *345*
Uterine Sarcoma *354*
Endometrial Stromal Sarcoma *358*
Technique of External Irradiation *360*
Techniques for HDR Brachytherapy *361*
References *362*

14. Radiation Treatment of Advanced or Recurrent Endometrial Cancer *367*
Eleanor E. R. Harris
Role of Radiation Therapy for Stage III–IV EC *368*
Radiation Therapy for Pelvic Recurrence *382*
Radiation Therapy for Medically Inoperable Patients *390*
References *397*

15. Systemic Therapies for Endometrial Carcinoma *407*
Brian M. Slomovitz and Karen H. Lu
Endometrioid Endometrial Carcinoma (EEC) *408*
Hormonal Therapy *413*
Uterine Papillary Serous Carcinoma (UPSC) *417*
Molecular Therapies *420*
Summary *421*
References *421*

16. Targeted Therapy of Endometrial Cancer *435*
David O. Holtz, Ronald Buckanovic, and George Coukos
Introduction *435*
Epidermal Growth Factor Receptors *436*
Transforming Growth Factors *440*
PTEN–PI3 kinase *441*
Angiogenesis *444*
Invasion and Metastasis *451*
Conclusions *454*
References *454*

17. Management of Uterine Sarcomas **471**
Gregory Sutton and Heidi J. Gray
Epidemiology and Incidence *471*
Prognostic Factors *473*
Surgical Staging of Uterine Sarcomas *474*
Adjuvant Chemotherapy in Early Uterine
    Sarcomas *477*
Adjuvant Radiotherapy in Uterine Sarcomas *479*
Palliative Chemotherapy in Uterine Sarcomas *480*
Hormonal Therapy in Uterine Sarcomas *485*
Multimodality Adjuvant Therapy *486*
References *487*

18. Hormone Replacement in the Patient with
    Uterine Cancer **495**
Kathleen Lin and Carolyn D. Runowicz
Conclusion *503*
References *504*

Index *507*

Contributors

Christina A. Bandera
Harvard Medical School, Brigham and Women's Hospital, Boston, Massachusetts, U.S.A.

Richard R. Barakat
Memorial Sloan-Kettering Cancer Center, New York, New York, U.S.A.

Genesis Bowen
Pennsylvania Hospital, Philadelphia, Pennsylvania, U.S.A.

Robert E. Bristow
The Johns Hopkins Medical Institutions, Baltimore, Maryland, U.S.A.

Ronald Buckanovec
Hospital of the University of Pennsylvania, Philadelphia, Pennsylvania, U.S.A.

Christina S. Chu
University of Pennsylvania Medical Center, Philadelphia, Pennsylvania, U.S.A.

Jay M. Cooper
University of Arizona School of Medicine, Phoenix, Arizona, U.S.A.

George Coukos
Hospital of the University of Pennsylvania, Philadelphia, Pennsylvania, U.S.A.

Suzy Davies
The University of New Mexico Health Sciences Center,
Albuquerque, New Mexico, U.S.A.

Lora Hedrick Ellenson
Weill Medical College of Cornell University New York
Hospital–Cornell Medical College, New York,
New York, U.S.A.

Paul J. Goodfellow
Washington University School of Medicine, St. Louis,
Missouri, U.S.A.

Heidi J. Gray
University of Pennsylvania Medical Center, Philadelphia,
Pennsylvania, U.S.A

Perry W. Grigsby
Washington University Medical Center, St. Louis, Missouri,
U.S.A.

Eleanor E. R. Harris
University of Pennsylvania, Philadelphia, Pennsylvania,
U.S.A

Michael R. Hendrickson
Stanford University Medical Center, Stanford, California,
U.S.A.

David O. Holtz
Hospital of the University of Pennsylvania, Philadelphia,
Pennsylvania, U.S.A.

Richard L. Kempson
Stanford University Medical Center, Stanford, California,
U.S.A.

Robert J. Kurman
The Johns Hopkins University School of Medicine
and The Johns Hopkins Hospitals, Baltimore, Maryland,
U.S.A.

Nicholas Lambrou
University of Miami School of Medicine, Miami, Florida,
U.S.A.

Kimberly K. Leslie
The University of New Mexico Health Sciences Center,
Albuquerque, New Mexico, U.S.A

Kathleen Lin
New York Presbyterian Hospital/New York Weill Cornell
Center, New York, New York, U.S.A.

Terry A. Longacre
Stanford University Medical Center, Stanford, California,
U.S.A.

Karen H. Lu
University of Texas, M.D. Anderson Cancer Center, Houston,
Texas, U.S.A.

Robert S. Mannel
University of Oklahoma, Oklahoma City, Oklahoma, U.S.A.

Luis Mendez
University of Miami School of Medicine, Miami, Florida,
U.S.A.

F.J. Montz
The Johns Hopkins Medical Institutions, Baltimore,
Maryland, U.S.A.

Manuel Penalver
University of Miami School of Medicine, Miami, Florida,
U.S.A.

Thomas Randall
Pennsylvania Hospital, Philadelphia, Pennsylvania,
U.S.A.

Brigitte M. Ronnett
The Johns Hopkins University School of Medicine and The
Johns Hopkins Hospital, Baltimore, Maryland, U.S.A.

Carolyn D. Runowicz
St. Luke's-Roosevelt Hospital Center and Women's Health
Service Line of Continuum Health Partners, Inc., New York,
New York, U.S.A.

Jeffrey D. Seidman
Washington Hospital Center, Washington, D.C., U.S.A.

Meenakshi Singh
University of Colorado Health Sciences Center, Denver, Colorado, U.S.A.

Brian M. Slomovitz
University of Texas, M.D. Anderson Cancer Center, Houston, Texas, U.S.A.

Harriet O. Smith
The University of New Mexico Health Sciences Center, Albuquerque, New Mexico, U.S.A.

Barbara J. Stegmann
Phoenix Integrated Residency in Obstetrics and Gynecology, Phoenix, Arizona, U.S.A.

Gregory Sutton
St. Vincent Hospitals and Health Services, Indianapolis, Indiana, U.S.A.

Joan L. Walker
University of Oklahoma, Oklahoma City, Oklahoma, U.S.A.

Richard J. Zaino
The Milton S. Hershey Medical Center, Pennsylvania State University, Hershey, Pennsylvania, U.S.A.

Cancer of the
UTERUS

1

Molecular Genetics of Uterine Malignancies

PAUL J. GOODFELLOW
Washington University School of Medicine,
St. Louis, Missouri, U.S.A.

INTRODUCTION

Cancers of the uterine corpus represent the most common gynecologic malignancy in the United States with an estimated
39,300 new cases in 2002 (1). The incidence in the United States
is among the highest worldwide (2) with the majority of uterine
cancers being adenocarcinomas. Sarcomas (leiomyosarcomas,
stromal sarcomas, and mixed malignant müllerian tumors), on
the other hand, make up a small fraction of the uterine cancers
in North America. Among the adenocarcinomas, the endometrioid subtype is the most common. Endometrioid adenocarcinomas are associated with a variety of risk factors, many of which
directly or indirectly influence estrogen levels, and as such have

an effect on endometrial proliferation. Exposure to exogenous estrogen, a family history of cancer, race, obesity, hypertension, low parity, and late menopause have all been associated with increased risk for endometrial cancer (3). Endometrioid adenocarcinomas frequently arise on a background of abnormal uterine proliferation or endometrial hyperplasia. In a large prospective study it was demonstrated that if untreated, patients with atypical endometrial hyperplasia had a high risk for developing endometrial carcinoma (4). It is now generally accepted that endometrial hyperplasias represent precursor lesions for endometrioid carcinoma. The endometrioid, estrogen-related tumors have been designated Type I endometrial carcinoma (5–7), and are histologically similar to the normal endometrium. Architectural complexity, cytologic atypia and stromal invasion are the hallmarks of endometrioid adenocarcinoma. In general, Type I tumors are more frequent in younger endometrial cancer patients, are often low-grade (well-differentiated), low-stage (confined to the uterus) tumors and hold a good prognosis.

The second major group of endometrial carcinomas— Type II carcinomas—generally have a poorer prognosis, appear unrelated to estrogenic stimulation, are of higher grade and stage, and manifest at a later age. The majority of Type II tumors are histologically classified as serous carcinoma, showing striking nuclear atypia and either a glandular or papillary architecture (8). The serous cancers of the endometrium usually appear on an atrophic endometrium, and it has recently been proposed that they arise from a histologically recognizable precursor referred to as endometrial intraepithelial carcinoma (9). This distinguishes them from the endometrioid tumors, which are often seen on hyperplastic endometrium. It is important to note that not all Type II tumors are uterine papillary serous carcinomas. There are other histologic variants including clear cell, mucinous, and other carcinomas that are potentially under-diagnosed because of lack of familiarity with these uncommon subtypes.

The differences in epidemiology, presentation, and behavior between Type I and Type II endometrial carcinomas are paralleled by differences in the molecular defects seen in these lesions. Most molecular studies have been focused on endometrioid or Type I tumors, largely because of the relative abundance of these cancers. In some studies different histologic subtypes have been combined, and as a consequence, differences between Type I and II may have been overlooked. What has become evident in recent years is that when the molecular defects seen in different histologic subtypes of uterine cancers are compared, there are mutations or molecular signatures that are characteristic of Type I and II carcinomas.

The genetics and biology of cancer have been reviewed recently (10,11). In this chapter the role that oncogenes, tumor suppressors, and DNA mismatch repair genes play in uterine cancers is discussed. We have entered into an era in which molecular and cancer genetics hold great promise for providing new insights into the fundamentals of cancer biology. A greater understanding of the molecular biology of uterine malignancies will bring new approaches to the prevention, detection, and treatment of these diseases.

GENETIC AND ENVIRONMENTAL FACTORS

Tumorigenesis is a multi-step process. Both environmental and genetic factors contribute to the development of uterine cancers, and it is generally accepted that an accumulation of genetic insults is necessary for tumor formation. Defects in three main classes of "cancer genes" are seen in uterine malignancies: activation of oncogenes, silencing of DNA repair genes, and inactivation of tumor suppressor genes. Most of these genetic alterations are somatic, having arisen in the cancer cell or its precursors. In some cases, inherited mutations contribute substantially to the disease process.

Mutation in a single copy of an oncogene is usually sufficient to bring about a change in cell growth. Tumor suppressor and DNA repair genes come into play when their functions are lost. Both copies of tumor suppressor or DNA repair genes are mutated or silenced in cancers. As defects in these three main classes of cancer-promoting genes accumulate, the growth properties of the mutant cell and its progeny change. For some tumors, there is a recognizable progression from normal to a precancerous state, and finally on to frank cancer. The concept of genotypic and phenotypic progression is illustrated in Figure 1.

Inherited Risk

The vast majority of women with uterine cancers have what would be typically be classified as "sporadic" disease. In such cases, inherited genetic factors play a small or negligible role in determining a woman's risk for developing endometrial

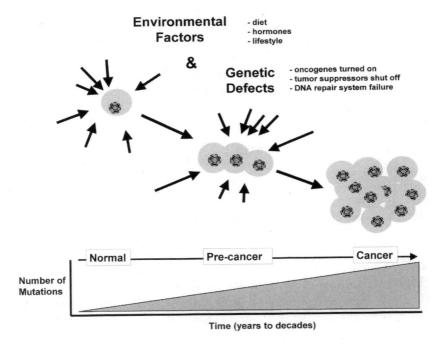

Figure 1. Genotypic and phenotypic progression in the development of a cancer. A predictable pattern of phenotypic progression is seen in some uterine adenocarcinomas. Atypical endometrial hyperplasia is a histologically recognized precursor of endometrioid adenocarcinomas and may be preceded by forms of hyperplasia that lack nuclear atypia. Endometrial intraepithelial carcinoma is a precursor to papillary serous cancers (12). Only a few of the genetic defects that result in uterine cancers are known, and even less is known about when specific mutations arise.

cancer. Environmental factors, perhaps the most important of which are hormonal, contribute substantially to the disease process but no more so than mutations and other changes in the genetic makeup of long-lived uterine cells.

The best understood inherited form of endometrial cancer occurs in the context of hereditary nonpolyposis colorectal cancer (HNPCC). HNPCC (or Lynch syndrome) is a dominantly inherited cancer susceptibility syndrome. Mutations in genes responsible for repair of DNA mismatches increase the risk among HNPCC family members for colon and a variety of other malignancies including endometrial, ovarian, urinary tract, and small bowel cancers (13–15). Endometrial carcinoma is the most common extracolonic malignancy in this disorder, and a female HNPCC mutation carrier has a lifetime risk for endometrial carcinoma that approaches 40% (16). Inherited mutations in four different mismatch repair genes have been shown to result in HNPCC: MLH1, MSH2, MSH6, and PMS2. A fifth DNA repair gene (MLH3) has also been implicated in HNPCC (17). Between 50% and 75% of patients with a clinical diagnosis of HNPCC (18,19) have mutations in a known DNA mismatch repair gene. At this time it is unclear whether there are additional yet unidentified HNPCC-causing genes.

Tumors that arise in individuals with HNPCC typically lack DNA mismatch repair. In these cancers both copies of a DNA repair gene are defective. One mutation is inherited and the second is somatic or acquired. The absence of DNA repair gene products (MLH1, MSH2, and MSH6) can be assessed by immunohistochemistry, or a general defect in DNA repair can be demonstrated through the analysis of repetitive sequences. Loss of mismatch repair function in the tumor leads to somatic DNA replication errors and a marked instability of microsatellite repeats. The so-called microsatellite instability (MSI) is seen in greater than 90% of colorectal cancers and approximately 75% of endometrial cancers in HNPCC family members with MLH1 and MSH2 mutations (20,21). MSH6 mutation appears to be associated with an overall lower rate of MSI in tumors and a high frequency of endometrial cancer or atypical endometrial hyperplasia in mutation carriers (22–25).

The clear association between DNA mismatch repair gene mutation and cancer risk led to clinical recommendations for surveillance (26). The benefits of colonic surveillance for members of HNPCC families has been documented, and colonoscopy at 18- to 24-month intervals beginning at age 25 to 30 is recommended (26). A recommendation for endometrial screening beginning between ages 25 and 30 has been made, but the optimal methods for screening and the clinical benefit of endometrial surveillance are not yet well established (26).

The criteria used to diagnose HNPCC are rather stringent, and in most families the three cardinal features of inherited cancer susceptibility are present: early age-of-onset, synchronous and metachronous cancers, and multiple closely related affected family members. By focusing on one of two of the features that are characteristic of genetic disease, several investigators have shown a further association between defects in DNA mismatch repair and endometrial carcinoma. Parc and colleagues studied tumors for MSI and family histories of endometrial cancer patients with early onset disease (27). Among the patients investigated were individuals who fulfilled the HNPCC diagnostic criteria and others who had relatives affected with colon cancer but who could not be classified as having HNPCC. DNA mismatch repair mutation analysis was not performed. In a study by Millar and colleagues (28) 40 women who had double primary cancers of the colorectum and endometrium were studied, with 7 of the 40 cases having a mutation in either MSH2 or MLH1. Six of the seven mutation-positive probands had a family history consistent with HNPCC. Although the study by Millar and colleagues pointed to a role for MSH2 in HNPCC risk and endometrial cancer, the MSH6 gene was not evaluated. As noted, mutations in MSH6 may be important in endometrial cancer–prone HNPCC families, and the frequency of HNPCC mutations in such families may be higher than currently appreciated (25). This observation could ultimately influence what approaches are taken to identify patients and families with HNPCC. Some groups have recommended that evaluating tumors for MSI might be useful in establishing a diagnosis of HNPCC (29,30). When the recommendations were made, however, the relationship between MSH6 mutation, endometrial cancer risk, and low levels of MSI was not apparent. For endometrial cancer–prone families, tumor MSI may not be such an important predictor of HNPCC. A population-based series reported by Cederquist et al. (2001) confirmed the risk for familial disease in patients with double primary cancers (colorectal and endometrial, or two colorectal carcinomas) and a higher risk for inherited susceptibility in cases with early-onset, MSI-positive tumors. The importance of considering MSH6 in cases with MSI-negative tumors was noted by these authors (31).

The study of rare inherited forms of cancer brought to light the overall importance of the loss of DNA mismatch repair in endometrial cancers (see below). The clinical implications of an inherited defect leading to endometrial cancers should not be underestimated. The endometrial cancer patient with inherited susceptibility is at a substantially increased risk for colorectal and other HNPCC-associated malignancies. Furthermore, her relatives are at increased risk for these tumors as well. Although only a small fraction of endometrial carcinoma patients are likely to have a DNA mismatch repair gene mutation, this group of women can serve as windows to families whose members would clearly benefit from intensified surveillance and/or intervention. Where the responsibility for identifying and caring for these at-risk family members lies is a matter of debate.

In addition to the HNPCC-associated inherited endometrial cancer, there have been reports of familial site-specific endometrial carcinoma (32,33). It seems likely that if such a disorder exists, it is very uncommon.

There is a single report of what may be familial inherited susceptibility to uterine sarcoma. Launonen and colleagues (2001) identified a region on the long arm of chromosome 1 that is linked to risk for uterine leiomyoma and renal carcinoma in two families (34). Two affected family members had uterine leiomyosarcomas. Clearly, if an inherited form of leiomyosarcoma exists, it is very rare. This region of chromosome 1 (1q42–q44) is not a frequent site of deletion in sporadic leiomyosarcomas (35,36) and the role that the 1q gene or genes plays in these tumors is uncertain.

Familial breast cancer susceptibility genes were suggested to increase risk for endometrial cancers (37,38). However, when Levine and colleagues assessed the constitutional DNA of 199 consecutive Ashkenazi Jewish patients with endometrial cancers, they saw no increase in three BRCA founder mutations (39). A recent study by Geisler and colleagues demonstrated an association between breast and uterine papillary serous carcinoma (40). In a consecutive series of 592 endometrial cancer patients, 37 women had synchronous or metachronous breast cancer. Whereas only 3% of the patients with endometrioid adenocarcinomas had breast cancer, 25% of the patients with uterine papillary serous carcinoma had breast cancers. This association may reflect genetic and/or environmental risk factors that link breast and uterine cancer.

The PTEN tumor suppressor gene is frequently mutated in sporadic endometrial tumors (see below). Inherited PTEN mutations are associated with Cowden Syndrome, an uncommon disorder in which affected females have high risk for thyroid and breast cancers (41,42). Mutation carriers are also at risk for multiple early-onset uterine leiomyoma (43). Although there are families in which PTEN mutation carriers have developed uterine cancers (44), an association between inherited PTEN mutation and increased risk for endometrial carcinoma has not been established.

In summary, a small fraction of women with uterine cancers develop disease because of a major inherited genetic susceptibility. The syndromes and genes associated with inherited uterine cancer are summarized in Table 1. The true incidence of "inherited" cancers of the uterine corpus is not known, but as many as 5% of women with endometrial cancer have features suggestive of an underlying genetic susceptibility. Despite the rarity of clear inherited forms of disease, it is important that physicians, patients, and relatives of cancer patients be aware that genetic risk for endometrial and other cancers exists. In families with inherited cancer susceptibility, appropriate cancer education and surveillance could lead to a reduction in cancer morbidity and mortality.

Sporadic Cancers: Acquired Genetic Changes

As noted previously, many changes in the genetic makeup of a cell are required for the onset of cancer. In this section some of the major defects seen in uterine cancers are reviewed and the impact that such changes have on the cell's behavior discussed. Rather than serving as a catalogue of all the molecular defects that have been reported for this group of malignancies, this section highlights the most common or best understood of the molecular changes seen in uterine cancers. Representatives of the three major classes of "cancer genes"—DNA repair genes, tumor suppressors, and oncogenes—are discussed.

DNA Mismatch Repair Defects

Uterine cancers acquire defects in DNA mismatch repair, with approximately 25% of endometrial cancers defective in DNA mismatch repair. This is not surprising in light of the fact that inherited mutations in DNA mismatch repair genes confer a high risk for the development of endometrial cancer. There are relatively few reports on defective DNA mismatch repair in uterine sarcomas and it appears to be far less frequent in these cancers than in endometrial carcinomas (45). The loss of normal DNA repair function is actually more frequent in endometrial cancers than any other common human malignancy. Defective DNA mismatch is more common in endometrioid adenocarcinomas than the other less frequently seen histologic variants (46–49). The inability to correct strand mispairing during replication leads to frequent deletion or insertion in repetitive DNA sequences and a molecular phenotype in tumors referred to as microsatellite instability (MSI). The MSI phenotype in endometrial cancers is illustrated in Figure 2.

When a cell loses its ability to repair DNA errors, it accumulates mutations at an accelerated rate. Loeb (50,51) proposed that acquiring a mutator phenotype might be an early and necessary step in tumor formation. It is widely accepted that in a population of tumor cells there is continuous selection for mutations that provide a competitive advantage. The frequency at which defective DNA mismatch repair is seen in

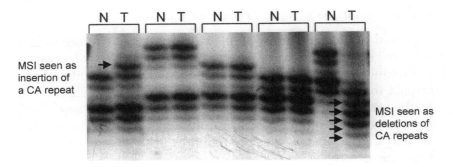

Figure 2. MSI in endometrioid endometrial carcinomas. Polymerase chain reaction amplification of D17S250 repeat sequences reveals defective DNA mismatch repair. Tumors with defective DNA repair show aberrant PCR products. Tumors with normal DNA repair, on the other hand, have the same DNA patterns as the patient's normal DNA. Normal cellular (N) and tumor (T) DNA from five patients are analyzed side by side. Arrowheads indicate abnormal PCR products in tumor DNA that result from mutations in repetitive sequences.

endometrial cancers (approximately 25%) suggests that loss of DNA repair confers a specific advantage to the tumor cells. The most straightforward explanation for the selective advantage is that loss of DNA repair provides the mutator phenotype, and with that a greater repertoire of gene mutations in a continuously evolving tumor cell population. In endometrial cancers, however, the genes that accumulate mutations because of the loss of DNA repair remain elusive (52). Although the PTEN tumor suppressor (see below) and several other genes may be particularly prone to mutations that would accumulate in cells lacking DNA mismatch repair (52–57), selection for loss of mismatch repair in endometrial cancer may go beyond the mutator phenotype. Recent work from Gradia et al. and Fishel and colleagues provides a second explanation for why loss of DNA mismatch repair may be so frequent in some tumor types (58–60). Mismatch repair proteins theoretically function as molecular sensors that connect signaling pathways and the nucleus to direct the repair of DNA damage or to elicit cell death (61). Loss of this molecular sensor function could provide the endometrial cancer cell with a growth and/or survival advantage.

Endometrial cancer MSI is most frequently associated with loss of the MLH1 mismatch repair protein (62,63). Approximately 75% of sporadic (nonfamilial) MSI-positive endometrial cancers have methylation of the MLH1 promoter (52,62,64). Methylation of key sequences in the 5' regulatory region of the MLH1 gene is a so-called "epigenetic" change that serves either to silence transcription or to maintain an inactive state once established. Somatic mutations in MLH1 and other DNA repair genes are infrequent in MSI-positive endometrial cancers (65–69).

MSI is an early event in endometrial tumorigenesis. The molecular phenotype is seen in atypical endometrial hyperplasia and simple hyperplasia (54,70–72). In a study of hyperplasia concomitant with carcinoma, Horowitz and colleagues (73) observed hyperplasias in which the MLH1 gene was methylated but did not show MSI. Immunohistochemical studies suggested that loss of MLH1 expression is an early event, occurring before the appearance of atypia (73). The observed methylation in MSI-negative tissues and loss of expression in proliferative but nonmalignant endometrium is reminiscent of the absence of MLH1 staining in normal colonic epithelium from patients with colorectal cancer (74).

The clinical implications of MLH1 analysis using immunohistochemical or DNA methods to detect precancerous lesions and to distinguish benign from precancerous proliferation in the endometrium is yet to be determined.

The relationship between the MSI phenotype and a variety of histopathologic and clinical features in endometrial cancers has been investigated. As noted, MSI is seen primarily in endometrioid (Type I) tumors. There is no consistent association between MSI and outcome in endometrial cancers. In some studies MSI is associated with a favorable prognosis, while in others it is of no prognostic significance or is associated with poor outcome (75–78). Studies in cancer cell lines with defective DNA mismatch repair and in colorectal cancer patients with MSI-positive tumors suggest that loss of mismatch repair could influence how the tumor cell responds to chemo- or radiation therapy (79–82). However, there have been no reports to date in which the relationship between DNA mismatch repair status and response to adjuvant therapies has been assessed in endometrial cancers.

Failures in other DNA repair processes are likely to contribute to the development of uterine cancers. It is appealing to suggest that defects in base-excision or double strand break repair come into play in uterine sarcomas or Type II endometrial adenocarcinomas that have normal DNA mismatch repair. DNA repair is an important factor in cancer cell response to many of the adjuvant therapies used to treat advanced or recurrent uterine cancers. A better understanding of DNA repair function in uterine cancers might help guide the development and use of DNA damaging agents for the treatment of these malignancies.

Tumor Suppressor Gene Defects

A number of tumor suppressors have been shown to contribute to the genesis of uterine cancers. The TP53 gene is mutated in a wide range of malignancies. Loss of TP53 in the cancer cell confers a survival advantage. Normal processes required for the detection of DNA damage, cell cycle arrest, and DNA repair depend upon TP53 function. Cancer cells that lack TP53 continue to divide despite the presence of DNA damage. Furthermore, cells lacking TP53 have a general apoptotic failure: Cancer cells that otherwise would undergo programmed cell death survive.

TP53 mutations are seen in both uterine adenocarcinomas and sarcomas. Approximately 50% of sarcomas have TP53 mutations (83,84). The frequency of TP53 mutation in adenocarcinomas varies with histologic subtype. Whereas most uterine serous carcinomas have TP53 mutations (85–87), the rate of mutation in endometrioid cancers is considerably lower, ranging from 10–30% (88,89). TP53 mutation is therefore an example of a molecular feature that distinguishes Type I and II cancers. Some investigators have argued that, in tumors that are defective in DNA mismatch repair, mutations in BAX, a promoter of cell death, might explain the low frequency of TP53 mutation. In particular, Type I tumors (endometrioid adenocarcinomas) with defects in DNA mismatch repair might be expected to acquire mutations in the coding sequence repeats of BAX. The observation that somatic frameshift mutations in BAX were seen in colon cancers with MSI provided a basis for the investigation of endometrial carcinomas (90). Frameshift mutations in BAX are indeed frequent in MSI-positive endometrial cancers (52,91). Studies by Catasus and colleagues, however, failed to provide evidence for consistent inactivation of both alleles or selection for BAX defects in endometrial carcinomas (92). Furthermore, in a study of 25 MSI-positive and 25 MSI-negative endometrioid adenocarcinomas matched for grade, stage, and patient race, the frequency of TP53 mutation was similar in the two groups of tumor (89), bringing into question the apparent inverse relationship between tumor MSI and TP53 mutation.

The PTEN tumor suppressor gene is arguably the most frequently mutated gene in uterine cancers (93). PTEN encodes a cytoplasmic protein/lipid phosphatase, the main substrate for which is phosphatidylinositol (3,4,5) triphosphate (PIP-3). Accumulation of PIP-3 at the cell membrane leads to recruitment of members of the Akt serine/theronine kinase family (94). Activation of Akt has effects on cell survival at the levels of apoptosis and the regulation of other genes (95,96). Not only is PTEN mutated in endometrial carcinoma, it also appears to be a very early event (54,97). Work from the laboratory of Mutter and colleagues (98,99) has shown that PTEN expression is absent in a large fraction of endometrioid adenocarcinomas and is also missing in abnormally proliferative glands. Interestingly, PTEN defects are more common in early stage disease than more advanced endometrial cancers. The prognostic significance of PTEN mutation and/or lack of expression in endometrial carcinoma and association with race, stage, and grade are unclear (100–102). The relationship between PTEN inactivation and defects in DNA mismatch repair (the MSI phenotype) are similarly unclear. Several investigators have suggested that PTEN mutations are more frequent in cancers with MSI

(53–56,103). The preponderance of mutations involved coding sequence repeats (strings of A_5 and A_6) in MSI-positive tumors seems to account for most mutations in PTEN. However, in one study, the frequency and distribution of PTEN mutation was similar in cancers with defects in DNA mismatch repair and mismatch repair–competent cancers matched for stage, grade, and race (104). One of the simplest explanations for the abundance of coding sequence repeat mutations in MSI-positive endometrial cancers is that repeat sequence mutations are secondary to defects in mismatch repair. The fact that not all cases with A_5 and A_6 repeat defects have a mutation in the second allele leaves open the question of whether all of these MSI-type mutations are functionally significant. Despite this uncertainty, PTEN is a key player in the development of uterine adenocarcinomas. In contrast to the high frequency of mutation that is seen in endometrioid adenocarcinomas, uterine sarcomas rarely show mutation in PTEN (105). PTEN is another example of a molecular lesion that distinguishes Type I and II cancers. The recent development of a mouse PTEN knockout animal has provided further evidence that PTEN function is important in protecting the endometrium from cancers. Mice lacking one copy of the PTEN gene develop endometrial hyperplasia (106).

A variety of other known and putative tumor suppressors have been studied in uterine cancers. Although mutations have been identified in some of these genes, or deletions of the chromosomal regions in which they lie has been seen in sizable fractions of the tumors studied, there are few candidates that are major contributors to the disease state. With these genes of uncertain significance, the overall rate of mutation is often low or varies substantially from one study to another, or the evidence for the gene's involvement is indirect. Indirect evidence for the involvement of a tumor suppressor is usually in the form of deletion of a large segment of the genome.

A tumor suppressor pathway recently recognized as important in endometrial carcinomas is the APC/beta-catenin (CTNNB1) signaling pathway. CTNNB1 is an example of a gene for which the reported rate of mutation varies considerably. Between 10% and 45% of endometrial adenocarcinomas have a mutation in CTNNB1. It is probable that confounding environmental or genetic factors lead to differences in rates of mutation seen in the various studies. In particular, the generally lower rate of mutation seen in Asian endometrial cancers suggests a role for other genetic or environmental effects. CTNNB1 mutation frequency does not seem to differ between cases with MSI (defective DNA mismatch repair) and those with normal DNA repair, suggesting that beta-catenin mutation is an important event overall in the genesis of endometrioid cancers (57,107–109). Immunohistochemical studies looking at the distribution of beta-catenin protein in the cancer cell reveal a higher frequency of defects in endometrioid tumors (110). Nuclear localization of beta-catenin is associated with mutation in the coding sequences and potentially MSI (107,111). However, in one study, the rate of CTNNB1 mutation was higher in tumors with normal DNA repair (57). At this time the absolute rates of mutation or disruption of the APC/beta-catenin signaling pathway in Type I and Type II cancers are not known.

The problems in interpreting the significance of indirect evidence for the involvement of tumor suppressors in uterine cancers are perhaps best addressed by a discussion of chromosome 10 deletions. Loss of heterozygosity (LOH) on the long arm of chromosome 10 is a frequent event in uterine cancers, with approximately 40% of cancers showing loss of a portion of 10q (112,113). It is presumed that deletion of a chromosomal region is selected in the cancer cell because it serves to inactivate a tumor suppressor. The PTEN tumor suppressor maps to 10q23 (114) and is an obvious target for allelic deletion. Not all chromosome 10 deletions, however, involve the PTEN region and not all uterine cancer with chromosome 10 LOH have PTEN mutations (53,115,116). These observations strongly support the notion that there is more than one suppressor on the long arm of chromosome 10 playing a role in uterine cancers. Careful evaluation of published LOH/deletion data suggests that there may be three tumor suppressor genes based on different regions and patterns of deletion in endometrioid tumors (115,117–119). A homeodomain gene, EMX2, was suggested as the candidate tumor suppressor mapping in the 10q25–q26 region (120). EMX2 mutations are infrequent in endometrial cancers (10%) and additional studies are required to determine whether loss of EMX2 contributes to the development of uterine adenocarcinomas. It is noteworthy that, like adenocarcinomas, uterine sarcomas show frequent deletion of sequences on the long arm of chromosome 10 (36). In contrast to endometrioid tumors, uterine sarcomas rarely have mutations in PTEN (105). Whether the same tumor suppressor on distal 10q is involved in both uterine adenocarcinomas and sarcomas is not known at this time. As additional tumor suppressor genes are identified and characterized, a clearer understanding of the relationships among the different types of uterine cancers will emerge.

Oncogenes

Activation of proto-oncogenes is a feature of many malignancies and not surprisingly, there have been numerous searches for oncogene mutations in uterine cancers. Amplification or overexpression of the HER-2/neu gene (HER2) is an independent prognostic indicator in breast carcinoma (121). Specific therapies for breast cancers that are based on HER2 status are now widely used (122). Given the similar role that estrogen plays in breast and endometrial cancers, it was logical that HER2 be investigated in uterine cancers. Despite numerous studies and different approaches to measuring HER2 levels, the relationships between HER2 and endometrial cancer remain obscure. In some studies, overexpression correlates with histologic subtype and advanced stage or grade (123–125). Other investigators have failed to observe such correlations between HER2 levels and histopathologic variables or outcome (126–129). Although HER2 overexpression is seen at modest frequency (usually less than 20%), the overall significance of oncogenic activation HER2 in uterine cancers is yet to be established.

Gain-of-function mutations in the KRAS2 member of the *ras* family are seen in 10–30% of uterine cancers (89,130–136). Point mutations in codons 12, 13, and 61 result in a *ras* protein that is constitutionally activated. KRAS2 mutations are seen in all histologic subtypes of endometrial carcinoma and uterine sarcomas. There is a tendency toward a higher frequency of KRAS2 mutation in endometrioid adenocarcinomas than serous carcinomas (46,137,138). Mutations are also seen in atypical hyperplasia, a precursor to endometrioid carcinoma, suggesting that *ras* activation is an early event in Type I tumors (72,131,132,134). The relationship between KRAS2 mutation and other clinical and histopathological features is unclear. Activated *ras* levels have been correlated with less well-differentiated tumors in some studies, but not in others (139–141). There are conflicting reports on the associations between KRAS2 mutation and outcome (142,143). Confounding genetic and environmental factors, coupled with the small sample sizes for many of the molecular studies likely explain the apparently contradictory results.

The relationship between defective DNA mismatch repair (MSI) and KRAS2 mutation in endometrial cancers is also uncertain. In colon tumors, there seems to be an inverse relationship between MSI and KRAS2 mutation (144,145). This may not, however, be the case in sporadic MSI-positive cancers (146). In sporadic endometrioid endometrial cancers matched for grade, stage, and patient race, the rate of KRAS2 mutation was the same in the MSI-positive and -negative cancers (89). In a smaller series of endometrioid adenocarcinomas, Lagarda and colleagues (138) saw an increase in the rate of KRAS2 mutation in MSI-positive tumors. By looking at methylation of MLH1 promoter in precancerous lesions and evaluating patterns of KRAS2 mutation, these authors concluded that KRAS2 and DNA repair defects occur early in endometrial tumorigenesis, and that methylation defects could account for the higher, more frequent KRAS2 mutation seen in MSI-positive tumors (138). This hypothesis that methylation-promoted mutation of KRAS2 is a feature of endometrial cancers has not been tested.

SUMMARY

The genetic defects that contribute to the development of uterine cancers are just beginning to be understood. A small number of genes and pathways have been implicated in the genesis of Type I endometrial cancers: These include loss of DNA mismatch repair, inactivation of the PTEN and TP53 tumor suppressor genes, and activation of the KRAS2 oncogene. Even fewer of the genes involved in the development of Type II carcinomas have been identified, perhaps owing in part to rarity of these tumors. TP53 mutation, however, appears to be a key factor in the development of Type II tumors. Differences in gene defects in Type I and II endometrial cancers may in part explain the very different presentation and behavior of these two tumor types (Fig. 3).

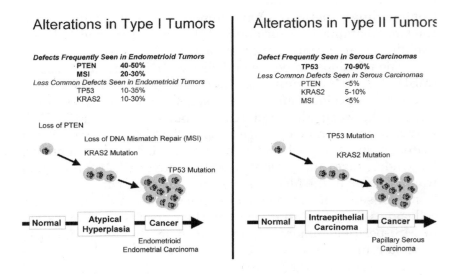

Figure 3 Gene defects in Type I and II endometrial cancers. The frequency and timing of four major gene defects are presented. PTEN mutation and MSI are common in Type I tumors (endometrioid endometrial cancers). Loss of PTEN is seen in atypical hyperplasia and may occur even earlier in the progression from histologically normal endometrium to cancer. MSI is also believed to be an early event based on studies of hyperplasias. Unlike Type I tumors, Type II tumors rarely have defects in PTEN and DNA mismatch repair. TP53 mutations are seen in most Type II endometrial cancers (uterine papillary serous carcinomas) and in the precursor lesion, intraepithelial endometrial carcinoma. Whereas most Type II cancers have a TP53 defect, TP53 mutation is less frequent in Type I cancers and appears to be a late event in tumor formation.

Better methods are constantly being devised for the collection, preservation, and analysis of tumor and other tissue specimens. These advances, coupled with new techniques for analysis of microquantities of DNA, RNA, and protein hold great promise for unravelling the secrets of the cancer cell. A more complete understanding of the genetic basis of uterine cancer development will pave the way for discovery of new approaches for the prevention, detection, and treatment of these malignancies.

REFERENCES

1. Ahmedin J, Thomas A, Murray T, Thun M. Cancer Statistics 2002. *CA Cancer J Clin* 2002; 52:23–47.

2. Kneale BLG, Giles GG. Endometrial cancer: trends in incidence and survival: a preventable disease? *Aust NZ J Obstet Gynaecol* 1993; 33:1–7.

3. Sherman ME, Sturgeon S, Brinton LA, et al. Risk factors and hormone levels in patients with serous and endometrioid uterine carcinomas. *Mod Pathol* 1997; 10:963–8.

4. Kurman RJ, Kaminski PF, Norris HJ. The behavior of endometrial hyperplasia a long-term study of "untreated" hyperplasia in 170 patients. *Cancer* 1985; 56:403–412.

5. Bokhman JV. Two pathogenetic types of endometrial carcinoma. *Gyn Oncol* 1983; 15:10–17.

6. Deligdisch L, Holinka CF. Endometrial carcinoma: two diseases? *Cancer Detection* Prevention 1987; 10:237–246.

7. Kurman RJ, Norris HJ. Blaustein's Pathology of the Female Genital Tract. In: Kurman RJ, ed. Endometrial Carcinoma. New York: Springer-Verlag, 1987:338–372.

8. Sherman ME, Bitterman P, Rosenshein NB, Delgado G, Kurman RJ. Uterine serous carcinoma. A morphologically diverse neoplasm with unifying clinicopathologic features. *Am J Surg Pathol* 1992; 16:600–10.

9. Ambros RA, Sherman ME, Zahn CM, Bitterman P, Kurman RJ. Endometrial intraepithelial carcinoma: a distinctive lesion specifically associated with tumors displaying serous differentiation. *Hum Pathol* 1995; 26:1260–1267.

10. Hanahan D, Weinberg RA. The hallmarks of cancer. *Cell* 2000; 100:57–70.

11. Knudson AG. Chasing the cancer demon. *Ann Rev Genetics* 2000; 34:1–19.

12. Hedrick L. Endometrial Cancer. In: Vogelstein K, ed. The Genetic Basis of Human Cancer: McGraw-Hill, 1998:621–629.

13. Lynch HT, Smyrk T. Hereditary nonpolyposis colorectal cancer (Lynch syndrome). An updated review. *Cancer* 1996; 78:1149–1167.

14. Mecklin JP, Jarvinen HJ. Clinical features of colorectal carcinoma in cancer family syndrome. *Dis Colon Rectum* 1986; 29:160–164.

15. Marra G, Boland CR. Hereditary nonpolyposis colorectal cancer: the syndrome, the genes, and historical perspectives. *J Nat Cancer Inst* 1995; 87:1114–1125.

16. Aarnio M, Mecklin JP, Aaltonen LA, Nystrom-Lahti M, Jarvinen HJ. Life-time risk of different cancers in hereditary non-polyposis colorectal cancer (HNPCC) syndrome. *Int J Cancer* 1995; 64:430–433.

17. Wu Y, Berends MJ, Sijmons RH, et al. A role for MLH3 in hereditary nonpolyposis colorectal cancer. *Nature Genetics* 2001; 29:137–138.

18. Vasen HF, Mecklin JP, Khan PM, Lynch HT. The International Collaborative Group on HNPCC. *Anticancer Res* 1994; 14:1661–1664.

19. Vasen HF, Watson P, Mecklin JP, Lynch HT, Khan PM. New clinical criteria for hereditary nonpolyposis colorectal cancer (HNPCC, Lynch syndrome) proposed by the International Collaborative Group on HNPCC. *Gastroenterol* 1999; 116:1453–1456.

20. Aaltonen LA, Peltomaki P, Leach FS, et al. Clues to the pathogenesis of familial colorectal cancer. *Science* 1993; 260:812–815.

21. Peltomäki P, Lothe RA, Aaltonen LA, et al. Microsatellite instability is associated with tumors that characterize the hereditary non-polyposis colorectal carcinoma syndrome. *Cancer Res* 1993; 53:5853–5855.

22. Miyaki M, Konishi M, Tanaka K, et al. Germline mutation of MSH6 as the cause of hereditary nonpolyposis colorectal cancer. *Nature Genetics* 1997; 17:271–272.

23. Wijnen J, Khan PM, Vasen H, et al. Hereditary nonpolyposis colorectal cancer families not complying with the Amsterdam criteria show extremely low frequency of mismatch-repair-gene mutations. *Am J Hum Genetics* 1997; 61:329–335.

24. Wagner A, Hendriks Y, Meijers-Heijboer EJ, et al. Atypical HNPCC owing to MSH6 germline mutations: analysis of a large Dutch pedigree. *J Med Genetics* 2001; 38:318–322.

25. Berends MJ, Wu Y, Sijmons RH, et al. Molecular and clinical characteristics of MSH6 variants: an analysis of 25 index carriers of a germline variant. *Am J Hum Genetics* 2002; 70:26–37.

26. Burke W, Petersen G, Lynch P, et al. Recommendations for follow-up care of individuals with an inherited predisposition to cancer. I. Hereditary nonpolyposis colon cancer. Cancer Genetics Studies Consortium. *JAMA* 1997; 277:915–919.

27. Parc YR, Halling KC, Burgart LJ, et al. Microsatellite instability and hMLH1/hMSH2 expression in young endometrial carcinoma patients: association with family history and histopathology. *Inter J Cancer* 2000:60–66.

28. Millar AL, Pal T, Madlensky L, et al. Mismatch repair gene defects contribute to the genetic basis of double primary cancers of the colorectum and endometrium. *Hum Mol Genetics* 1999; 8:823–829.

29. Boland CR, Thibodeau SN, Hamilton SR, et al. A national cancer institute workshop on microsatellite instability for cancer detection and familial predisposition: development of international criteria for the determination of microsatellite instability in colorectal cancer. *Cancer Res* 1998; 58:5248–5257.

30. Calistri D, Presciuttini S, Buonsanti G, et al. Microsatellite instability in colorectal-cancer patients with suspected genetic predisposition. *Int J Cancer* 2000; 89:87–91.

31. Cederquist K, Golovleva I, Emanuelsson M, Stenling R, Gronberg H. A population based cohort study of patients with multiple colon and endometrial cancer: correlation of

microsatellite instability (MSI) status, age at diagnosis and cancer risk. *Int J Cancer* 2001; 91:486–491.

32. Sandles LG, Shulman LP, Elias S, et al. Endometrial adenocarcinoma: genetic analysis suggesting heritable site-specific uterine cancer. *Gynecol Oncol* 1992; 47:167–171.

33. Boltenberg A, Furgyik S, Kullander S. Familial cancer aggregation in cases of adenocarcinoma corporis uteri. *Acta Obstet Gynecol* Scandinavia 1990; 69:249–258.

34. Launonen V, Vierimaa O, Kiuru M, et al. Inherited susceptibility to uterine leiomyomas and renal cell cancer. Proceedings of the National Academy of Science U.S.A. 2001; 98:3387–3392.

35. Levy B, Mukherjee T, Hirschhorn K. Molecular cytogenetic analysis of uterine leiomyoma and leiomyosarcoma by comparative genomic hybridization. *Cancer Genetics Cytogenet* 2000; 121:1–8.

36. Quade BJ, Pinto AP, Howard DR, Peters WA, 3rd, Crum CP. Frequent loss of heterozygosity for chromosome 10 in uterine leiomyosarcoma in contrast to leiomyoma. *Am J Pathol* 1999; 154:945–950.

37. Tulinius H, Egilsson V, Olafsdottir GH, Sigvaldason H. Risk of prostate, ovarian, and endometrial cancer among relatives of women with breast cancer. *Br Med J* 1992; 305:855–857.

38. Anderson DE, Badzioch MD. Familial effects of prostate and other cancers on lifetime breast cancer risk. *Breast Cancer Res Treat* 1993; 28:107–113.

39. Levine DA, Lin O, Barakat RR, et al. Risk of endometrial carcinoma associated with BRCA mutation. *Gynecol Oncol* 2001; 80:395–398.

40. Geisler JP, Sorosky JI, Duong HL, et al. Papillary serous carcinoma of the uterus: increased risk of subsequent or concurrent development of breast carcinoma. *Gynecol Oncol* 2001; 83:501–503.

41. Liaw D, Marsh DJ, Li J, et al. Germline mutations of the PTEN gene in Cowden disease, an inherited breast and thyroid cancer syndrome. *Nature Genetics* 1997; 16:64–67.

42. Nelen MR, van Staveren WC, Peeters EA, et al. Germline mutations in the PTEN/MMAC1 gene in patients with Cowden disease. *Hum Mol Genetics* 1997; 6:1383–1387.

43. Eng C, Parsons R. Cowden Sydrome. In: Vogelstein, Kinzler, eds. The Genetic Basis of Human Cancer: McGraw-Hill, 1998:519–525.

44. Lynch ED, Ostermeyer EA, Lee MK, et al. Inherited mutations in PTEN that are associated with breast cancer, Cowden disease, and juvenile polyposis. *Am J Hum Genetics* 1997; 61:1254–1260.

45. Risinger JI, Umar A, Boyer JC, Berchuck A, Kunkel TA, Barrett JC. Microsatellite instability in gynecological sarcomas and in hMSH2 mutant uterine sarcoma cell lines defective in mismatch repair activity. *Cancer Res* 1995; 55:5664–5669.

46. Lax SF, Kendall B, Tashiro H, Slebos RJ, Hedrick L. The frequency of p53, K-ras mutations, and microsatellite instability differs in uterine endometrioid and serous carcinoma: evidence of distinct molecular genetic pathways. *Cancer* 2000; 88:814–824.

47. Tashiro H, Lax SF, Gaudin PB, Isacson C, Cho KR, Hedrick L. Microsatellite instability is uncommon in uterine serous carcinoma. *Am J Pathol* 1997; 150:75–79.

48. Caduff RF, Johnston CM, Svoboda-Newman SM, Poy EL, Merajver SD, Frank TS. Clinical and pathological significance of microsatellite instability in sporadic endometrial carcinoma. *Am J Pathol* 1996; 148:1671–1678.

49. Catasus L, Machin P, Matias-Guiu X, Prat J. Microsatellite instability in endometrial carcinomas: clinicopathologic correlations in a series of 42 cases. *Human Pathol* 1998; 29:1160–1164.

50. Loeb LA. Mutator phenotype may be required for multistage carcinogenesis. *Cancer Res* 1991; 51:3075–3079.

51. Loeb LA. A mutator phenotype in cancer. *Cancer Res* 2001; 61:3230–3239.

52. Gurin CC, Federici MG, Kang L, Boyd J. Causes and consequences of microsatellite instability in endometrial carcinoma. *Cancer Res* 1999; 59:462–466.

53. Tashiro H, Blazes MS, Wu R, et al. Mutations in PTEN are frequent in endometrial carcinoma but rare in other common gynecological malignancies. *Cancer Res* 1997; 57:3935–3940.

54. Levine RL, Cargile CB, Blazes MS, van Rees B, Kurman RJ, Ellenson LH. PTEN mutations and microsatellite instability in complex atypical hyperplasia, a precurser to lesion to uterine endometrioid carcinoma. *Cancer Res* 1998; 58:3254–3258.

55. Risinger JI, Hayes K, Maxwell GL, et al. PTEN mutation in endometrial cancers is associated with favorable clinical and pathologic characteristics. *Clin Cancer Res* 1998; 4:3005–3010.

56. Bussaglia E, del Rio E, Matias-Guiu X, Prat J. PTEN mutations in endometrial carcinomas: a molecular and clinicopathologic analysis of 38 cases. *Human Pathol* 2000; 31:312–317.

57. Mirabelli-Primdahl L, Gryfe R, Kim H, et al. Beta-catenin mutations are specific for colorectal carcinomas with microsatellite instability but occur in endometrial carcinomas irrespective of mutator pathway. *Cancer Res* 1999; 59:3346–3351.

58. Gradia S, Acharya S, Fishel R. The human mismatch recognition complex hMSH2–hMSH6 functions as a novel molecular switch. *Cell* 1997; 91:995–1005.

59. Fishel R. Mismatch repair, molecular switches, and signal transduction. *Genes & Dev* 1998; 12:2096–2101.

60. Fishel R. Signaling mismatch repair in cancer. *Nature Med* 1999; 5:1239–1241.

61. Fishel R. The selection for mismatch repair defects in hereditary nonpolyposis colorectal cancer: revising the mutator hypothesis. *Cancer Res* 2001; 61:7369–7374.

62. Simpkins SB, Bocker T, Swisher EM, et al. MLH1 promoter methylation and gene silencing is the primary cause of microsatellite instability in sporadic endometrial cancers. *Hum Mol Genetics* 1999; 8:661–666.

63. Chiaravalli AM, Furlan D, Facco C, et al. Immunohistochemical pattern of hMSH2/hMLH1 in familial and sporadic colorectal, gastric, endometrial and ovarian carcinomas with instability in microsatellite sequences. *Virchows Arch* 2001; 438:39–48.

64. Esteller M, Levine R, Baylin SB, Ellenson LH, Herman JG. MLH1 promoter hypermethylation is associated with the microsatellite instability phenotype in sporadic endometrial carcinomas. *Oncogene* 1998; 16:2413–2417.

65. Kobayashi K, Matsushima M, Koi S, et al. Mutational analysis of mismatch repair genes, hMLH1 and hMSH2, in sporadic endometrial carcinomas with microsatellite instability. *Jpn J Cancer Res* 1996; 87:141–145.

66. Katabuchi H, van Rees B, Lambers AR, et al. Mutations in DNA mismatch repair genes are not responsible for microsatellite instability in most sporadic endometrial carcinomas. *Cancer Res* 1995; 55:5556–5560.

67. Kowalski LD, Mutch DG, Herzog TJ, Rader JS, Goodfellow PJ. Mutational analysis of MLH1 and MSH2 in 25 prospectively-acquired RER+ endometrial cancers. *Genes Chrom Cancer* 1997; 18:219–227.

68. Basil JB, Swisher EM, Herzog TJ, et al. Mutational analysis of the PMS2 gene in sporadic endometrial cancers with microsatellite instability. *Gynecol Oncol* 1999; 74:395–399.

69. Swisher EM, Mutch DG, Herzog TJ, et al. Analysis of MSH3 in endometrial cancers with defective DNA mismatch. *J Soc Gynecol Invest* 1998; 5:210–216.

70. Jovanovic AS, Boynton KA, Mutter GL. Uteri of women with endometrial carcinoma contain a histopathological spectrum of monoclonal putative precancers, some with microsatellite instability. *Cancer Res* 1996; 56:1917–1921.

71. Mutter GL, Boynton KA, Faquin WC, Ruiz RE, Jovanovic AS. Allelotype mapping of unstable microsatellites established direct lineage continuity between endometrial precancer and cancer. *Cancer Res* 1996; 56:4483–4486.

72. Cohn DE, Mutch DG, Herzog TJ, et al. Genotypic and phenotypic progression in endometrial tumorigenesis: determining when defects in DNA mismatch repair and KRAS2 occur. *Genes Chrom Cancer* 2001; 32:295–301.

73. Horowitz N, Pinto K, Mutch D, et al. MSI, MLH1 promoter methylation and loss of mismatch repair in endometrial cancer and concomitant atypical hyperplasia. *Gynecol Oncol* 2002; submitted.

74. Nakagawa H, Nuovo GJ, Zervos EE, et al. Age-related hyper-methylation of the 5' region of MLH1 in normal colonic mucosa is associated with microsatellite-unstable colorectal cancer development. *Cancer Res* 2001; 61:6991–6995.

75. Maxwell GL, Risinger JI, Alvarez AA, Barrett JC, Berchuck A. Favorable survival associated with microsatellite instability in endometrioid endometrial cancers. *Obst Gynecol* 2001; 97:417–422.

76. MacDonald ND, Salvesen HB, Ryan A, Iversen OE, Akslen A, Jacobs IJ. Frequency and prognostic impact of microsatellite instability in a large population-based study of endometrial carcinomas. *Cancer Res* 2000; 60:1750–1752.

77. Basil JB, Goodfellow PJ, Rader JS, Mutch DG, Herzog TJ. Clinical significance of microsatellite instability in endometrial cancer. *Cancer* 2000; 89:1758–1764.

78. Fiumicino S, Ercoli A, Ferrandina G, et al. Microsatellite instability is an independent indicator of recurrence in sporadic stage I-II endometrial adenocarcinoma. *J Clin Oncol* 2001; 19:1008–1014.

79. Aebi S, Kurdi-Haidar B, Gordon R, et al. Loss of DNA mismatch repair in acquired resistance to Cisplatin. *Cancer Res* 1996; 56:3087–3090.

80. Karran P, Bignami M. Self-destruction and tolerance in resistance of mammalian cells to alkylation damage. *Nucleic Acids Res* 1992; 20:2933–2940.

81. Davis TW, Wilson-Van Patten C, Meyers M, et al. Defective expression of the DNA mismatch repair protein, MLH1, alters G2–M cell cycle checkpoint arrest following ionizing radiation. *Cancer Res* 1998; 58:767–778.

82. Elsaleh H, Joseph D, Grieu F, et al. Association of tumour site and sex with survival benefit from adjuvant chemotherapy in colorectal cancer. *Lancet* 2000; 355:1745–1750.

83. Jeffers MD, Farquharson MA, Richmond JA, McNicol AM. p53 immunoreactivity and mutation of the p53 gene in smooth muscle tumours of the uterine corpus. *J Pathol* 1995; 177:65–70.

84. Zhai YL, Nikaido T, Orii A, Horiuchi A, Toki T, Fujii S. Frequent occurrence of loss of heterozygosity among tumor suppressor genes in uterine leiomyosarcoma. *Gynecol Oncol* 1999; 75:453–459.

85. Tashiro H, Isacson C, Levine R, Kurman RJ, Cho KR, Hedrick L. p53 gene mutations are common in uterine serous carcinoma and occur early in their pathogenesis. *Am J Pathol* 1997; 150:177–185.

86. Kihana T, Hamada K, Inoue Y, et al. Mutation and allelic loss of the p53 gene in endometrial carcinoma. *Cancer* 1995; 76:72–78.

87. Kohler MF, Berchuck A, Davidoff AM, et al. Overexpression and mutation of p53 in endometrial carcinoma. *Cancer Res* 1992; 52:1622–1627.

88. Honda T, Kato H, Imamura T, et al. Involvement of p53 gene mutations in human endometrial carcinomas. *Int J Cancer* 1993; 53:963–967.

89. Swisher EM, Peiffer-Schneider S, Mutch DG, et al. Differences in patterns of TP53 and KRAS2 mutations in a large series of endometrial carcinomas with or without microsatellite instability. *Cancer* 1999; 85:119–126.

90. Rampino N, Yamamoto H, Ionov Y, et al. Somatic framshift mutations in the BAX gene in colon cancers of the microsatellite mutator phenotype. *Science* 1997; 275:967–969.

91. Schwartz S, Jr., Yamamoto H, Navarro M, Maestro M, Reventos J, Perucho M. Frameshift mutations at mononucleotide repeats in caspase-5 and other target genes in endometrial and gastrointestinal cancer of the microsatellite mutator phenotype. *Cancer Res* 1999; 59:2995–3002.

92. Catasus L, Matias-Guiu X, Machin P, et al. Frameshift mutations at coding mononucleotide repeat microsatellites in endometrial carcinoma with microsatellite instability. *Cancer* 2000; 88:2290–2297.

93. Ali IU, Schriml LM, Dean M. Mutational spectra of PTEN/MMAC1 gene: a tumor suppressor with lipid phosphatase activity. *J Nat Cancer Inst* 1999; 91:1922–1932.

94. Datta SR, Brunet A, Greenberg ME, Ali IU, Schriml LM, Dean M. Cellular survival: a play in three Akts. *Genes & Devel* 1999; 13:2905–2927.

95. Kennedy SG, Kandel ES, Cross TK, Hay N. Akt/Protein kinase B inhibits cell death by preventing the release of cytochrome c from mitochondria. *Mol Cell Biol* 1999; 19:5800–5810.

96. Brunet A, Bonni A, Zigmond MJ, et al. Akt promotes cell survival by phosphorylating and inhibiting a Forkhead transcription factor. *Cell* 1999; 96:857–868.

97. Maxwell GL, Risinger JI, Gumbs C, et al. Mutation of the PTEN tumor suppressor gene in endometrial hyperplasias. *Cancer Res* 1998; 58:2500–2503.

98. Mutter GL, Lin MC, Fitzgerald JT, et al. Altered PTEN expression as a diagnostic marker for the earliest endometrial precancers. *J Nat Cancer Inst* 2000; 92:924–930.

99. Mutter GL, Ince TA, Baak JP, et al. Molecular identification of latent precancers in histologically normal endometrium. *Cancer Res* 2001; 61:4311–4314.

100. Maxwell GL, Risinger JI, Hayes KA, et al. Racial disparity in the frequency of PTEN mutations, but not microsatellite instability, in advanced endometrial cancers. *Clin Cancer Res* 2000; 6:2999–3005.

101. Salvesen HB, MacDonald N, Ryan A, et al. PTEN methylation is associated with advanced stage and microsatellite instability in endometrial carcinoma. *Int J Cancer* 2001; 91:22–26.

102. Minaguchi T, Yoshikawa H, Oda K, et al. PTEN mutation located only outside exons 5, 6, and 7 is an independent predictor of favorable survival in endometrial carcinomas. *Clin Cancer Res* 2001; 7:2636–2642.

103. Yoshinaga K, Sasano H, Furukawa T, et al. The PTEN, BAX, and IGFIIR genes are mutated in endometrial atypical hyperplasia. *Jpn J Cancer Res* 1998; 89:985–990.

104. Cohn DE, Basil JB, Mutch DG, et al. Absence of PTEN repeat tract mutation in endometrial cancers with microsatellite instability. *Soc Gynecol Oncol* 2000 Annual Meeting 2000; 79:101–106.

105. Lancaster JM, Risinger JI, Carney ME, Barrett JC, Berchuck A. Mutational analysis of the PTEN gene in human uterine sarcomas. *Am J Obst Gynecol* 2001; 184:1051–1053.

106. Stambolic V, Tsao MS, Macpherson D, Suzuki A, Chapman WB, Mak TW. High incidence of breast and endometrial neoplasia resembling human cowden syndrome in *pten* +/- mice. *Cancer Res* 2000; 60:3605–3611.

107. Ikeda T, Yoshinaga K, Semba S, et al. Mutational analysis of the CTNNB1 (beta-catenin) gene in human endometrial cancer: frequent mutations at codon 34 that cause nuclear accumulation. *Oncol Rep* 2000; 7:323–326.

108. Kobayashi K, Sagae S, Nishioka Y, Tokino T, Kudo R. Mutations of the beta-catenin gene in endometrial carcinomas. *Jpn J Cancer Res* 1999; 90:55–59.

109. Fukuchi T, Sakamoto M, Tsuda H, Maruyama K, Nozawa S, Hirohashi S. Beta-catenin mutation in carcinoma of the uterine endometrium. *Cancer Res* 1998; 58:3526–3528.

110. Palacios J, Catasus L, Moreno-Bueno G, Matias-Guiu X, Prat J, Gamallo C. Beta- and gamma-catenin expression in endometrial carcinoma. Relationship with clinicopathological features and microsatellite instability. *Virchows Arch* 2001; 438:464–469.

111. Saegusa M, Okayasu I. Frequent nuclear beta-catenin accumulation and associated mutations in endometrioid-type endometrial and ovarian carcinomas with squamous differentiation. *J Pathol* 2001; 194:59–67.

112. Jones MH, Koi S, Fujimoto I, Hasumi K, Kato K, Nakamura Y. Allelotype of uterine cancer by analysis of RFLP and microsatellite polymorphisms: Frequent loss of heterozygosity on chromosome amrs 3p, 9q, 10q, and 17p. *Genes, Chromo & Cancer* 1994; 9:119–123.

113. Peiffer SL, Herzog TJ, Tribune DJ, Mutch DG, Gersell DJ, Goodfellow PJ. Allelic loss of sequences from the long arm of chromosome 10 and replication errors in endometrial cancers. *Cancer Res* 1995; 55:1922–1926.

114. Steck PA, Pershouse MA, Jasser SA, et al. Identification of a candidate tumour suppressor gene, MMAC1, at chromosome

10q23.3 that is mutated in multiple advanced cancers. *Nature Genetics* 1997; 15:356–362.

115. Peiffer-Schneider S, Noonan FC, Mutch DG, et al. Mapping an endometrial cancer tumor suppressor gene at 10q25 and development of a bacterial clone contig for the consensus deletion interval. *Genomics* 1998; 52:9–16.

116. Simpkins SB, Peiffer-Schneider S, Mutch DG, Gersell D, Goodfellow PJ. PTEN mutations in endometrial cancer with 10qLOH: additional evidence for the involvement of multiple tumor suppressors. *Gynecol Oncol* 1998; 71:391–395.

117. Nagase S, Sato S, Tezuka F, Wada Y, Yajima A, Horii A. Deletion mapping on chromosome 10q25–q26 in human endometrial cancer. *Br J Cancer* 1996; 74:1979–1983.

118. Nagase S, Yamakawa H, Sato S, Yajima A, Horii A. Identification of a 790–kilobase region of common allelic loss in chromosome 10q25–q26 in human endometrial cancer. *Cancer Res* 1997; 57:1630–1633.

119. Palmieri G, Manca A, Cossu A, et al. Microsatellite analysis at 10q25–q26 in Sardinian patients with sporadic endometrial carcinoma: identification of specification patterns of genetic alteration. *Cancer* 2000; 89:1773–1782.

120. Noonan FC, Mutch DG, Ann Mallon M, Goodfellow PJ. Characterization of the homeodomain gene EMX2: sequence conservation, expression analysis, and a search for mutations in endometrial cancers. *Genomics* 2001; 76:37–44.

121. Slamon DJ, Clark GM, Wong SG, et al. Human breast cancer: correlation of relapse and survival with amplification of the HER-2/neu oncogene. *Science* 1987; 235:177–182.

122. Slamon DJ, Leyland-Jones B, Shak S, et al. Use of chemotherapy plus a monoclonal antibody against HER2 for metastatic breast cancer that overexpresses HER2. *N Engl J Med* 2001; 344:783–792.

123. Berchuck A, Rodriguez G, Kinney RB, Soper JT, Dodge RK, Clarke-Pearson DL, Bast RC. Overexpression of HER-2/neu in endometrial cancer is associated with advanced stage disease. *Am J Obstet Gynecol* 1991; 164:15–21.

124. Khalifa MA, Mannel RS, Haraway SD, Walker J, Min KW. Expression of EGFR, HER-2/neu, P53, and PCNA in endometrioid, serous papillary, and clear cell endometrial adenocarcinomas. *Gynecol Oncol* 1994; 53:84–92.

125. Monk BJ, Chapman JA, Johnson GA, Brightman B K, Wilczynski SP, Schell MJ, Fan H. Correlation of C-myc and HER-2/neu amplification and expression with histopathologic variables in uterine corpus cancer. *Am J Obstet Gynecol* 1994; 171:1193–8.

126. Bigsby RM, Li AX, Bomalaski J, Stehman FB, Look KY, Sutton GP. Immunohistochemical study of HER-2/neu, epidermal growth factor receptor, and steroid receptor expression in normal and malignant endometrium. *Obstet Gynecol* 1992; 79:95–100.

127. Hetzel DJ, Wilson TO, Keeney GL, Roche PC, Cha SS, Podratz KC. HER-2/*neu* expression: A major prognostic factor in endometrial cancer. *Gynecol Oncol* 1992; 47:179–185.

128. Gassel AM, Backe J, Krebs S, Schon S, Caffier H, Muller-Hermelink HK. Endometrial carcinoma: immunohistochemically detected proliferation index is a prognosticator of long-term outcome. *J Clin Pathol* 1998; 51:25–29.

129. Coronado PJ, Vidart JA, Lopez-asenjo JA, et al. P53 overexpression predicts endometrial carcinoma recurrence better than HER-2/neu overexpression. *Eur J Obstet Gynecol Reprod Biol* 2001; 98:103–108.

130. Enomoto T, Inoue M, Perantoni AO, et al. K-ras activation in premalignant and malignant epithelial lesions of the human uterus. *Cancer Res* 1991; 51:5308–5314.

131. Enomoto T, Fujita M, Inoue M, et al. Alterations of the p53 tumor suppressor gene and its association with activation of the c-K-*ras*-2 protooncogene in premalignant and malignant lesions of the human uterine endometrium. *Cancer Res* 1993; 53:1883–1888.

132. Duggan BD, Felix JC, Muderspach LI, Tsao JL, Shibata DK. Early mutational activation of the c-Ki-ras oncogene in endometrial carcinoma. *Cancer Res* 1994; 54:1604–1607.

133. Ignar-Trowbridge D, Risinger JI, Dent GA, et al. Mutations of the Ki-ras oncogene in endometrial carcinoma. *Am J Obstet Gynecol* 1992; 167:227–232.

134. Sasaki H, Nishii H, Takahashi H, et al. Mutation of the Ki-ras protooncogene in human endometrial hyperplasia and carcinoma. *Cancer Res* 1993; 53:1906–1910.

135. Hill MA, Gong C, Casey TJ, et al. Detection of K-ras mutations in resected primary leiomyosarcoma. *Cancer Epidemiol Biomarkers Prev* 1997; 6:1095–1100.

136. Wada H, Enomoto T, Fujita M, et al. Molecular evidence that most but not all carcinosarcomas of the uterus are combination tumors. *Cancer Res* 1997; 57:5379–5385.

137. Caduff RF, Johnston CM, Frank TS. Mutations of the Ki-ras oncogene carcinoma of the endometrium. *Am J Pathol* 1995; 146:182–188.

138. Lagarda H, Catasus L, Arguelles R, et al. K-ras mutations in endometrial carcinomas with microsatellite instability. *J Pathol* 2001; 193:193–199.

139. Long CA, O'Brien TJ, Sanders MM, Bard DS, Quirk JG, Jr. ras oncogene is expressed in adenocarcinoma of the endometrium. *Am J Obstet Gynecol* 1988; 159:1512–1516.

140. Scambia G, Catozzi L, Benedetti-Panici P, et al. Expression of ras p21 oncoprotein in normal and neoplastic human endometrium. *Gynecol Oncol* 1993; 50:339–346.

141. Tsuda H, Jiko K, Yajima M, et al. Frequent occurrence of c-Ki-ras gene mutations in well differentiated endometrial adenocarcinoma showing infiltrative local growth with fibrosing stromal response. *Int J Gynecol Pathol* 1995; 14:255–259.

142. Ito K, Watanabe K, Nasim S, et al. K-ras point mutations in endometrial carcinoma: effect on outcome is dependent on age of patient. *Gynecol Oncol* 1996; 63:238–246.

143. Semczuk A, Berbec H, Kostuch M, Cybulski M, Wojcierowski J, Baranowski W. K-ras gene point mutations in human endometrial carcinomas: correlation with clinicopathological features and patients' outcome. Journal of *Cancer Res Clin Oncol* 1998; 124:695–700.

144. Ionov Y, Peinado MA, Malkhosyan S, Shibata D, Perucho M. Ubiquitous somatic mutations in simple repeated sequences reveal a new mechanism for colonic carcinogenesis. *Nature* 1993; 363:558–561.

145. Thibodeau SN, Bren G, Schaid D. Microsatellite instability in cancer of the proximal colon. *Science* 1993; 260:816–819.

146. Konishi M, Kikuchi-Yanoshita R, Tanka K, et al. Molecular nature of colon tumors in hereditary nonpolyposis colon cancer, familial polyposis and sporadic colon cancer. *Gastroenterol* 1996; 111:307–317.

2

Endometrial Cancer in the Hereditary Nonpolyposis Colorectal Cancer Syndrome

CHRISTINA A. BANDERA

Harvard Medical School,
Brigham and Women's Hospital,
Boston, Massachusetts, U.S.A.

INTRODUCTION

Endometrial carcinoma is the most common gynecologic cancer with approximately 40,000 cases diagnosed in 2004 in the United States (1). Approximately 5% of these are hereditary cancers. The majority of hereditary endometrial cancers occur within families designated as hereditary nonpolyposis colorectal cancer or HNPCC carriers. There are several autosomal dominant genes that, when mutated, can cause this familial syndrome. These genes are involved in DNA repair, and are often collectively called the mismatch repair (MMR) genes. Though the syndrome is named after colon cancer, endometrial cancer is also extremely common in this syndrome, and some studies suggest that female carriers of the abnormal HNPCC genes are more likely to develop endometrial cancer than colon cancer (discussed later in this chapter). This syndrome was initially described by Aldred Warthin in 1895 when the striking family history of his seamstress, who died of endometrial cancer, came to his attention. In 1913, he published a paper describing this remarkable kindred, which included 10 cases of endometrial cancer and 7 cases of stomach cancer in 48 descendants of a man who died of cancer of the stomach or intestine (2). Multiple cases of colorectal cancer were noted in subsequent generations of this family (3).

The HNPCC syndrome is also commonly called the Lynch Syndrome II, after Henry Lynch who systematically characterized this syndrome in the 1960s (4). Lynch Syndrome I refers to families in which colorectal cancer is the only malignancy identified. During the 1990s, genes responsible for the HNPCC phenotype were identified, and protocols for screening and prevention, including prophylactic surgery, were developed. Gynecologists diagnosing and treating women with endometrial cancer have an important role to play in identifying HNPCC families and referring them for counseling and appropriate screening.

CLINICAL AND PATHOLOGIC FEATURES OF HNPCC-RELATED CANCERS

Endometrial Cancer

Endometrial cancer is extremely common in female carriers of HNPCC gene mutations with studies reporting a frequency of 22–60% (5–8). One study from the United Kingdom found that women had a relative risk of 42% of developing endometrial cancer compared to a 30% risk of developing colorectal cancer. Therefore, for women carrying HNPCC gene mutations, endometrial cancer is at least as big a threat as colorectal cancer. The frequency of endometrial cancer may be dependent on the exact mutation in the family. For example, with a mutation in the MLH1 gene, the risk of endometrial cancer by age 50 is 42% compared with a risk of 61% for women with a mutation in the MSH2 gene (8).

Some studies show an early age of diagnosis of HNPCC-related endometrial cancer compared with sporadic endometrial cancer, with approximately one-half of cases developing before age 50 (9).

In contrast to colorectal cancer, it appears that endometrial cancer associated with HNPCC is indistinguishable from sporadic endometrial cancer in terms of histology. Furthermore, though literature reports a slightly poorer prognosis of HNPCC-associated endometrial cancer compared to sporadic cancers of the same stage, these differences are not statistically significant (9,10).

Ovarian Cancer

Approximately 12% of women carriers of HNPCC gene mutations will develop ovarian cancer by age 70 (11), compared with a general population risk of only 1%. HNPCC-related ovarian cancer occurs at an earlier age compared to sporadic ovarian cancer, with one series of 80 cases reporting a mean age of diagnosis of 42 (12). Evaluation of the same series of 80 cases found that invasive HNPCC ovarian cancers are commonly well or moderately differentiated. Given the deadly nature of this disease, it is important to offer screening and counseling about the risk of ovarian cancer to all women from HNPCC families.

Colorectal Cancer

Mutations in HNPCC genes account for 3–5% of all cases of colorectal cancer. The features of colorectal cancer in HNPCC families are well characterized. The rate of colorectal cancer development in HNPCC gene mutation carriers is high; it is estimated that approximately 74% of men and 30% of women carrying HNPCC mutations will develop colorectal cancers (6), although the higher frequency of colorectal cancer in men is not understood. These cancers tend to be right-sided colon malignancies that occur at an average age of 40 years old, 30 years earlier than the average age of patients with sporadic colorectal cancer. Frequently, multiple primary sites of cancer may be identified in the colon at the same time (synchronous tumors) or several years apart (metachronous tumors).

The characteristics of colorectal cancer associated with HNPCC are different from those seen in familial adenomatous polyposis (FAP), which accounts for less than 1% of colorectal cancers. In FAP, adenomatous polyps are profuse throughout the gastrointestinal (GI) tract, and most patients develop colorectal cancer by age 40. It is recommended that patients with FAP undergo prophylactic colectomy. Other manifestations of FAP include desmoid tumors and osteomas. Patients with FAP are identified clinically on the basis of diffuse polyps. In HNPCC, polyps are rare, tend to appear flat rather than polypoid, and tend to be more aggressive than adenomatous polyps in FAP or the general population.

The histology of colorectal cancer associated with HNPCC mutations is poorly differentiated or undifferentiated in 10% of cases, compared to 0.5% of sporadic colorectal cancers. Furthermore, these cancers often produce a large amount of mucin, and may be associated with infiltration by CD3$^+$ T cells (13).

Interestingly, HNPCC colorectal cancers appear to have a better prognosis than sporadic colorectal cancer, even when studies adjust for stage (14,15).

Other Malignancies

Other malignancies considered part of the HNPCC syndrome include cancer of the urinary tract (kidney and ureter), stomach, biliary tract, brain, and small intestine. The risk of developing one of these malignancies in the presence of an HNPCC mutation ranges from 3.7% to 13%. The frequencies of these cancers may vary according to the HNPCC gene that is mutated and other population risk factors (16). For example, a comparison of Korean and Dutch families with identical mutations revealed an increased frequency of gastric cancer in the Korean families. Presumably, this is due to environmental factors such as diet, which also accounts for the higher rate of sporadic gastric cancer in parts of Asia.

GENETIC BASIS OF HNPCC

The genetic basis of HNPCC was elucidated in the early 1990s. Mutations in several genes are associated with the syndrome. Though on different chromosomes, all the genes are associated with the process of DNA mismatch repair (MMR). Malfunction of this process results in the loss of a cell's ability to repair errors made during DNA replication. The accumulation of DNA mutations within a cell leads to progression to a cancerous phenotype.

In addition to creating mutations in functional genes, the inability to repair DNA leads to a phenomenon called microsatellite instability (MSI). Microsatellites are simple, repetitive sequences located throughout the genome. MSI is the result of DNA insertions or deletions that are easily identified in the laboratory using genetic screening techniques. It is found in 90% of HNPCC colorectal cancer, but only 15–20% of sporadic colorectal cancer. Similarly, the overwhelming majority of HNPCC-related endometrial cancers are associated with MSI, compared to less than 1/3 of sporadic endometrial cancers (17). Therefore, the identification of MSI in DNA extracted from cancer is highly suggestive of the presence of an HNPCC mutation. The functional significance of MSI is unclear; however, MSI appears to be more common in HNPCC individuals who are Caucasian and have early stage disease. The presence or absence of MSI does not appear to correlate with survival (18).

The most common HNPCC gene mutations occur in the MSH2 and MLH1 genes located on chromosomes 2 and 3, respectively. These genes account for 90% of HNPCC kindred in equal proportions. Interestingly, loss of MLH1 and MSH2 protein expression has been identified in the cancer precursor endometrial hyperplasia, suggesting that this loss is an early event in endometrial carcinogenesis (19).

Other genes that are associated with the HNPCC syndrome include PMS1, PMS2, and MSH6. One of the rarer
HNPCC genes, MSH6, does not appear to be associated with
MSI, suggesting that MSI is not necessary for HNPCC-
related colorectal and endometrial cancers to develop (20).
In fact, this gene has been associated with metachronous
endometrial and colorectal primary cancers. There are many
families with the HNPCC phenotype for whom no mutation
is identifiable in known HNPCC genes. This suggests that
additional genes are involved in the DNA repair pathway
that is critical for protection against HNPCC-related malignancies (21).

IDENTIFYING THE HNPCC SYNDROME

Clinical Diagnosis

The large number of genes associated with the HNPCC
hereditary cancer syndrome makes it impractical to initiate
mutation screening in low risk individuals. Therefore, before
proceeding with genetic testing, a clinical diagnosis of
HNPCC should be made. Several clinical criteria for identifying HNPCC kindred have been suggested, including the
Amsterdam Criteria in 1999 (22), the Revised Amsterdam
Criteria in 1999 (23), the Japanese Criteria in 1996 (24), the
Mount Sinai Criteria (25), the ICG-HNPCC Study Criteria
(26), and the Bethesda Criteria (27). The first Amsterdam
Criteria failed to take into account extra-colonic cancers, and
its accuracy was somewhat dependent on information from a
large kindred. Subsequent criteria sought to increase the sensitivity of identifying HNPCC kindred. The Bethesda Criteria
is focused on identifying HNPCC through the clinicopathologic characteristics of an individual, rather than evaluating
an entire family group.

At present, most clinicians use a combination of the
Amsterdam I, Amsterdam II, and Bethesda criteria in their
practice (Table 1). For the purpose of the non-oncologist, it is
important to consider the number of relatives with any malignancy associated with HNPCC mutations. Referral to a
genetic counselor is warranted if three or more relatives

(including at least one first degree relative) have a history of colorectal, endometrial, ovarian, small bowel, or urinary tract cancer. When these cancers are diagnosed below the age of 45, it further raises the suspicion of a familial syndrome.

Genetic Testing

Confirming the diagnosis of HNPCC with genetic testing will not alter the treatment of a given patient's disease. However, this information may be used to direct further screening and prophylaxis against other cancers in the patient, as well as in his or her family members.

There are currently three commercially available tests available to aid in identifying HNPCC individuals. These tests should be covered by insurance for high-risk individuals. The first test is MSI screening, performed on DNA extracted from the cancer. Either fresh tumor or paraffin-embedded tumor may be used for MSI characterization. Five genetic loci are typically examined, and the tumor is classified as MSI negative, low MSI, or high MSI. At present, MSI testing is only recommended for colorectal cancer screening, since there is a lack of data to support its use for screening endometrial cancer.

The second test available for HNPCC screening is germ line testing for MSH2 and MLH1 mutations through DNA sequencing. Usually, this test is performed using DNA extracted from a blood sample, and may be performed on individuals with or without cancer.

The third genetic HNPCC test is a diagnostic tool, which is not currently widely used. This procedure involves screening fecal material for MSI. Stool that tests positive for MSI may be indicative of a malignancy.

Testing Recommendations and Interpretation of Results

The American Cancer Association has suggested that germ line DNA testing for mutations in the MSH2 and MLH1 genes should be offered to any patient whose family meets the first three Bethesda criteria. For other patients meeting "modified Bethesda criteria" (Table 1), there are several options. The

Table 1. Clinical Criteria for Diagnosis of HNPCC

Classification System	Strengths and Weaknesses
Amsterdam I Patient must meet **all** of the following criteria: • Familial adenomatous polyposis should be excluded • Three or more relatives with histologically confirmed colorectal cancer, one of whom is a first-degree relative of the other two • Colorectal cancer involves at least two generations • One or more colorectal cancers is diagnosed before the age of 50	• First attempt at standard definition of HNPCC family • Failed to consider extracolonic cancers in definition • Sensitivity dependent on large family
Amsterdam II Patients must meet **all** of the following criteria: • Familial adenomatous polyposis should be excluded • Three or more relatives with a histologically confirmed HNPCC-associated cancer (includes cancer of the colorectum, endometrium, small bowel, ureter or renal pelvis), one of whom is a first-degree relative of the other two • Colorectal cancer involving at least two generations • One or more colorectal cancer cases diagnosed before the age of 50	• Includes extracolonic cancers • Sensitivity dependent on large family
Bethesda Criteria Patient may meet **any** of the following criteria: • Individuals with cancer in families who meet the Amsterdam Criteria • Individuals with two HNPCC-related cancers, including synchronous or metachronous colorectal cancers or associated extracolonic cancers including endometrial, ovarian, gastric, hepatobiliary, small bowel, and transitional cell carcinoma of renal pelvis or ureter • Individuals with colorectal cancer and a first-degree relative with colorectal cancer and/or HNPCC-related extracolonic cancer and/or a colorectal adenoma; one of the cancers diagnosed at age <45 years, and the adenoma diagnosed at age <40 years	• Less restrictive than Amsterdam systems • Focused on specific patient rather than on entire family

Table 1. *(Continued)*

Classification System	Strengths and Weaknesses
Bethesda Criteria (*continued*) • Individuals with colorectal cancer or endometrial cancer diagnosed at age <45 years • Individuals with right-sided colorectal cancer with an undifferentiated pattern (solid/cribiform) on histology diagnosed at age <45 years (solid/cribiform defined as poorly differentiated or undifferentiated carcinoma composed of irregular, solid sheets of large eosinophilic cells and containing small gland-like spaces) • Individuals with signet-ring cell type colorectal cancer diagnosed at age <45 years (signet-ring cell type is defined as tumor composed of >50% signet-ring cells) • Individuals with colorectal adenomas diagnosed at age <40 years	

least expensive option involves obtaining DNA from a colorectal cancer and testing it for MSI. Since over 90% of the HNPCC colorectal cancers are associated with MSI, this is a powerful screening tool. If the MSI screening is high, then further testing for germ line MSH2/MLH1 mutations may be performed. If no mutation is found, then the test is inconclusive. In cases where no tumor is available for MSI testing, screening for MSH2/MLH1 mutations may be performed. However, testing the cancer patient is more informative than screening family members without cancer, since their chance of inheriting an abnormal gene is only 50%. When an HNPCC-associated mutation is identified, screening should be offered to all at-risk family members. Patients who decline testing should be counseled and offered clinical screening and prophylactic strategies as if they have a mutation.

The implications of a negative test result are often difficult to explain to the layperson. If a negative germ line genetic screen is identified in an individual who has a family member with a known HNPCC mutation, then the individual has not inherited the mutation, and his/her risk is no higher than baseline for the general population. On the other hand, if no individual in the family is known to carry a mutation, then negative screening for MSH2/MLH1 does not rule out the presence of another mutation in the family. If the family meets the Amsterdam Criteria, especially if MSI has been identified, then members of the family should be counseled that might be likely harboring an HNPCC mutation even if testing for MSH2/MLH1 is negative.

Indeterminate test results occasionally occur when performing germ line mutation screening for MSH2/MLH1 mutations. Usually these are missense mutations involving a single base pair substitution not located in translated regions of the gene. The significance of these mutations is unknown. If it is possible to perform testing on multiple members of the family with and without cancer, then it may be possible to determine whether the mutation correlates with the development of cancer.

COUNSELING REGARDING SCREENING AND PREVENTION

Screening for Gynecologic Cancers (Table 2)

The screening recommendations for uterine cancer are controversial. Since endometrial cancer has been diagnosed as early as 25 years of age in HNPCC families, abnormal bleeding at any age should be evaluated by biopsy and possibly dilatation and curettage of the uterus. The American Cancer Society recommends gynecologic surveillance for women from HNPCC families beginning at age 35 (1), while other experts have suggested surveillance beginning at age 25 (28). Recommended screening for women from HNPCC families includes yearly ultrasound and endometrial biopsy done with an aspirator instrument in the office, though no evidence of the efficacy of this protocol exists (29). In fact, one study offering yearly ultrasound screening failed to identify any uterine cancers through scans, though two endometrial cancers were identified through abnormal uterine bleeding during the study period (30). Screening by endometrial biopsy might identify cancers before the symp-

Table 2. Surveillance for Women from HNPCC Families

Site	Procedure	Lower Age Limit (Work-up Symptoms at Any Age)	Interval
Endometrial cancer	• Endometrial biopsy • Ultrasound	30–35 years old	Yearly
Ovarian cancer	• Ultrasound • CA125	30–35 years old	Yearly
Colorectal cancer	• Colonoscopy	20–25 years old	1–3 years
Stomach (if runs in family)	• Gastroscopy or upper GI	30–35 years old	1–2 years
Urinary tract (if runs in family)	• Ultrasonography urine cytology	30–35 years old	1–2 years

tom of bleeding occurs, but whether this translates into a survival advantage is again unclear.

Though ovarian cancer is less common than endometrial cancer in the HNPCC syndrome, screening may be more critical because of the poor cure rate of the disease. Unfortunately, screening protocols for early detection of ovarian cancer are inadequate. Patients are generally offered ultrasound and CA125 screening with the caveat that these tests rarely identify disease at an early curable stage. Efforts to improve screening protocols for ovarian cancer using a panel of cancer markers are actively being pursued (31).

Screening for Colorectal Cancer (Table 2)

Screening members of HNPCC families for colorectal cancer is critical. Surveillance recommendations include colonoscopy every 1–3 years beginning at age 20–25 (29). Treatment of adenomatous polyps is clearly beneficial, since most of these polyps in HNPCC patients will develop into cancers.

Screening for Other Cancers (Table 2)

As with gynecologic cancers, appropriate surveillance for other non-colorectal cancers is unclear. If gastric cancer or genitourinary cancers are present in family members, then it is reasonable to initiate screening every 1–2 years beginning at age 30–35 (29). This screening may include endoscopy or barium swallow studies and urine cytology.

Lifestyle

Endometrial cancer associated with HNPCC is not associated with obesity, the most common risk factor for sporadic endometrial cancer. Obesity is thought to stimulate sporadic endometrial cancer through the increased circulating estrogen produced by the conversion of adrenal androstendione to estrone in fat cells. Though HNPCC-related endometrial cancer does not appear to be hormonally stimulated, it is reasonable to recommend weight reduction to patients at risk as part of a general health strategy, and to minimize possible cofactors in the pathogenesis of endometrial cancer.

Chemoprevention

It is thought that the use of oral contraceptives reduces endometrial cancer due to progesterone inhibition of the endometrium (32). Furthermore, these medications also appear to be associated with a decreased risk of ovarian cancer. Whether hormonal suppression is effective against HNPCC-related cancers is unknown; however, if a patient is considering oral contraceptives, chemoprevention may be an added benefit.

Prophylactic Surgery

Gynecologic Cancer

Women from HNPCC families should be counseled about the option of prophylactic hysterectomy with removal of ovaries and tubes. Though endometrial cancer has a high cure rate, removing the uterus will reduce the stress, discomfort, and worry associated with endometrial screening. Removal of the ovaries will minimize the risk of ovarian cancer, which, though relatively rare in HNPCC patients, is more likely to be deadly. Hysterectomy with removal of ovaries may be performed via a laparotomy or vaginally. When performing a vaginal hysterectomy, we recommend detaching the ovaries using the laparoscope to ensure that the ovaries are completely removed.

The ideal age for prophylactic hysterectomy with removal of tubes and ovaries has not been established for the HNPCC group of patients. Certainly, waiting until childbearing is complete is appropriate, though cases of endometrial cancer in HNPCC families have been reported as early as age 25. The safety of hormone replacement in these patients after prophylactic surgery has not been established. However, since the HNPCC cancers do not appear to be hormonally stimulated, estrogen supplementation is unlikely to increase the risk of other HNPCC-related cancers.

Finally, any HNPCC patient undergoing colon surgery should be offered a prophylactic hysterectomy with removal of tubes and ovaries. This additional procedure is unlikely to add significant morbidity to the primary operation.

Colorectal Cancer

The most successful method to prevent colon cancer in the HNPCC syndrome is prophylactic surgery. Some patients may consider total colectomy. Certainly, when a colorectal cancer is identified, patients may opt for total colectomy rather than hemicolectomy to prevent metachronous disease. Even after total colectomy, continued screening for rectal cancer with proctoscopy is necessary.

CONCLUSION

Endometrial cancer is the second most common cancer in HNPCC families, with some studies showing a higher frequency of endometrial cancer than colon cancer in women from these kindred. All women who present with endometrial cancer, especially those presenting under the age of 45, should undergo preliminary screening for HNPCC by taking a thorough family history. Those patients meeting the Amsterdam or Bethesda Criteria should be offered counseling regarding genetic testing, screening regimens, chemoprevention, and prophylactic surgery.

REFERENCES

1. Cancer Facts and Figures 2004. In: Atlanta, GA: American Cancer Society, 2004.

2. Warthin A. Hereditary with reference to carcinoma. *Arch Intern Med* 1913; 12:546–555.

3. Lynch HT, Krush AJ. Cancer family "G" revisited: 1895–1970. *Cancer* 1971; 27 (6):1505–1511.

4. Lynch HT, Smyrk T. Hereditary nonpolyposis colorectal cancer (Lynch syndrome). An updated review. *Cancer* 1996; 78(6):1149–67.

5. Aarnio M, Sankila R, Pukkala E, Salovaara R, Aaltonen LA, de la Chapelle A, et al. Cancer risk in mutation carriers of DNA-mismatch-repair genes. *Int J Cancer* 1999; 81(2):214–218.

6. Dunlop MG, Farrington SM, Carothers AD, Wyllie AH, Sharp L, Burn J, et al. Cancer risk associated with germline DNA mismatch repair gene mutations. *Hum Mol Genet* 1997; 6(1):105–110.

7. Watson P, Vasen HF, Mecklin JP, Jarvinen H, Lynch HT. The risk of endometrial cancer in hereditary nonpolyposis colorectal cancer. *Am J Med* 1994; 96(6):516–520.

8. Vasen HF, Wijnen JT, Menko FH, Kleibeuker JH, Taal BG, Griffioen G, et al. Cancer risk in families with hereditary nonpolyposis colorectal cancer diagnosed by mutation analysis. *Gastroenterology* 1996; 110(4):1020–1027.

9. Vasen HF, Watson P, Mecklin JP, Jass JR, Green JS, Nomizu T, et al. The epidemiology of endometrial cancer in hereditary nonpolyposis colorectal cancer. *Anticancer Res* 1994; 14(4B):1675–1678.

10. Boks DE, Trujillo AP, Voogd AC, Morreau H, Kenter GG, Vasen HF. Survival analysis of endometrial carcinoma associated with hereditary nonpolyposis colorectal cancer. *Int J Cancer* 2002; 102(2):198–200.

11. Aarnio M, Mecklin JP, Aaltonen LA, Nystrom-Lahti M, Jarvinen HJ. Life-time risk of different cancers in hereditary non-polyposis colorectal cancer (HNPCC) syndrome. *Int J Cancer* 1995; 64(6):430–433.

12. Watson P, Butzow R, Lynch HT, Mecklin JP, Jarvinen HJ, Vasen HF, et al. The clinical features of ovarian cancer in hereditary nonpolyposis colorectal cancer. *Gynecol Oncol* 2001; 82(2):223–228.

13. Jass JR. Pathology of hereditary nonpolyposis colorectal cancer. *Ann N Y Acad Sci* 2000; 910:62–73; discussion 73–74.

14. Sankila R, Aaltonen LA, Jarvinen HJ, Mecklin JP. Better survival rates in patients with MLH1–associated hereditary colorectal cancer. *Gastroenterology* 1996; 110(3):682–687.

15. Watson P, Lin KM, Rodriguez-Bigas MA, Smyrk T, Lemon S, Shashidharan M, et al. Colorectal carcinoma survival among hereditary nonpolyposis colorectal carcinoma family members. *Cancer* 1998; 83(2):259–266.

16. Park JG, Park YJ, Wijnen JT, Vasen HF. Gene-environment interaction in hereditary nonpolyposis colorectal cancer with implications for diagnosis and genetic testing. *Int J Cancer* 1999; 82(4):516–519.

17. de Leeuw WJ, Dierssen J, Vasen HF, Wijnen JT, Kenter GG, Meijers-Heijboer H, et al. Prediction of a mismatch repair gene defect by microsatellite instability and immunohistochemical analysis in endometrial tumours from HNPCC patients. *J Pathol* 2000; 192(3):328–335.

18. Basil JB, Goodfellow PJ, Rader JS, Mutch DG, Herzog TJ. Clinical significance of microsatellite instability in endometrial carcinoma. *Cancer* 2000; 89(8):1758–1764.

19. Berends MJ, Hollema H, Wu Y, van Der Sluis T, Mensink RG, ten Hoor KA, et al. MLH1 and MSH2 protein expression as a pre-screening marker in hereditary and non-hereditary endometrial hyperplasia and cancer. *Int J Cancer* 2001; 92(3):398–403.

20. Charames GS, Millar AL, Pal T, Narod S, Bapat B. Do MSH6 mutations contribute to double primary cancers of the colorectum and endometrium? *Hum Genet* 2000; 107(6):623–629.

21. Cederquist K, Golovleva I, Emanuelsson M, Stenling R, Gronberg H. A population based cohort study of patients with multiple colon and endometrial cancer: correlation of microsatellite instability (MSI) status, age at diagnosis and cancer risk. *Int J Cancer* 2001; 91(4):486–491.

22. Vasen HF, Mecklin JP, Khan PM, Lynch HT. The International Collaborative Group on Hereditary Non-Polyposis Colorectal Cancer (ICG-HNPCC). *Dis Colon Rectum* 1991; 34(5):424–425.

23. Vasen HF, Watson P, Mecklin JP, Lynch HT. New clinical criteria for hereditary nonpolyposis colorectal cancer (HNPCC, Lynch syndrome) proposed by the International Collaborative group on HNPCC. *Gastroenterology* 1999; 116(6):1453–1456.

24. Fujita S, Moriya Y, Sugihara K, Akasu T, Ushio K. Prognosis of hereditary nonpolyposis colorectal cancer (HNPCC) and the role of Japanese criteria for HNPCC. *Jpn J Clin Oncol* 1996; 26(5):351–355.

25. Bapat BV, Madlensky L, Temple LK, Hiruki T, Redston M, Baron DL, et al. Family history characteristics, tumor microsatellite instability and germline MSH2 and MLH1 mutations in hereditary colorectal cancer. *Hum Genet* 1999; 104(2):167–176.

26. Park JG, Vasen HF, Park KJ, Peltomaki P, Ponz de Leon M, Rodriguez-Bigas MA, et al. Suspected hereditary nonpolyposis colorectal cancer: International Collaborative Group on Hereditary Non-Polyposis Colorectal Cancer (ICG-HNPCC) criteria and results of genetic diagnosis. *Dis Colon Rectum* 1999; 42(6):710–715; discussion 715–716.

27. Wijnen JT, Vasen HF, Khan PM, Zwinderman AH, van der Klift H, Mulder A, et al. Clinical findings with implications for genetic testing in families with clustering of colorectal cancer. *N Engl J Med* 1998; 339(8):511–518.

28. Brown GJ, St John DJ, Macrae FA, Aittomaki K. Cancer risk in young women at risk of hereditary nonpolyposis colorectal cancer: implications for gynecologic surveillance. *Gynecol Oncol* 2001; 80(3):346–349.

29. Identifying and managing risk for hereditary Nonpolyposis colorectal cancer and endometrial cancer (HNPCC). In: American Medical Association, 2001; pp. 1–27.

30. Dove-Edwin I, Boks D, Goff S, Kenter GG, Carpenter R, Vasen HF, et al. The outcome of endometrial carcinoma surveillance by ultrasound scan in women at risk of hereditary nonpolyposis colorectal carcinoma and familial colorectal carcinoma. *Cancer* 2002; 94(6):1708–1712.

31. Bandera CA, Ye B, Mok SC. New technologies for the identification of markers for early detection of ovarian cancer. *Curr Opin Obstet Gynecol* 2003; 15(1):51–55.

32. Dayal M, Barnhart KT. Noncontraceptive benefits and therapeutic uses of the oral contraceptive pill. *Semin Reprod Med* 2001; 19(4):295–303.

3

Steroid Hormone Receptors in the Normal Endometrium and in Endometrial Cancer

KIMBERLY K. LESLIE AND SUZY DAVIES

The University of New Mexico Health Sciences Center,
Albuquerque, New Mexico, U.S.A.

MEENAKSHI SINGH

University of Colorado Health Sciences Center, Denver, Colorado, U.S.A.

HARRIET O. SMITH

The University of New Mexico Health Sciences Center,
Albuquerque, New Mexico, U.S.A.

INTRODUCTION: ENDOMETRIAL CANCER AND THE LINK TO STEROID HORMONES AND STEROID RECEPTORS

Endometrial carcinogenesis is related to overexposure to estrogen that is not modulated by the differentiating effects of progesterone and potentially other steroid hormones including androgens and glucocorticoids. The endometrium is one of the most estrogen-sensitive tissues in the body and responds to estrogens with rapid cell growth: Unopposed estrogen stimulation can lead to endometrial hyperplasia, cellular atypia, and endometrial cancer. Initial studies indicating that the proliferation of the endometrium was under hormonal control employed tritiated thymidine incorporation as a measure of DNA synthesis in animal models. These original data have now been supplemented by detailed investigations that show that estrogens act upon the endometrium through estrogen receptors (ERs) resulting in the induction of growth factors such as the epidermal growth factor (EGF) (1), its receptor (EGFR) (2), insulin-like growth factor-1 (IGF-1) (3), and growth-enhancing protooncogenes, such as *c-fos* and *c-myc* (4). ERs induce progesterone receptors (PRs) through which progesterone exerts differentiating effects on the glandular epithelium and opposes the growth-promoting effects of estrogen. Androgen receptors (ARs) and glucocorticoid receptors (GRs) are also expressed in the endometrium and in endometrial tumors and may be involved in endometrial differentiation (5,6).

HORMONE RECEPTORS IN THE NORMAL ENDOMETRIUM

With respect to endometrial proliferation and differentiation, by far the best-studied steroid hormones are estrogen and progesterone. ERs are expressed in both the glandular eplithelium and the stroma in increasing concentrations as the proliferative phase of the cycle progresses. At ovulation, ERs are down-regulated in response to progesterone production from the ovary. PRs are also induced in increasing concentrations during the proliferative phase, in part due to rising estradiol levels that induce PRs through ERs. A complete explanation of receptor isoforms is presented later in the chapter; however, briefly, the A isoform of PR (PRA) predominates over the B isoform (PRB) throughout the menstrual cycle, particularly in the stroma (7). However, PRBs are induced more dramatically by estradiol, most particularly in the glandular epithelium. During the secretory phase of the menstrual cycle, ERs and PRs are gradually down-regulated in the glandular epithelium, but PRs are still expressed in the stroma where progesterone is critical for ongoing proliferation and the secretory response (Fig. 1).

GRs are expressed in human and rodent endometrium, and ARs have been identified in the human and rodent ovary and uterus (8). ARs are induced by estrogen and down-regulated by testosterone (9). Other investigators suggest that estradiol plus testosterone most strongly induces ARs (10). Progesterone has also been implicated in the induction of ARs in the endometrium (11), most likely when it is combined with estrogen (10). ARs are present in the glandular epithelium and to a greater extent in the stroma of the endometrium. The receptors are induced during the proliferative phase of the cycle, are present in stable

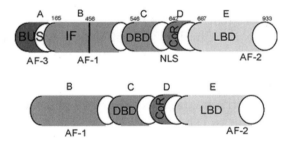

Functional Domains of Progesterone Receptor A and B

Figure 1. Functional domains of progesterone receptor A and B. The A and B isoforms of PR arise from alternative promoters from the same gene. The B isoform (upper figure) is identical in sequence to the A isoform (lower figure) with the exception of the first 164 amino acids at the N-terminus, termed the B upstream segment (BUS). The domains are divided into functional units A–E. IF = an inhibitory function area unmasked by the absence of BUS; DBD = the DNA binding domain; CoR = a hinge region known to bind to receptor co-modulators; LBD = the ligand (hormone) binding domain; AF 1–3 = activation functions required for gene transactivation and protein/protein interactions. The numbers noted above indicate the amino acids.

amounts during the early secretory phase, and lost in the late secretory phase of the menstrual cycle (12). Androgens act through ARs in the endometrial stroma to induce the expression of prolactin, a marker for endometrial differentiation, which is also induced by progesterone through PRs (13). Androgen also inhibits the effects of estrogen, limiting proliferation in the epithelium and the stroma (5). ARs are expressed in 40–88% of endometrial cancers (14).

HORMONAL EFFECTS AND HORMONE RECEPTORS IN ENDOMETRIAL CANCER

Numerous lines of clinical evidence link endometrial cancer with unopposed estrogen stimulation. High rates of endometrial cancer occur in young women with polycystic ovary syndrome and other hyperestrogenic states, and estrogen-only hormone replacement results in a clear increase in the rate of endometrial cancer (15) that is completely reversed by the addition of a progestin (16). Only 1 year of unopposed estrogen treatment results in 20% of the patients developing endometrial hyperplasia. Ten percent of women with complex hyperplasia will develop endometrial cancer, and over 20% of women with complex hyperplasia and cellular atypia will develop endometrial cancer (17). A recent study of "low-potency" estrogen to relieve urogenital symptoms in Swedish women again confirmed the link between estrogen and endometrial cancer. Oral estriol, 1–2 mg daily, increased the relative risk of endometrial cancer and atypical endometrial hyperplasia. The odds ratios for at least 5 years of use compared with never use were 3.0 (95% confidence interval, 2.0–4.4) for cancer and 8.3 (95% confidence interval, 4.0–17.4) for atypical hyperplasia (18). Fortunately, with the institution of combined estrogen plus progestin hormone replacement therapy, the incidence of endometrial cancer has declined among users to rates below the general population (16).

The role of progesterone in the glandular epithelium of the endometrium is primarily antagonistic to estrogen-mediated cell proliferation (19); this is in contrast to the breast, where progesterone mediates both proliferative and antiproliferative effects (20,21). Therefore, the study of progestin action in the endometrium has particular importance because the epithelium relies on progesterone to induce cell differentiation and to counter uncontrolled growth. While progestins have been used with great success to reverse pre-malignant endometrial hyperplasia, they are not consistently effective in the treatment of endometrial cancer. Progestins have been used traditionally in the treatment of recurrent or metastatic endometrial adenocarcinoma and are still under investigation by the Gynecologic Oncology Group as a major therapeutic arm in clinical trials. However, the overall response rate ranges from only 20–40% (22) and is of short duration in most cases. This is somewhat disappointing considering the observation that fully 90% of pre-malignant lesions are completely reversed.

A critical question that must be addressed is why, unlike non-malignant hyperplastic disorders of the endometrium, so many endometrial cancers fail to respond to the growth limiting effects of progestins. A possible explanation is that endometrial cancers down-regulate PRs and, when present, PRs are down-regulated by progestins given as therapy. In fact, expression of PRs has been positively correlated with a good prognosis and response to progestin treatment. The overall response rate has been reported to be 72% in patients with PR-rich tumors but only 12% in patients with PR-poor lesions (23). More than 90% of endometrial carcinomas express high levels of ERs, whereas PR levels vary. Even in the presence of ERs, some tumors do not contain PRs (24). As PRs are normally up-regulated by estrogens via ERs, this implies that failure to induce PRs may be a factor in the genesis and/or progression of endometrial cancer. Loss of PR expression is likely to be the primary cause of progestin resistance in endometrial cancer, and tumors that re-grow after an initial period of regression in response to progestin down-regulate PR expression (25).

The known variation in PR expression in endometrial cancer is complicated by the fact that such tumors are extremely heterogeneous, and each tumor may be composed of multiple sub-populations of cells with high or low responsiveness to progestins (26) and varying levels of PR expression. Interestingly, tumor heterogeneity and response to progestins is not necessarily predicted by the state of tumor differentiation (26), so even well-differentiated cancers are not predictably sensitive to progestin treatment. Even in cancers demonstrating high total PR levels, progestin treatment may leave small sub-populations of cells with low PR expression unaffected, leading to eventual treatment failures.

LIGAND BINDING ASSAYS AND IMMUNOHISTOCHEMISTRY TO DETERMINE STEROID RECEPTOR STATUS

Ligand binding assays for steroid receptors as well as immunohistochemistry (IHC) have been used to determine protein levels in endometrial tumors. Most studies from the last decade use IHC, which is well accepted as a modality to localize and semi-quantitate ERs and PRs in paraffin-embedded endometrial tumor tissues as shown in (Fig. 2). IHC allows the evaluation of multiple regions of the tumor and can be used to distinguish ERs and PRs in the glands as well as the surrounding stroma, thereby providing a significant advantage over ligand binding assays (27).

Numerous studies support the finding that high ER and PR levels are associated with a well differentiated tumor phenotype. Initial work was done by the ligand binding method on protein extracts from tumors. McCarty et al. studied 58 patients for histologic grade and ligand binding activity for ERs and PRs (28). Eighty-five percent of the well differentiated lesions demonstrated high levels of ERs and PRs, whereas only 13% of poorly differentiated tumors had detectable levels of ERs or PRs. Following 114 patients with endometrial cancer, Ehrlich et al. demonstrated a reduction in PRs with poorly differentiated tumors as well as a statistical correlation between the response of the patient to progestin treatment and the presence of PRs (29). Improved response to therapy for patients with high ERs and PRs was also documented by other ligand binding studies (30,31) as well as by Carcangiu et al. (32) and Chambers et al. (33) in some of the first major reports of IHC

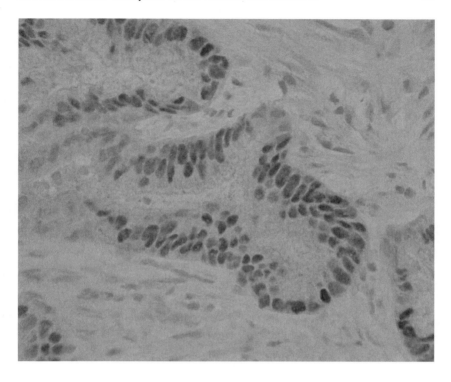

Figure 2A. ER by immunohistochemistry in endometrial cancer tissue. The staining is nuclear.

for ERs and PRs in endometrial cancers. In these studies, receptor status was determined by IHC as well as by traditional ligand binding assays on 183 tumor specimens. The correlation was very good between the techniques, and the best predictor of a good outcome was high ER levels by IHC. An early paper that distinguished between hormone responsive tumors (Type I) and non-hormone responsive tumors (Type II) demonstrated the loss of PRs in type II tumors by ligand binding (34). Even in early stage and grade tumors, loss of PRs has been reported to be a predictor for adverse clinical outcome (35,36). ER status by IHC was correlated with survival in a study of 78 cases of endometrial cancer (37). High PR and ER levels were found to be predictive of survival and low PR levels to be predictive of

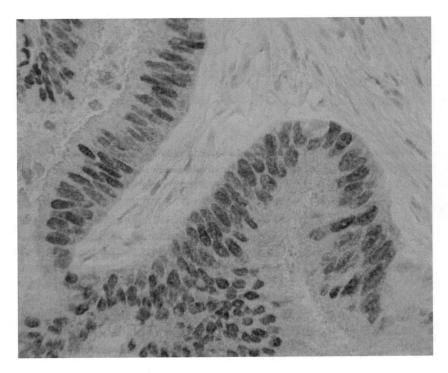

Figure 2B. PR by immunohistochemistry in endometrial cancer using an antibody that recognizes PRA with greater affinity than PRB. The staining is mainly nuclear.

lymph node metastasis in two similar IHC studies from the same laboratory (38,39). In spite of the apparent usefulness of identifying receptor status in endometrial tumors as a predictor of hormonal responsiveness and good clinical outcome, recent data cast doubt on whether receptor status is an independent predictor of recurrence. Indeed, Fanning et al. (40) studied 62 endometrial cancers for ERs, PRs, p53, HER-2/neu, *c-myc*, and additional proteins considered to be markers for proliferation. They determined that none of the proteins identified by IHC were independently able to predict recurrence over and above the surgical stage and grade of the tumor (40). This suggests that more investigations are indicated, including an analysis of

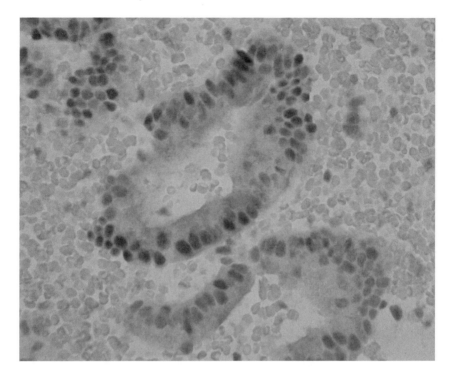

Figure 2C. PRB by immunohistochemistry in endometrial cancer using an antibody to the unique N terminus of PRB. Note the light cytoplasmic staning indicative of the location of this receptor in both the cytoplasm and the nucleus of the glandular epithelial cells.

receptor isoforms, to more firmly establish the clinical usefulness of receptor identification in endometrial cancers.

CROSS-TALK AND EXPRESSION IN ENDOMETRIAL GLANDS AND STROMA

The endometrium is composed of two cell types, the glandular epithelium and the stroma. Endometrial cancers arise most commonly in the glandular epithelium. However, the glands and stroma communicate directly, and it is likely that abnormal interactions between the two tissues may occur in the process of endometrial carcinogenesis (41). The epithelial glands and the stroma both express ERs and PRs, and expression in both tissue types is likely to be necessary to induce normal growth and differentiation of the glandular epithelium. For example, reconstitution experiments using stromal and epithelial cells from ER knock-out (ERKO) and normal mice demonstrate that epithelial cell proliferation in the mouse is mediated via ER action from the stroma (41–43). In addition, stromal PR levels are much higher than epithelial levels at the time of implantation, making it clear that progesterone's effects at critical stages in endometrial function are mediated through the stroma (44). It is predicted that some aspects of epithelial cell differentiation in response to progesterone may be mediated through stromal PRs (45). Therefore, evaluation of receptor expression in the stroma as well as the glands may provide insight into the process of carcinogenesis and to the responsiveness of the tumor to progestin therapy.

GENOMIC EFFECTS OF SRS

Estrogen, progesterone, glucocorticoids, and androgens act via genomic and non-genomic pathways to control cell function and proliferation. The genomic pathway leads directly to the transcription of hormone-dependent genes and is the principal and best-studied mode of action. Gene expression profiling in response to steroid hormones through their cognate receptors has provided new information on the large number of pathways controlled by these factors. Cytokines, cell adhesion molecules, growth factors and their receptors, signaling molecules, pro- and anti-apoptotic factors, DNA binding proteins, enzymes, other classes of transcription factors, and cell cycle regulators are now known to be under hormonal control (46–59). Hormone-dependent gene transcription results from the binding of the steroid hormones as ligands to specific nuclear receptors (60). ERs, PRs, GRs, and ARs are members of the super-family of steroid and thyroid hormone receptors (61). They are best characterized as nuclear transcription factors responsible for binding to DNA, recruiting a protein complex of co-modulators as well as the basal transcriptional unit, and initiating the expression of hormone-dependent proteins (62).

The functional domains of the receptors (shown for PRs in Fig. 1), consist of an N-terminus A/B domain, a DNA binding domain (DBD), a ligand (hormone) binding domain (LBD), and a carboxy terminus. The A/B domain is not highly conserved but contains important activation functions (AFs) responsible for protein–protein interactions with co-activators and co-repressors that impart a positive or a negative transcriptional conformation on the receptor complex (63). The most highly conserved region of the receptor family is the DBD. It contains numerous basic amino acids arranged into two zinc fingers responsible for recognizing and binding to specific DNA response elements in the promoters of hormone-dependent genes. The LBD is located near the carboxyl terminus. Amino acid sequences among family members are heterogeneous within the LBD to allow different ligands to bind to the otherwise similar family members. In addition, the LBD contains a hormone-dependent AF involved in protein–protein interactions.

RECEPTOR ISOFORMS

Two isoforms of PRs, PRA and PRB, are expressed in humans, and both are likely to be required for endometrial differentiation. PRA encodes a 90 kD protein, and PRB encodes a 120 kD protein. Both forms arise from alternative promoters on the same gene and can form homo- (A/A, B/B) or hetero- (A/B) dimers. Dimerization between two individual PRA and/or PRB molecules is required to form the functional transciption factor unit on DNA. Studies by Clarke and Southerland (19) have demonstrated that, while both isoforms are present in the glands and the stroma, PRA may be the primary form present in the stroma, and PRB predominates in the glandular epithelium (64). The isoforms are identical except that PRB has a longer N-terminus consisting of 164 amino acids not present in PRA and containing a third activation function (AF-3), as shown in Figure 1. The sequences down-stream from the N-terminus of PRB are identical between the A and B isoforms, including a DNA binding domain (DBD), a hinge region including the nuclear localization sequence (NLS) and a region to which co-modulators bind (Co-R), and the ligand binding domain (LBD) including activation function-2 (AF-2).

The unique N-terminus of PRB with AF-3 encoded therein has conferred different functional characteristics on the isoforms: PRB is a stronger transcriptional activator of many genes compared to PRA (65–67), but PRA apparently counters estrogen action directly by inhibiting ER function in a dominant negative manner (68). In endometrial cancer cell lines, both isoforms function to enhance differentiation, with PRA inducing cell senescence and PRB inducing a secretory phenotype. Both isoforms sensitize endometrial cancer cells to apoptosis and inhibit the cell cycle at the G1 to S transition (46). However, with respect to growth inhibition, PRB appears to be the principal effector in human endometrial cancer cells grown in vitro (55). PRB is lost in poorly differentiated endometrial cancer cell lines such as Hec50 and KLE, suggesting that this isoform is important to maintain endometrial differentiation (65,66), and endometrial cancers appear to down-regulate PRA and PRB (69) or only PRA (70). The data appear to be somewhat different in mice models, where PRB can induce proliferation in the absence of PRA (71). Female knock-out mice deficient in both isoforms of PR, as well as those deficient in only the A isoform, demonstrate significant endometrial hyperplasia (72). In this model, progesterone treatment causes endometrial proliferation through PRB in the absence of PRA. While these studies are of interest and require further consideration, differences between rodents and humans must be taken into account. Rodents do not develop endometrial cancers, and the proliferative effects of progestin through PRB do not appear to be malignant in this model, indicating differences between the potential of endometrial cells to respond to hormone stimulation between the species. Also, rodents do not produce progesterone except during pregnancy. Hence, the endometrium does not require the monthly production of progesterone from the ovary to induce differentiation and to limit estrogen's proliferative effects as do humans. It is therefore not surprising that PR may have different functions in rodents compared to humans. Nevertheless, the functions of PRA compared to PRB are still under investigation, and the possibility that PRB can be a proliferative signal for the endometrial epithelium in humans as well as rodents has not been ruled out.

Further studies on the expression of receptor isoforms such as PRA relative to PRB and other hormone-dependent genes that may be potential biomarkers are warranted to clarify the role of receptor expression and recurrence. Studies now indicate that commercially available antibodies may not recognize PRA and PRB with equal affinity by IHC despite findings to the contrary using immunoblotting. Mote et al. have found that PRB is not recognized by many commonly used antibodies, and this raises the possibility that PRB expression may have been under-reported in the past (73). Therefore, studies to evaluate differential expression of receptor isoforms and their association with clinical outcome will be important for the future understanding of hormone action in endometrial cancer.

Like PRs, ERs are of two types, ERα and ERβ. ERα was the first of the two to be recognized, cloned, and studied. ERα is a 65kD protein encoded on chromosome 6. ERβ is reported to be the predominant ER in the endometrium (74) and induces numerous growth-promoting genes. ERβ is a 53 kD protein that was cloned from the rat prostate several years ago (74), and unlike the PR isoforms, ERα and ERβ are encoded by different genes. ERβ is 95% identical to ERα in the DBD, but only 55% identical in the LBD; however, both receptors bind estrogens at the LBD. As is predicted by the high DBD homology, ERα and ERβ both bind to estrogen DNA response elements. The transcriptionally active form of ER is a ligand-bound dimer; ERα and ERβ can form homo- and heterodimers (ERα–ERα; ERα–ERβ; ERβ–ERβ). Very little is yet known about ERβ with respect to what genes are differentially regulated compared to ERα, or the functional differences of the different dimeric forms. In addition, antibodies that distinguish between the two ER forms have only recently become available. Studies of ERα compared to ERβ expression in endometrial tumors are just now being performed.

Although currently in debate in the literature (75), ARs have been reported to be expressed in two isoforms, the longer B protein (110 kD) and the shorter A protein (87 kD), the product of an N-terminus truncation (76). In vitro data suggest that the two forms are functionally equivalent in cell lines with respect to activation by androgens and anti-androgens on synthetic DNA promoters, but additional data on the gene expression profiles induced by the two forms would be helpful to confirm these initial findings (77). Alterations in the expression of AR isoforms has been reported in colon cancer (78), with the A isoform predominating over the B and raising the possibility that, like PR, AR isoform expression may be disturbed in the process of carcinogenesis.

GRs are transcribed and translated into a number of isoforms. Therefore, GRs, like PRs and ARs, exist in at least two isoforms as a result of alternative transcription and translation from the same gene. The two principal proteins that result are the 94 kD GRA and the 91 kD GRB. Studies now indicate that the two isoforms differ in their ability to activate transcription on consensus glucocorticoid DNA response elements, with the shorter isoform GRB twice as efficient at inducing transcription as the longer GRA (79). Interestingly, the DNA response elements for PRs and GRs are identical in their consensus form; however, the actual sequences in hormone-responsive gene promoters vary and may direct whether the gene is controlled by progestins through PRs or by glucocorticoids through GRs (53). Interestingly, the shorter GRB resides in the cell nucleus in the absence of ligand, whereas GRA requires ligand for nuclear localization (79). This is reminiscent of observations in endometrial cancer cells, where the shorter form of PR, PRA, is nuclear even in the absence of ligand (Leslie, unpublished observations), whereas the longer isoform, PRB, requires ligand or phosphorylation by MAP kinase for nuclear localization. The similarities between PR and GR isoforms are in distinction to the ER isoforms. ERα and -β are transcribed from different genes and diverge significantly in structure over much of the molecules. The exceptions being the ligand and DNA binding domains where the homology is high, indicating that the receptors bind to similar DNA response elements and are activated by the same family of ligands, i.e., estrogens.

NON-GENOMIC EFFECTS OF STEROID HORMONES THROUGH MEMBRANE AND CYTOSOLIC RECEPTORS

Non-genomic functions within the cytosol and at the cell membrane are also attributed to steroid hormones. The best studied thus far is estrogen acting through ERs and other receptors (80), but ARs are also reported to be present in the membrane cellular fraction (81), indicating that the findings for estrogen may also relate to other steroid hormones. Recent evidence suggests that there are at least two non-genomic pathways to estrogen action in the membrane. First, the classic ERα protein has been localized to the membrane as well as the nucleus. These data suggest that estrogens activate ERs at the membrane, resulting in rapid cellular effects that may control ion fluxes and signaling pathways (82,83). Second, recent findings indicate that estrogens, and to a lesser extent, partial estrogens and anti-estrogens such as tamoxifen and ICI 182780, respectively, can bind a novel membrane G-protein receptor, GPR-30 (84,85). Interestingly, the transcription of GPR-30 is under the control of progesterone in breast cancer cells, and is involved in progesterone as well as estrogen control of cell proliferation (86–88). GPR-30 controls the activation of EGFR and downstream signaling events including Ras phosphorylation. The effects of Ras activation include the phosphorylation of proteins, such as PI3 kinase, that ultimately control apoptosis, and others, such as MAP kinases, that phosphorylate and activate a myriad of transcription factors, including the hormone receptors themselves, members of the AP-1 family, and proto-oncogenes such as c-Myc. Protein kinases C and A are also activated by non-genomic pathways of estrogen action, and these are involved in the control of intracellular calcium and pH.

Membrane PRs and GRs have also been hypothesized to exist because progesterone and corticosteroids have a number of very rapid cellular effects, on the order of seconds and minutes, that could not occur as a result of transcription, which takes hours. A progesterone-binding protein distinct from the nuclear receptor has been identified in porcine vascular smooth muscle cells (89). Most recently, a new family of membrane progesterone binding proteins with similarities to G protein-coupled receptors have been cloned from the spotted seatrout, the mouse, pig, zebrafish, Xenopus, and the human (90,91). These bind progestins with high affinity and are saturable, indicating their function as specific receptors through which progestins may exert rapid membrane and cytoplasmic effects. Classic GRs have been identified in the membranes of lymphoma cells (92), and cytoplasmic GRs and PRs may cross talk with signal transduction pathways that could initiate or enhance responses in conjunction with membrane bound growth factor receptors or G-protein receptors. Both GRs and PRs shuttle in and out of the nucleus, and PRB, for example, exists mainly in the cytoplasm in the absence of ligand in breast cancer cells (93) and in endometrial cancer cells (Leslie, unpublished observations). PRB is driven into the nucleus in the presence of progesterone or EGF by two distinct mechanisms, indicating that growth factor signaling as well as hormonal ligands may activate hormone receptors and set the stage for steroid receptor activity in the nucleus (93).

Hence, the understanding of hormone effects now encompasses the nuclear receptors as activators of transcription as classically described, as well as cytosolic and membrane receptors (membrane-bound ERs, ARs, GRs, GPR-30, G-protein like receptors for progesterone, and possibly others) through which moment-by-moment ion fluxes, signal transduction pathways, apoptosis, as well as the activity of other transcription factors are controlled.

REFERENCES

1. Huet-Hudson YM, et al. Estrogen regulates the synthesis of epidermal growth factor in mouse uterine epithelial cells. *Mol Endocrinol* 1990; 4(3):510–523.

2. Lingham RB, Stancel GM, Loose-Mitchell DS. Estrogen regulation of epidermal growth factor receptor messenger ribonucleic acid. *Mol Endocrinol* 1988; 2(3):230–235.

3. Murphy LJ, Murphy LC, Friesen HG. Estrogen induces insulin-like growth factor-I expression in the rat uterus. *Mol Endocrinol* 1987; 1(7):445–450.

4. Weisz A, Bresciani F. Estrogen induces expression of *c-fos* and *c-myc* protooncogenes in rat uterus. *Mol Endocrinol* 1988; 2(9):816–824.

5. Brenner RM, Slayden OD, Critchley HO. Anti-proliferative effects of progesterone antagonists in the primate endometrium: a potential role for the androgen receptor. *Reproduction* 2002; 124(2):167–172.

6. Tuckerman EM, et al. Do androgens have a direct effect on endometrial function? An in vitro study. *Fertil Steril* 2000; 74(4):771–779.

7. Mote PA, et al. Heterogeneity of progesterone receptors A and B expression in human endometrial glands and stroma. *Hum Reprod* 2000; 15 Suppl 3:48–56.

8. Hirai M, et al. Androgen receptor mRNA in the rat ovary and uterus. *J Steroid Biochem Mol Biol* 1994; 49(1):1–7.

9. Fujimoto J, et al. Biological implications of estrogen and androgen effects on androgen receptor and its mRNA levels in human uterine endometrium. *Gynecol Endocrinol* 1995; 9(2):149–55.

10. Adesanya-Famuyiwa OO, et al. Localization and sex steroid regulation of androgen receptor gene expression in rhesus monkey uterus. *Obstet Gynecol* 1999; 93(2):265–270.

11. Slayden OD, et al. Progesterone antagonists increase androgen receptor expression in the rhesus macaque and human endometrium. *J Clin Endocrinol Metab* 2001; 86(6):2668–2679.

12. Mertens HJ, et al. Androgen receptor content in human endometrium. *Eur J Obstet Gynecol Reprod Biol* 1996; 70(1):11–13.

13. Narukawa S, et al. Androgens induce prolactin production by human endometrial stromal cells in vitro. *J Clin Endocrinol Metab* 1994; 78(1):165–168.

14. Brys M, et al. Androgen receptor (AR) expression in normal and cancerous human endometrial tissues detected by RT-PCR and immunohistochemistry. *Anticancer Res* 2002; 22(2A):1025–1031.

15. Antunes CM, et al. Endometrial cancer and estrogen use. Report of a large case-control study. *N Engl J Med* 1979; 300(1):9–13.

16. Persson I, et al. Risk of endometrial cancer after treatment with oestrogens alone or in conjunction with progestogens: results of a prospective study. *Br Med J* 1989; 298(6667):147–151.

17. Kurman RJ, Kaminski PF, Norris HJ. The behavior of endometrial hyperplasia. A long-term study of "untreated" hyperplasia in 170 patients. *Cancer* 1985; 56(2):403–412.

18. Weiderpass E, et al. Low-potency oestrogen and risk of endometrial cancer: a case-control study. *Lancet* 1999. 353(9167):1824–1828.

19. Clarke CL, Sutherland RL. Progestin regulation of cellular proliferation. *Endocr Rev* 1990; 11(2):266–301.

20. Anderson TJ, et al. Oral contraceptive use influences resting breast proliferation. *Hum Pathol* 1989; 20(12):1139–1144.

21. Longacre TA Bartow SA. A correlative morphologic study of human breast and endometrium in the menstrual cycle. *Am J Surg Pathol* 1986; 10(6):382–393.

22. Deppe G. Chemotherapy of endometrial carcinoma. In Deppe G, ed. Chemotherapy of gynecologic *Cancer*. Liss: New York, 1984, pp. 139–150.

23. Ehrlich CE, et al. Steroid receptors and clinical outcome in patients with adenocarcinoma of the endometrium. *Am J Obstet Gynecol* 1988; 158(4):796–807.

24. Polczaski CE, Satyaswaroop PG, Mortel R. Hormonal interactions in gynecologic malignancies. In: Hoskins WJ, Perez CA, Young RC, Ed. *Principles and Practice of Gynecologic Oncology*, Lippincott-Raven: Philadelphia, 1997, pp. 211–229.

25. Satyaswaroop PG. Development of a preclinical model for hormonal therapy of human endometrial carcinomas. *Ann Med* 1993; 25(2):105–111.

26. Siracky J, et al. Cell proliferation kinetics and nuclear morphology in endometrial cancer under progesteron treatment. *Neoplasma* 1978; 25(5):535–539.

27. Soper JT, et al. Estrogen and progesterone receptor content of endometrial carcinomas: comparison of total tissue versus cancer component analysis. *Gynecol Oncol* 1990; 36(3):363–368.

28. McCarty KS, Jr, et al. Correlation of estrogen and progesterone receptors with histologic differentiation in endometrial adenocarcinoma. *Am J Pathol* 1979; 96(1):171–183.

29. Ehrlich CE, Young PC, Cleary RE. Cytoplasmic progesterone and estradiol receptors in normal, hyperplastic, and carcinomatous endometria: therapeutic implications. *Am J Obstet Gynecol* 1981; 141(5):539–546.

30. Ingram SS, et al. The predictive value of progesterone receptor levels in endometrial cancer. *Int J Radiat Oncol Biol Phys* 1989; 17(1):21–27.

31. Kauppila AJ, et al. Prediction of clinical outcome with estrogen and progestin receptor concentrations and their relationships to clinical and histopathological variables in endometrial cancer. *Cancer Res* 1986; 46(10):5380–5384.

32. Carcangiu ML, et al. Immunohistochemical evaluation of estrogen and progesterone receptor content in 183 patients with endometrial carcinoma. Part I: Clinical and histologic correlations. *Am J Clin Pathol* 1990; 94(3):247–254.

33. Chambers JT, et al. Immunohistochemical evaluation of estrogen and progesterone receptor content in 183 patients with endometrial carcinoma. Part II: Correlation between biochemical and immunohistochemical methods and survival. *Am J Clin Pathol* 1990; 94(3):255–260.

34. Deligdisch L, Holinka CF. Progesterone receptors in two groups of endometrial carcinoma. *Cancer* 1986; 57(7):1385–1388.

35. Tornos, C et al. Aggressive stage I grade 1 endometrial carcinoma. *Cancer* 1992; 70(4):790–798.

36. Creasman WT. Prognostic significance of hormone receptors in endometrial cancer. *Cancer* 1993; 71(4 Suppl):1467–1470.

37. Pertschuk LP, et al. Estrogen receptor immunocytochemistry in endometrial carcinoma: a prognostic marker for survival. *Gynecol Oncol* 1996; 63(1):28–33.

38. Iwai K, et al. Prognostic significance of progesterone receptor immunohistochemistry for lymph node metastases in endometrial carcinoma. *Gynecol Oncol* 1999; 72(3):351–359.

39. Fukuda K, et al. Prognostic significance of progesterone receptor immunohistochemistry in endometrial carcinoma. *Gynecol Oncol* 1998; 69(3):220–225.

40. Fanning J, et al. Immunohistochemical evaluation is not prognostic for recurrence in fully staged high-risk endometrial cancer. *Int J Gynecol Cancer* 2002; 12(3):286–289.

41. Cooke PS, et al. Stromal estrogen receptors mediate mitogenic effects of estradiol on uterine epithelium. *Proc Natl Acad Sci USA* 1997; 94(12):6535–65340.

42. Cooke PS, et al. Mechanism of estrogen action: lessons from the estrogen receptor-alpha knockout mouse. *Biol Reprod* 1998; 59(3):470–475.

43. Buchanan DL, et al. Role of stromal and epithelial estrogen receptors in vaginal epithelial proliferation, stratification, and cornification. *Endocrinol* 1998; 139(10):4345–4352.

44. Wathes DC, et al. Regulation of oxytocin, oestradiol and progesterone receptor concentrations in different uterine regions by oestradiol, progesterone and oxytocin in ovariectomized ewes. *J Endocrinol* 1996; 151(3):375–393.

45. Rider V, Kimler BF, Justice WM. Progesterone-growth factor interactions in uterine stromal cells. *Biol Reprod* 1998; 59(3):464–469.

46. Dai D, et al. Progesterone inhibits human endometrial cancer cell growth and invasiveness: down-regulation of cellular adhesion molecules through progesterone B receptors. *Cancer Res* 2002; 62(3):881–886.

47. Mutter GL, et al. Global expression changes of constitutive and hormonally regulated genes during endometrial neoplastic transformation. *Gynecol Oncol* 2001; 83(2):177–185.

48. Richer JK, et al. Differential gene regulation by the two progesterone receptor isoforms in human breast cancer cells. *J Biol Chem* 2002; 277(7):5209–5218.

49. Salleh MN, Caldwell J, Carmichael PL. A comparison of gene expression changes in response to diethylstilbestrol treatment in wild-type and p53+/–hemizygous knockout mice using focused arrays. *Toxicology* 2003; 185(1–2):49–57.

50. Levenson AS, et al. Molecular classification of selective oestrogen receptor modulators on the basis of gene expression profiles of breast cancer cells expressing oestrogen receptor alpha. *Br J Cancer* 2002; 87(4):449–456.

51. Levenson AS, et al. Gene expression profiles with activation of the estrogen receptor alpha-selective estrogen receptor modulator complex in breast cancer cells expressing wild-type estrogen receptor. *Cancer Res* 2002; 62(15):4419–4426.

52. Kramer PR, Wray S. 17–Beta-estradiol regulates expression of genes that function in macrophage activation and cholesterol homeostasis. *J Steroid Biochem Mol Biol* 2002; 81(3):203–216.

53. Wan Y, Nordeen SK. Overlapping but distinct gene regulation profiles by glucocorticoids and progestins in human breast cancer cells. *Mol Endocrinol*, 2002; 16(6):1204–1214.

54. Wan Y, Nordeen SK. Identification of genes differentially regulated by glucocorticoids and progestins using a Cre/loxP-mediated retroviral promoter-trapping strategy. *J Mol Endocrinol*, 2002; 28(3):177–192.

55. Smid-Koopman E, et al. Distinct functional differences of human progesterone receptors A and B on gene expression and growth regulation in two endometrial carcinoma cell lines. *J Soc Gynecol Inves* 2003; 10(1):49–57.

56. Kao LC, et al. Global gene profiling in human endometrium during the window of implantation. *Endocrinol* 2002; 143(6):2119–1238.

57. Naciff JM, et al. Gene expression profile induced by 17alpha-ethynyl estradiol, bisphenol A, and genistein in the developing female reproductive system of the rat. *Toxicol Sci* 2002; 68(1):184–99.

58. Rockett JC, et al. DNA arrays to monitor gene expression in rat blood and uterus following 17beta-estradiol exposure: bio-

monitoring environmental effects using surrogate tissues. *Toxicol Sci* 2002; 69(1):49–59.

59. Weston GC, Haviv I, Rogers PA. Microarray analysis of VEGF-responsive genes in myometrial endothelial cells. *Mol Hum Reprod* 2002; 8(9):855–863.

60. Jensen EV, DeSombre ER. Estrogen-receptor interaction. *Science* 1973; 182(108):126–134.

61. Evans RM. The steroid and thyroid hormone receptor super-family. *Science* 1988; 240(4854):889–895.

62. Onate SA, et al. Sequence and characterization of a coactivator for the steroid hormone receptor superfamily. *Science* 1995; 270(5240):1354–1357.

63. McDonnell DP, Chang CY, Norris JD. Development of peptide antagonists that target estrogen receptor-cofactor interactions. *J Steroid Biochem Mol Biol* 2000; 74(5):327–335.

64. Mote PA, et al. Colocalization of progesterone receptors A and B by dual immunofluorescent histochemistry in human endometrium during the menstrual cycle. *J Clin Endocrinol Metab* 1999; 84(8):2963–2971.

65. Kumar NS, et al. Selective down-regulation of progesterone receptor isoform B in poorly differentiated human endometrial cancer cells: implications for unopposed estrogen action. *Cancer Res* 1998; 58(9):1860–1865.

66. Leslie KK, et al. Differential expression of the A and B isoforms of progesterone receptor in human endometrial cancer cells. Only progesterone receptor B is induced by estrogen and associated with strong transcriptional activation. *Ann N Y Acad Sci* 1997; 828:17–26.

67. Jacobsen BM, et al. New human breast cancer cells to study progesterone receptor isoform ratio effects and ligand-independent gene regulation. *J Biol Chem* 2002; 277(31):27793–27800.

68. Vegeto E, et al. Human progesterone receptor A form is a cell- and promoter-specific repressor of human progesterone receptor B function [see comments]. *Mol Endocrinol* 1993; 7(10):1244–1255.

69. Arnett-Mansfield RL, et al. Relative expression of proges-terone receptors A and B in endometrioid cancers of the endometrium. *Cancer Res* 2001; 61(11):4576–4582.

70. Fujimoto J, et al. Expression of progesterone receptor form A and B mRNAs in gynecologic malignant tumors. *Tumour Biol* 1995; 16(4):254–260.

71. Mulac-Jericevic B, et al. Subgroup of reproductive functions of progesterone mediated by progesterone receptor-B isoform. *Science* 2000; 289(5485):1751–1754.

72. Lydon JP, et al. Mice lacking progesterone receptor exhibit pleiotropic reproductive abnormalities. *Genes Dev* 1995; 9(18):2266–2278.

73. Mote PA, et al. Detection of progesterone receptor forms A and B by immunohistochemical analysis. *J Clin Pathol* 2001; 54(8):624–630.

74. Kuiper GG, et al. Cloning of a novel receptor expressed in rat prostate and ovary. *Proc Natl Acad Sci USA* 1996; 93(12):5925–5930.

75. Gregory CW, He B, Wilson EM. The putative androgen recep-tor-A form results from in vitro proteolysis. *J Mol Endocrinol*, 2001; 27(3):309–319.

76. Tilley WD, et al. Characterization and expression of a cDNA encoding the human androgen receptor. *Proc Natl Acad Sci USA* 1989; 86(1):327–331.

77. Gao T, McPhaul MJ. Functional activities of the A and B forms of the human androgen receptor in response to androgen receptor agonists and antagonists. *Mol Endocrinol* 1998; 12(5):654–663.

78. Catalano MG, et al. Altered expression of androgen-receptor isoforms in human colon-cancer tissues. *Int J Cancer* 2000; 86(3):325–330.

79. Yudt MR, Cidlowski JA. The glucocorticoid receptor: coding a diversity of proteins and responses through a single gene. *Mol Endocrinol*, 2002; 16(8):1719–1726.

80. Ho KJ, Liao JK. Nonnuclear actions of estrogen. *Arterioscler Thromb Vasc Biol* 2002; 22(12):1952–1961.

81. McCann JP, et al. Subcellular distribution and glycosylation pattern of androgen receptor from sheep omental adipose tissue. *J Endocrinol* 2001; 169(3):587–593.

82. Harvey BJ, et al. Non-genomic convergent and divergent signalling of rapid responses to aldosterone and estradiol in mammalian colon. *Steroids* 2002; 67(6):483–491.

83. Singleton DW, et al. Nongenomic activity and subsequent *c-fos* induction by estrogen receptor ligands are not sufficient to promote deoxyribonucleic acid synthesis in human endometrial adenocarcinoma cells. *Endocrinol* 2003; 144(1):121–128.

84. Filardo EJ. Epidermal growth factor receptor (EGFR) transactivation by estrogen via the G-protein-coupled receptor, GPR30: a novel signaling pathway with potential significance for breast cancer. *J Steroid Biochem Mol Biol* 2002; 80(2):231–238.

85. Filardo EJ, et al. Estrogen action via the G protein-coupled receptor, GPR30: stimulation of adenylyl cyclase and cAMP-mediated attenuation of the epidermal growth factor receptor-to-MAPK signaling axis. *Mol Endocrinol* 2002; 16(1):70–84.

86. Ahola TM, et al. Progestin and G protein-coupled receptor 30 inhibit mitogen-activated protein kinase activity in MCF-7 breast cancer cells. *Endocrinol* 2002; 143(12):4620–4626.

87. Ahola TM, et al. G protein-coupled receptor 30 is critical for a progestin-induced growth inhibition in MCF-7 breast cancer cells. *Endocrinol* 2002; 143(9):3376–3384.

88. Ahola TM, et al. Progestin upregulates G-protein-coupled receptor 30 in breast cancer cells. *Eur J Biochem* 2002; 269(10):2485–2490.

89. Falkenstein E, et al. Full-length cDNA sequence of a progesterone membrane-binding protein from porcine vascular smooth muscle cells. *Biochem Biophys Res Commun* 1996; 229(1):86–89.

90. Zhu Y, et al. Cloning, expression, and characterization of a membrane progestin receptor and evidence it is an intermediary in meiotic maturation of fish oocytes. *Proc Natl Acad Sci USA* 2003; 100(5):2231–2236.

91. Zhu Y, Bond J, Thomas P. Identification, classification, and partial characterization of genes in humans and other vertebrates homologous to a fish membrane progestin receptor. *Proc Natl Acad Sci USA* 2003; 100(5):2237–2242.

92. Chen F, Watson CS, Gametchu B. Association of the glucocorticoid receptor alternatively-spliced transcript 1A with the presence of the high molecular weight membrane glucocorticoid receptor in mouse lymphoma cells. *J Cell Biochem* 1999; 74(3):430–46.

93. Qiu M, et al. Mitogen-activated protein kinase regulates nuclear association of human progesterone receptors. *Mol Endocrinol* 2003; 17(4):628–642.

4

The Effects of Tamoxifen on the Endometrium

RICHARD R. BARAKAT

Memorial Sloan-Kettering Cancer Center,
New York, New York, U.S.A.

INTRODUCTION

Tamoxifen, a nonsteroidal antiestrogen, was first approved by the Food and Drug Administration for the treatment of patients with breast cancer in 1978. Large clinical trials involving over 75,000 patients have demonstrated an improved recurrence-free and overall survival benefit in both pre- and postmenopausal women. Long-term adjuvant tamoxifen is the endocrine treatment of choice for selected patients with breast cancer, and there are currently large-scale trials to evaluate its role as a chemopreventative agent in healthy women at risk for breast cancer. One of the most significant

79

complications of long-term tamoxifen use is the possible development of endometrial cancer.

The indications for tamoxifen use have broadened to include long-term adjuvant therapy as well as preventive therapy for selected high-risk women. Consequently, a large number of women, including healthy young patients with no history of cancer, will be subjected to the long-term effects of tamoxifen. This chapter reviews the current literature regarding tamoxifen use in breast cancer patients and associated uterine neoplasia and explores the role of screening for endometrial cancer in tamoxifen-treated breast cancer patients.

ENDOMETRIAL CARCINOMA

Following the initial report by Killackey et al. (1) of endometrial cancer occurring in three breast cancer patients receiving antiestrogens, numerous other cases of tamoxifen-associated uterine cancers have been reported (2–14). The anecdotal nature of many of these small series suggests an association between tamoxifen treatment for breast cancer and the subsequent development of endometrial cancer, but fail to provide conclusive evidence for it. Perhaps the strongest data initially implicating tamoxifen use and the subsequent development of endometrial cancer were published in 1989 by Fornander et al. (4). The authors reviewed the frequency of new primary cancers as recorded in the Swedish Cancer Registry for a group of 1846 post-menopausal women with early breast cancer who were included in a randomized trial of adjuvant tamoxifen. They noted a 6.4-fold increase in the relative risk of endometrial cancer in 931 tamoxifen-treated patients, compared to 915 patients in the control group. The dose of tamoxifen in this study was 40 mg/d, and the greatest cumulative risk of developing endometrial cancer was after 5 years of tamoxifen use.

Fisher et al. (12) published the most compelling data to date regarding the association between tamoxifen use and the development of endometrial cancer in their report of the findings of the National Surgical Adjuvant Breast and Bowel

Project (NSABP) B-14 trial. Data regarding the rates of endometrial and other cancers were analyzed on 2843 patients with node-negative, estrogen receptor-positive, invasive breast cancer randomly assigned to placebo or tamoxifen (20 mg/d) and on 1220 tamoxifen-treated patients registered in NSABP B-14 subsequent to randomization. Two of the 1424 patients assigned to receive placebo developed endometrial cancer; however, both had subsequently received tamoxifen for treatment of breast cancer recurrence. Fifteen patients randomized to tamoxifen treatment developed endometrial cancer; one of these patients never actually accepted tamoxifen therapy. Eight additional cases of uterine cancer occurred in the 1220 tamoxifen-treated patients. Seventy-six percent of the endometrial cancers occurred in women age 60 or older. The mean duration of tamoxifen therapy was 35 months, with 36% of the endometrial cancers developing within 2 years of therapy and 6 occurring less than 9 months after treatment was initiated, suggesting that some of the cancers may have been present prior to starting tamoxifen therapy. The average annual hazard rate for endometrial cancer in the placebo group was 0.2/1000 and 1.6/1000 for the randomized tamoxifen-treated group. The relative risk of an endometrial cancer occurring in the randomized, tamoxifen-treated group was 7.5. Similar results were seen in the 1220 registered patients who received tamoxifen.

Any conclusions regarding the risks of tamoxifen treatment inducing endometrial cancer must weigh the benefits of tamoxifen in reducing breast cancer recurrence and new contralateral breast cancers. In the B-14 trial, the cumulative rate per 1000 participants of breast cancer relapse was reduced from 227.8 in the placebo group to 123.5 in the randomized tamoxifen-treated group. In addition, the cumulative rate of contralateral breast cancer was reduced from 40.5 to 23.5, respectively, in the two groups. Taking into account the increased cumulative rate of endometrial cancer, there was a 38% reduction in the 5-year cumulative hazard rate in the tamoxifen-treated group. These results led the authors to conclude that the benefit of tamoxifen therapy for breast cancer outweighs the potential increase in endometrial cancer.

Recent results from three large Scandinavian breast cancer trials have further confirmed the relationship between tamoxifen use and the development of endometrial cancer (15). These studies, which included a total of 4914 patients with a median follow-up of 8 to 9 years, were analyzed for the occurrence of second primary cancers. There were statistically significant increases in endometrial cancers among the tamoxifen-treated patients (RR = 4.1). In addition, the authors also noted a significant increase in colorectal cancer (RR = 1.9) and stomach cancers (RR = 3.2) in the tamoxifen-treated group. The association between tamoxifen and gastrointestinal cancers needs to be confirmed by other studies.

HISTOLOGY OF TAMOXIFEN-ASSOCIATED UTERINE CANCER

The etiology of tamoxifen-associated endometrial neoplasia has not been established. There are, however, some metabolites of tamoxifen that may act primarily as estrogen agonists, and some investigators favor this mechanism as a possible hypothesis for the development of endometrial neoplasia. Metabolite E is formed by the removal of the aminoethane side chain from tamoxifen. This compound is a weak estrogen agonist that binds the estrogen receptor with low affinity (16). The presence of a hydroxyl group in this compound destabilizes the ethylene bond, allowing isomerization of the compound to its E isomer, a potent estrogen agonist. The clinical significance of metabolite E is controversial, as it has not been detected in the serum of tamoxifen-treated breast cancer patients and its role in endometrial neoplasia remains speculative. It is well established that unopposed estrogen administration is associated with an increased risk of developing endometrial carcinoma. These tend to be predominantly early-stage, low-grade, minimally invasive lesions that have a favorable prognosis (17). If the effect of tamoxifen on the endometrium is that of a weak estrogen agonist, one could expect associated endometrial cancers to have clinical characteristics comparable to those associated with unopposed estrogen. A report from the Yale Tumor Registry by Magriples et al. (8) suggested that uterine cancers occurring in breast cancer patients on tamoxifen may behave more aggressively and carry a worse prognosis. The authors identified 53 patients with invasive or in situ breast cancer who subsequently developed uterine cancer. Fifteen of the patients had received adjuvant tamoxifen at a dose of 40 mg/d for a mean of 4.2 years, while 38 had not received tamoxifen. The mean patient age was 72.3 years for tamoxifen users, which was not statistically different from those not receiving tamoxifen (68.5 years). The interval between the diagnosis of breast and endometrial cancer was significantly lower in the tamoxifen-treated group compared to those not receiving tamoxifen (5.3 vs. 12.3 years). Sixty-seven percent of the uterine cancers occurring in the tamoxifen-treated patients had high-grade lesions (grade 3 adenocarcinoma) or high-risk histologies (papillary serous, clear cell, mixed mesodermal tumor), compared to 28% of those developing in the 38 breast cancer patients who had not received tamoxifen. In addition, patients in the tamoxifen-treated group were statistically more likely to die of endometrial cancer (33.3% vs. 2.6%). These findings led the authors to conclude that "women receiving tamoxifen as treatment for breast cancer are at risk for high-grade endometrial cancers that have a poor prognosis" (8). In addition, the presence of a high percentage of poor-prognosis histologies, including poorly differentiated adenocarcinoma, papillary serous, and clear-cell cancers, along with mixed mesodermal tumors in the tamoxifen-treated group, led the authors to speculate that the mechanism of tamoxifen-induced endometrial neoplasia may be different than exogenous estrogen, which is associated with more favorable histologies.

Silva et al. (18) reviewed the data from M.D. Anderson Cancer Center of 72 breast cancer patients who subsequently developed malignant uterine neoplasms. Fifty-seven patients had not received tamoxifen as part of their treatment, while 15 patients had. Among tamoxifen-treated patients, 33% of the tumors had papillary serous histology, which was significantly higher than the 7% incidence occurring in patients who had not received tamoxifen. However, the authors did not mention the type or duration of chemotherapy given to either group of patients for treatment of their breast cancer. A high incidence of leiomyosarcomas was noted in both tamoxifen-treated and untreated patients (14% vs. 17%), which is much higher than the 1% to 2% incidence of sarcomas that one would expect to find. Other reports of uterine sarcomas occurring in tamoxifen-treated breast cancer patients have been published, but these essentially consist of anecdotal case reports.

Several other studies (11–13,19), however, have not been able to confirm that tamoxifen use is associated with the development of high-risk endometrial cancers (Table 1) (20). Barakat et al. (13), at the Memorial Sloan-Kettering Cancer Center, reported their findings on 73 patients with a history of breast cancer who subsequently developed uterine cancer. Twenty-three (32%) had received tamoxifen for at least 1 year, with a median duration of use of 4.5 years, while 50 (68%) did not receive tamoxifen. There was no significant difference in the FIGO stage or grade of the uterine cancers occurring in those patients who had received tamoxifen compared with nonusers. Five women (22%) from the tamoxifen group died of uterine cancer, as did 13 (26%) of those who did not receive tamoxifen. The authors concluded that there was no difference in the stage, grade, or histologic subtype of corpus cancers that develop in breast cancer patients based on tamoxifen use.

Other authors have reported similar results. Fornander et al. (19) reported on the clinicopathologic findings of endometrial cancers occurring as second primaries in 931 tamoxifen-treated patients with early breast cancer from the Stockholm Adjuvant Tamoxifen Trial (4). The median duration of tamoxifen use was 24 months, given at a dose of 40 mg/d. On histologic review of these cancers, 82% were FIGO stage I, and all were histologic grade 1 or 2. Out of 931 patients, 17 developed endometrial cancer. Three of these patients (18%) died due to endometrial cancer. Similar findings were also reported by van Leeuwen et al. (11), and in the results of the NSABP B-14 trial (12), which confirmed that uterine cancers occurring in tamoxifen-treated breast cancer

Table 1. Clinicopathologic Data from Recent Series Reporting on Tamoxifen-Associated Uterine Cancer

Author	Magriples (8)	Barakat (13)	Silva (18)	Fisher (12)	Fornander (19)	van Leeuwen (11)	Total (%)
No. Pts.	15	23	15	25	17	23	118
FIGO Stage							
I	7	15	10	21	14	17	84 (71.2%)
II	0	2	1	1	2	3	9 (7.6%)
III	2	5	2	1	0	0	10 (8.5%)
IV	0	1	1	1	1	0	4 (3.4%)
Unstaged	6	0	1	1	0	3	11 (9.3%)
Histology							
Endometrioid	9	17	3	18	16	17	80 (67%)
High-risk[a]	6	6	12	7	1	6	38 (33%)
Grade (adeno carcinoma)							
Low (grade 1–2)	5	13	3	18	15	Not given	54 (74.0%)
High (grade 3)	10	4	0	5	0	Not given	19 (26.0%)
Deaths from uterine cancer	5 (33%)	5 (22%)	1 (7%)	4 (16%)	3 (18%)	0 (0%)	18 (15.3%)

[a]Includes papillary serous, clear cell, sarcoma.
(Modified from Ref. 20.)

patients are not associated with a higher incidence of adverse histologic features.

THE ROLE OF SCREENING

The published data would appear to support an association between tamoxifen and the development of both benign and malignant endometrial neoplasia. The increased risk of endometrial cancer associated with tamoxifen use will lead to increased morbidity in breast cancer patients, but this does not appear to outweigh the significant advantage that tamoxifen confers by controlling breast cancer. This issue is clear for the patient with a diagnosis of breast cancer; of greater concern is the possible implication of using tamoxifen in healthy women considered to be at high risk for developing breast cancer based on family history. Large-scale trials of tamoxifen as a chemopreventative agent are currently underway in England and the United States. Whether the postulated reduction in breast cancer outweighs the risk of endometrial cancer in this population remains to be determined.

Although the expected annual risk of developing endometrial cancer while taking tamoxifen is approximately 2/1000 as defined by the NSABP B-14 trial (12), many patients worry a great deal about developing a second cancer. Clinicians caring for these patients often sense this anxiety and in an effort to alleviate some of this anxiety, may subject their patients to screening procedures in an attempt to detect endometrial cancers earlier and thereby improve outcome. Although the chance of detecting endometrial cancer is very low, the patient may benefit from the reassurance that a negative test provides. To date, however, there is no evidence that any form of screening for endometrial cancer in tamoxifen-treated patients will provide such reassurance.

Transvaginal sonography (TVS) may provide a noninvasive means of screening the endometrium in tamoxifen-treated breast cancer patients by evaluating endometrial thickening, which may be indicative of pathology. There is, however, no clear definition of an abnormal endometrial stripe. As reported by Lahti et al. (9), if a cutoff of ≥ 5 mm was used to define an abnormal endometrial echo, 22 (51.2%) patients had no abnormal endometrial pathology. Kedar et al. (21) reported a predictive value of 100% (16/16) for atypical hyperplasia or polyps with an endometrial stripe of ≥ 8 mm. These findings suggested that premalignant changes could be detected with TVS, and the use of ultrasound and/or endometrial sampling to screen for endometrial neoplasia needed to be evaluated in large prospective trials before recommendations for screening could be made. Care must be taken, however, to avoid overinterpreting the ultrasonographic findings of the endometrium in tamoxifen-treated patients. Goldstein (22) reported on five postmenopausal tamoxifen-treated patients who on routine surveillance with vaginal-probe ultrasonography were described as having heterogeneous, bizarre-appearing endometria with multiple sonolucent areas suggestive of a polyp. Because of concerns regarding tamoxifen use and endometrial neoplasia, the first patient was referred for a curettage and hysteroscopy. Minimal tissue was obtained and hysteroscopic evaluation revealed a smooth atrophic endometrium. When the abnormal sonographic appearance persisted, the patient underwent a sonohysterogram, which involves the instillation of 3–10 ml of saline at the time of sonography. The fluid enhancement revealed that the changes originally interpreted as endometrial were actually subendometrial in origin. Four additional patients with similar abnormal sonographic findings were actually found to have subendometrial abnormalities on sonohysterogram. It is unclear what these abnormal areas represent, as none of the patients have undergone hysterectomy, although it was speculated that they may represent adenomyomatous-like changes.

In a study by Love et al. (23), the authors highlight the pitfalls of screening for endometrial abnormalities using TVS on this population by demonstrating that although 41% of tamoxifen-treated patients had abnormal endometrial thickness, no cancers were detected in this group. Gerber et al. (24) prospectively evaluated the role of TVS for endometrial screening in 247 tamoxifen-treated patients. Patients underwent TVS every 6 months for up to 5 years. The mean endometrial thickness was 3.5 mm prior to treatment and increased to a maximum of 9.5 mm, which was significantly thicker compared to 98 controls. Fifty-two asymptomatic patients with a thickened endometrial stripe underwent hysteroscopy, and dilation and curettage (D&C), resulting in four perforations. The majority of patients had atrophy, nine had polyps, four had hyperplasia, and one cancer was detected. Twenty of the screened patients reported abnormal bleeding, and two of these had cancer. Using a cutoff of 10 mm as abnormal in the tamoxifen-treated patients, TVS was associated with a high false-positive rate. Based on the increased iatrogenic morbidity and only one asymptomatic endometrial cancer, the authors concluded that routine endometrial screening with TVS is not indicated in the tamoxifen-treated patient.

Some have proposed annual endometrial sampling, although this is not without its difficulties. Gal et al. (25) were unable to perform outpatient endometrial biopsies with a Novak curette in 44% of 89 postmenopausal patients due to atrophic changes. The question arises as to whether these patients should be subjected to the inherent morbidity of a fractional D&C under general anesthesia. As reported by Gibson et al. (26), all cases of endometrial carcinoma detected by D&C in tamoxifen-treated breast cancer patients presented with abnormal bleeding, suggesting that a watch-and-wait attitude may be appropriate. Another frequently used method of screening the endometrium in this group of patients is the office endometrial biopsy (EMB). Barakat et al. (27) studied 111 evaluable patients who underwent semiannual endometrial biopsies utilizing a Pipelle endometrial biopsy device (Unimar; Wilmington, CT) for 2 years, then annually for an additional 3 years. A total of 635 endometrial biopsies were performed (mean, 5.8), with a median surveillance time of 36 months. Five hundred and forty-four (85.7%) revealed benign endometrium; 82 (12.9%) of the biopsies revealed tissue insufficient for diagnosis. This was assumed to reflect atrophic endometrium, if, in the investigator's opinion, the pipelle had been successfully introduced into the endometrial cavity. No further evaluation was done unless the patient developed abnormal bleeding. Nine patients (1.4%) had abnormal biopsies that led to further evaluation, usually consisting of a D&C with hysteroscopy. In total, 14 (12.6%) of the 111 patients underwent a D&C for an abnormal EMB, persistent bleeding, or for evaluation of adnexal masses at the time of laparoscopy. Findings at D&C included: complex hyperplasia (1), abnormal histiocytes (1), simple hyperplasia (2), polyps (4), endocervical polyp (1), and decidualization secondary to progesterone. Although three of the sampled patients (2.7%) required hysterectomy, only one had pathology detected by endometrial biopsy, and this patient had complex hyperplasia only. The authors concluded that, although office endometrial biopsies can be used to monitor the endometrium in the majority (95%) of patients, the utility of these tests in terms of cancer screening appears limited. Only one of these had pathology detected by endometrial biopsy, and no cancers were detected.

What, if any, recommendations can be made regarding the need for screening for endometrial cancer in breast cancer patients on tamoxifen? The ultimate goal of any cancer screening program is to detect disease at an earlier stage, when it is more curable. Since tamoxifen-associated endometrial cancers appear to have a similar stage, grade, and histology as endometrial cancers occurring in the general population (13), their prognosis is generally good and early detection will probably not improve outcome significantly. Since the annual risk of endometrial cancer is 2/1000 in this population, and approximately 15% of these cancers will result in the patient's death (20), annual screening could potentially decrease mortality in only $0.002 \times 0.15 = 0.0003$, or 0.03%, of all tamoxifen-treated patients. Since approximately 80,000 women begin tamoxifen treatment annually, the cost to undertake screening for endometrial cancer in this population may be prohibitively high.

Breast cancer patients on tamoxifen are anxious about developing a second cancer. Rather than feeding into this anxiety by ordering a battery of screening tests with unproven efficacy, clinicians should educate their patients regarding the actual risk and outcome of endometrial cancers that may develop while on tamoxifen. These patients should be instructed to alert their physician about any abnormal vaginal bleeding, including spotting or abnormal vaginal discharge. All women with breast cancer, whether they are receiving tamoxifen or not, should undergo an annual gynecologic evaluation. Endometrial sampling with or without a TVS should be reserved for patients with any sign of abnormal vaginal bleeding.

REFERENCES

1. Killackey MA, Hakes TB, Pierce VK. Endometrial adenocarcinoma in breast cancer patients receiving antiestrogens. *Cancer Treat Rep* 1985; 69:237–238.

2. Hardell L. Tamoxifen as risk factor for carcinoma of corpus uteri (letter). *Lancet* 1988; 2:563.

3. Neven P, De Muylder X, Van Belle Y, Vanderick G, DeMuylder E. Tamoxifen and the uterus and endometrium (letter). *Lancet* 1989; 1:375.

4. Fornander T, Rutqvist LE, Cedermark B, Glas U, Mattsson A, Silfversward C, Skoog L, Somell A, Theve T, Wilking N. Adjuvant tamoxifen in early breast cancer: occurrence of new primary cancers. *Lancet* 1989; 1:117–120.

5. Atlante G, Pozzi M, Vincenzoni C, Vocaturo G. Four case reports presenting new acquisitions on the association between breast and endometrial cancer. *Gynecol Oncol* 1990; 37:378–380.

6. Mathew A, Chabon AB, Kabakow B, Drucker M, Hirschman RJ. Endometrial carcinoma in five patients with breast cancer on tamoxifen therapy. *NY State J Med* 1990; 90:207–208.

7. Malfetano JH. Tamoxifen-associated endometrial carcinoma in postmenopausal breast cancer patients. *Gynecol Oncol* 1990; 39:82–84.

8. Magriples U, Naftolin F, Schwartz PE, Carcangiu ML. High-grade endometrial carcinoma in tamoxifen-treated breast cancer patients. *J Clin Oncol* 1993; 11:485–490.

9. Lahti E, Blanco G, Kauppila A, Apaja-Sarkkinen M, Taskinen PJ, Laatikainen T. Endometrial changes in postmenopausal

breast cancer patients receiving tamoxifen. *Obstet Gynecol* 1993; 81:660–664.

10. Seoud MA-F, Johnson J, Weed JC. Gynecologic tumors in tamoxifen-treated women with breast cancer. *Obstet Gynecol* 1993; 82:165–169.

11. van Leeuwen FE, Benraadt J, Coebergh JW, Kiemeney LA, Gimbrere CH, Otter R, Schouten LJ, Damhuis RA, Bontenbal M, Diepenhorst FW. Risk of endometrial cancer after tamoxifen treatment of breast cancer. *Lancet* 1994; 343:448–452.

12. Fisher B, Costantino JP, Redmond CK, Fisher ER, Wickerham DL, Cronin WM. Endometrial cancer in tamoxifen-treated breast cancer patients: findings from the National Surgical Adjuvant Breast and Bowel Project (NSABP) B-14. *J Natl Cancer Inst* 1994; 86:527–537.

13. Barakat RR, Wong G, Curtin JP, Vlamis V, Hoskins WJ. Tamoxifen use in breast cancer patients who subsequently develop corpus cancer is not associated with a higher incidence of adverse histologic features. *Gynecol Oncol* 1994; 55: 164–168.

14. Assikis VJ, Jordan VC. Gynecologic effects of tamoxifen and the association with endometrial carcinoma. *Int J Gynecol Obstet* 1995; 49:241–257.

15. Rutqvist LE, Johansson H, Signomklao T, Johansson U, Fornander T, Wilking N. Adjuvant tamoxifen therapy for early stage breast cancer and second primary malignancies. *J Natl Cancer Inst* 1995; 87:645–651.

16. Wolf DM, Jordan VC. Gynecologic complications associated with long-term adjuvant tamoxifen therapy for breast cancer. *Gynecol Oncol* 1992; 45:118–128.

17. Elwood JM, Boyes DA. Clinical and pathological features and survival of endometrial cancer patients in relation to prior use of estrogens. *Gynecol Oncol* 1980; 10:173–187.

18. Silva EG, Tornos CS, Follen-Mitchell M. Malignant neoplasms of the uterine corpus in patients treated for breast carcinoma: the effects of tamoxifen. *Int J Gynecol Pathol* 1994; 13:248–258.

19. Fornander T, Hellstrom A-C, Moberger B. Descriptive clinico-pathologic study of 17 patients with endometrial cancer dur-

ing or after adjuvant tamoxifen in early breast cancer. *J Natl Cancer Inst* 1993; 85:1850–1855.

20. Barakat RR: The effect of tamoxifen on the endometrium. *Oncology* 1995; 9:129–139.

21. Kedar RP, Bourne TH, Powles TJ, Collins WP, Ashley SE, Cosgrove DO, Campbell S. Effects of tamoxifen on uterus and ovaries of postmenopausal women in a randomised breast cancer prevention trial. *Lancet* 1994; 343:1318–1321.

22. Goldstein SR. Unusual ultrasonographic appearance of the uterus in patients receiving tamoxifen. *Am J Obstet Gynecol* 1994; 170:447–451.

23. Love CD, Muir BB, Scrimgeour JB, Leonard RC, Dillon P, Dixon JM. Investigation of endometrial abnormalities in asymptomatic women treated with tamoxifen and an evaluation of the role of endometrial screening. *J Clin Oncol* 1999; 17:2050–2054.

24. Gerber B, Krause A, Muller H, Reimer T, Kulz T, Makovitzky J, Kundt G, Friese K. Effects of adjuvant tamoxifen on the endometrium in postmenopausal women with breast cancer: a prospective long-term study using transvaginal ultrasound. *J Clin Oncol* 2000; 18:3464–3470.

25. Gal D, Kopel S, Bashevkin M, Lebowicz J, Lev R, Tancer ML. Oncogenic potential of tamoxifen on endometria of postmenopausal women with breast cancer: preliminary report. *Gynecol Onco* 1991; 42:120–123.

26. Gibson LE, Barakat RR, Venkatraman ES, Hoskins WJ. Endometrial pathology at dilatation and curettage in breast cancer patients: comparison of tamoxifen users and nonusers. *Cancer J Sci Am* 1996; 2:35–36.

27. Barakat RR, Gilewski TA, Almadrones L, Saigo PE, Venkatraman E, Hudis C, Hoskins WJ. Effect of adjuvant tamoxifen on the endometrium in women with breast cancer: a prospective study using office endometrial biopsy. *J Clin Oncol* 2000; 18:3459–3463.

5

Pathology of Endometrial Hyperplasia and Carcinoma

BRIGITTE M. RONNETT
The Johns Hopkins University School of Medicine and
The Johns Hopkins Hospital, Baltimore, Maryland, U.S.A.

JEFFREY D. SEIDMAN
Washington Hospital Center, Washington, D.C., U.S.A.

RICHARD J. ZAINO
The Milton S. Hershey Medical Center, Pennsylvania State University,
Hershey, Pennsylvania, U.S.A.

LORA HEDRICK ELLENSON
Weill Medical College of Cornell University New York Hospital–Cornell
Medical College, New York, New York, U.S.A.

ROBERT J. KURMAN
The Johns Hopkins University School of Medicine and
The Johns Hopkins Hospital, Baltimore, Maryland, U.S.A.

CLASSIFICATION

In the past two decades, clinicopathological, immunohistochemical, and molecular genetic studies have provided data to
allow for the development of a dualistic model of endometrial

93

carcinogenesis. In this model, there are two types of endometrial carcinoma that have been designated Type I and Type II
(Table 1). Factors associated with unopposed estrogenic stimulation, such as obesity and exogenous hormone use, as well
as the presence of endometrial hyperplasia, are related to the
development of the most common form of endometrial carcinoma; that is, the endometrioid subtype that represents the
Type I carcinomas (1). More recent studies have confirmed
this association by demonstrating elevated serum estrogen
levels in patients with endometrioid carcinoma. It also has
been recognized that some forms of endometrial carcinoma
appear to be unrelated to hormonal factors and hyperplasia
(2). Serous carcinoma is the prototypic endometrial carcinoma
that is not related to estrogenic stimulation and represents
the Type II carcinoma. Most of the other subtypes of endometrial carcinoma can be classified as variants of either Type I
or II on the basis of clinicopathologic and immunohistochemical features. Thus, other low-grade carcinomas, which are
associated with endometrial hyperplasia and estrogenic stimulation, such as mucinous or low-grade endometrioid with
squamous differentiation, are Type I carcinomas. In contrast,

Table 1 Pathogenetic Forms of Endometrial Carcinoma

	Type I	Type II
Unopposed estrogen	Present	Absent
Menopausal status	Pre- and perimenopausal	Postmenopausal
Precursor lesion	Atypical hyperplasia	Endometrial intraepithelial carcinoma
Tumor grade	Low	High
Myometrial invasion	Variable, often minimal	Variable, often deep
Histologic subtypes	Endometrioid	Serous and clear cell
Behavior	Indolent	Aggressive
Genetic alterations	PTEN mutation Microsatellite instability K-ras mutation	p53 mutation

(From: Ref. 58.)

most clear cell carcinomas share features with serous carcinoma and are thus considered Type II carcinoma. Some carcinomas display mixed patterns; for example, endometrioid and
serous carcinoma. It is likely that, in these neoplasms,
endometrioid carcinomas develop a serous component as a
progressive step in tumorigenesis. In a similar fashion, it is
conceivable that carcinosarcomas (malignant mesodermal
mixed tumors, MMMTs) evolve from endometrioid or serous
carcinomas. Thus, the proposed dualistic origin of endometrial carcinoma is a model that best explains the development
of these tumors with diverse morphological appearances. As
in all biological systems, there may be rare or unusual examples that cannot be accounted for using this model.

A modified version of the recent World Health
Organization (WHO) and International Society of
Gynecological Pathologists (ISGYP) classification of endometrial carcinoma is shown in Table 2 (3). This classification has
certain limitations. The WHO classification uses the term
"papillary" in the designation of serous carcinoma. Although
most uterine serous carcinomas do demonstrate papillary
growth, a papillary pattern can be seen in other carcinomas
as well, including the villoglandular subtype of endometrioid
carcinoma, mucinous, and clear cell carcinomas. Thus, papil-

Table 2 Classification of Endometrial Carcinoma[a]

Endometrioid adenocarcinoma
Villoglandular
Secretory
Ciliated cell
Endometrioid adenocarcinoma with squamous differentiation
Serous carcinoma
Clear cell carcinoma
Mucinous carcinoma
Squamous carcinoma
Mixed types of carcinoma
Undifferentiated carcinoma

[a]This classification is modified from the World Health Organization and
International Society of Gynecological Pathologists Histologic Classification of
endometrial carcinoma (3).

lary growth is not specifically associated with serous differ-entiation. In addition, some serous carcinomas display a glan-dular pattern and lack a papillary component. Hence, the use of the term "papillary" in designating subtypes of endometrial carcinoma can lead to confusion and should be avoided. Carcinosarcomas are classified as mixed epithelial and non-epithelial tumors in the WHO classification of uterine tumors, but as epithelial tumors in the ovarian tumor classi-fication. This inconsistency reflects the confusion over the his-togenesis and classification of carcinosarcomas in different anatomic sites. Recent molecular genetic data support the concept that both components in these biphasic tumors are clonally derived from a transformed epithelial cell. Accordingly, many investigators now consider these neo-plasms as metaplastic carcinomas.

PRECURSORS OF ENDOMETRIAL CARCINOMA

In this dualistic model two types of precursor lesions are pro-posed for the two pathways of endometrial carcinogenesis. Atypical hyperplasia (AH) is recognized as the precursor for the endometrioid type of endometrial carcinoma and endome-trial intraepithelial carcinoma (EIC) has been proposed as the precursor for serous carcinoma, the most common non-endometrioid subtype of endometrial carcinoma.

Precursors of Type I Carcinomas

Endometrial hyperplasia is defined as a proliferation of glands of irregular size and shape with an increase in the gland/stroma ratio compared with proliferative endometrium. The process is generally diffuse but may also be focal. Endometrial hyperplasia is subdivided into two broad cate-gories, hyperplasia without cytological atypia and hyperpla-sia with cytological atypia (atypical hyperplasia). These pro-liferative lesions are classified further into simple or complex according to the extent of glandular complexity and crowding. Thus, both types of hyperplasia, non-atypical and atypical, are classified further as either simple or complex based on the degree of glandular crowding. Fewer than 2% of hyperplasias without cytological atypia progress to carcinoma, whereas 23% of hyperplasias with cytological atypia (atypical hyperplasia) progress to carcinoma. For practical purposes, it is reasonable to classify non-invasive proliferative lesions of the endometrium as either hyperplasia without atypia or atypical hyperplasia.

Patients with endometrial hyperplasia typically have abnormal bleeding. Hyperplasia develops as a result of unopposed estrogenic stimulation and consequently most patients with hyperplasia have a history of either persistent anovulation or exogenous unopposed estrogen usage. Most hyperplasias that occur in perimenopausal women are associated with anovulation. Postmenopausal women who develop hyperplasia usually are on unopposed estrogen hormone replacement therapy. In these women, the hyperplasia is almost invariably manifested by abnormal bleeding.

Hyperplastic endometrium is not distinctive grossly. A diagnosis of hyperplasia depends on the histological pattern and not on the volume of tissue. A small volume of tissue may reflect inadequate sampling. Microscopically, hyperplasia is characterized by an increased gland/stroma ratio and a variety of abnormal architectural patterns. Glands typically vary in size and shape. Dilatation and outpouching of glandular epithelium into the stroma characterize the lesser degrees of architectural abnormalities (Fig. 1). With increasing degrees of architectural abnormality, glands become complex and branched with irregular outlines and papillary infoldings into the lumens. In addition, with increased proliferation glands become crowded, compressing the intervening stroma, resulting in "back-to-back" glandular crowding (Fig. 2). Thus, complex hyperplasia is composed of crowded glands with little intervening stroma (4). Usually the glandular outlines are highly complex but at times are tubular. Epithelial stratification and mitotic activity generally parallel the architectural complexity, but sometimes they are discordant. Mitotic activity is variable. Even in highly complex hyperplasia with marked stratification, mitotic figures may be inconspicuous. Cells of a hyperplasia lacking nuclear atypia contain oval,

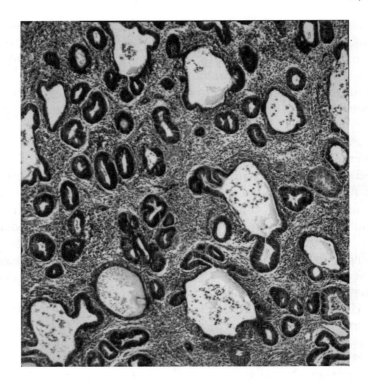

Figure 1 Simple endometrial hyperplasia. An increased gland/stroma ratio and cystically dilated glands with outpouchings are characteristic

basally oriented, bland nuclei with smooth, uniform contours resembling those in normal proliferative glands.

The most important feature in the evaluation of endometrial hyperplasia is the presence or absence of nuclear atypia. Cells with nuclear atypia are stratified and show loss of polarity and an increase in the nuclear/cytoplasmic ratio. The nuclei are enlarged, irregular in size and shape, with coarse chromatin clumping, a thickened irregular nuclear membrane, and prominent nucleoli (Fig. 3). Nuclei tend to be round as compared with the oval nuclei of proliferative endometrium and hyperplasia without atypia. Nuclear atypia is variable, both qualitatively and quantitatively. Not all

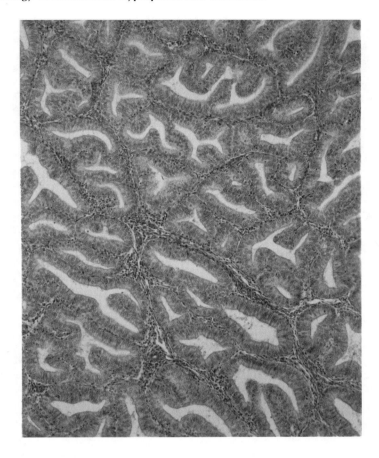

Figure 2 Complex endometrial hyperplasia: Markedly crowded glands are surrounded by a reduced amount of stroma. The glands display complex branching patterns.

glands contain atypical cells and, within an individual gland, some cells are atypical and others are not. Rare atypical cells should be ignored but if cellular atypia is evident without a diligent search, the diagnosis of atypical hyperplasia should be made. Grading atypia as mild, moderate, or severe is subjective and not reproducible. The architectural features of atypical simple and complex hyperplasia are similar to their non-atypical counterparts.

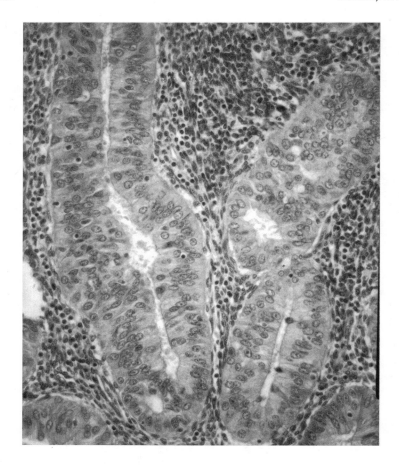

Figure 3 Atypical endometrial hyperplasia: Cytologic atypia in the epithelium lining these glands is manifested by nuclear rounding, prominent nucleoli, pseudostratification, and loss of polarity.

Complex atypical hyperplasia must be distinguished from well-differentiated adenocarcinoma. Most endometrial carcinomas are readily identified, but it may be difficult to distinguish some well-differentiated carcinomas from atypical hyperplasia. The two conditions can be separated if specific criteria are used to reduce the subjectivity of the appraisal. The stroma interacts with invasive carcinoma

(5,6) and the morphologic changes it undergoes can serve as a means of identifying carcinoma. The stromal and epithelial alterations associated with invasive carcinoma are referred to collectively as endometrial stromal invasion. There are three useful criteria, any of which identifies stromal invasion: (1) an irregular infiltration of glands associated with an altered fibroblastic stroma (desmoplastic response); (2) a confluent glandular pattern in which individual glands, uninterrupted by stroma, merge at times creating a cribriform pattern, and (3) an extensive papillary pattern. A process manifesting the latter two features of invasion must be sufficiently extensive to involve one-half (or 2 mm) of a low-power field that is 4 mm in diameter to have value in predicting the presence of a biologically significant carcinoma in the uterus (7,8). This criterion, however, should not be applied too rigidly in view of the potential of missing a carcinoma in small samples. If unequivocal evidence of stromal invasion is present in an area measuring less than one-half a low-power field, a diagnosis of well-differentiated carcinoma should be made. Reproducibility studies have shown that interobserver agreement is lowest for the diagnostic category of atypical hyperplasia, indicating that further refinement of the histologic criteria used to make the diagnosis of atypical hyperplasia is needed. Following is more detailed description of the three criteria for stromal invasion:

1. The altered stroma that reflects invasion contains parallel, densely arranged fibroblasts with more fibrosis than normal endometrial stroma and disrupts the usual glandular pattern (Figs. 4 and 5). The stromal cells are more spindle-shaped than are the stromal cells of proliferative endometrium, with more elongated nuclei.

2. Confluent glandular aggregates without intervening stroma reflect stromal invasion. Confluent patterns are characterized by glandular configurations in which individual glands are not surrounded by stroma. Instead, glands appear to merge into one another to form a complex labyrinth. Some prolifera-

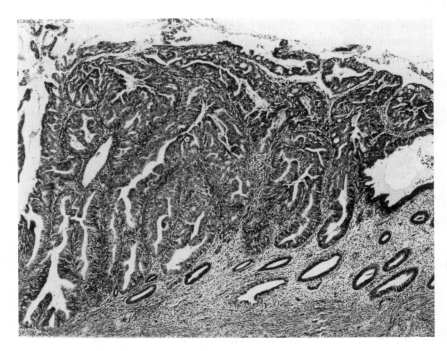

Figure 4 Well-differentiated endometrioid adenocarcinoma: A complex glandular architecture associated with an altered stroma is present. The endometrial basalis is preserved, and there is no myometrial invasion

   tions are cribriform, resulting from proliferation and
   bridging of epithelium.
3. Complex papillary patterns represent stromal invasion if multiple, branching, thin fibrous processes
   lined by epithelium are present. At times these may
   create a villoglandular pattern. Epithelial papilla-
   tions lacking a fibrovascular core do not qualify as a
   feature of invasion.

   In the past, the presence of masses of squamous epithelium replacing the endometrial stroma was considered a feature of invasion (7). Masses of squamous epithelium with
minimal nuclear atypia that extensively replace the
endometrium (over a 2 mm area) reflect stromal invasion only

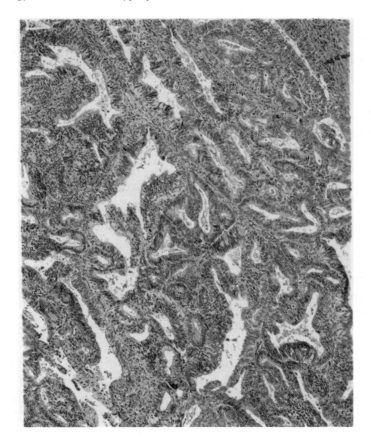

Figure 5 Well differentiated endometrioid adenocarcinoma: Complex back-to-back glands haphazardly infiltrate a desmoplastic stroma.

if they are associated with a desmoplastic response or a confluent glandular pattern.

When stromal invasion is absent in curettings, carcinoma is found in the uterus in only 17% of cases, and all the carcinomas are well differentiated and either confined to the endometrium or only superficially invasive. If stromal invasion is present in curettings, residual carcinoma is found in the uterus in half; more than one-third of the carcinomas are moderately or poorly differentiated, and a fourth of them

Table 3 Findings at Hysterectomy After Curettage Diagnosis of Atypical Hyperplasia versus Well-Differentiated Adenocarcinoma

| | | Of the Carcinomas | |
Curettage Findings	Carcinoma Present in Hysterectomy	Grade	Myometrial Invasion
Atypical hyperplasia	17%	1 (100%)	None (53%) Inner third (47%)
Well-differentiated adenocarcinoma	50%	1 (66%) 2/3 (34%)	None (28%) Inner third (48%) Mid/outer third (24%)

(From Ref. 7.)

invade deeply into the myometrium (Table 3). The absence of stromal invasion provides the basis for distinguishing atypical hyperplasia from a biologically significant, well-differentiated carcinoma (7,9). Two more recent studies, however, found higher frequencies of endometrial carcinoma (43% and 50%) in hysterectomy specimens following a diagnosis of atypical hyperplasia (10,11). Of the carcinomas detected in both studies, 43% were stage 1C or greater.

A retrospective analysis of 170 patients with endometrial hyperplasia in curettings who were followed (mean, 13.4 years) without a hysterectomy being performed for at least 1 year showed that only 2 (2%) of 122 patients with hyperplasia lacking cytological atypia, one with simple and one with complex hyperplasia, progressed to carcinoma. The two cases of hyperplasia that progressed underwent an alteration to atypical hyperplasia before developing into carcinoma. In contrast, 11 (23%) of the 48 women with atypical hyperplasia progressed to carcinoma ($p = 0.001$). Eight percent of patients with simple atypical hyperplasia and 29% of patients with complex atypical hyperplasia progressed to carcinoma (Table 4). The presence of glandular complexity and crowding superimposed on atypia, therefore, appears to place the patient at greater risk than does cytological atypia alone. The differences in progression to carcinoma among the four subgroups, however, were not statistically significant. Thus, cytological atypia is the most useful feature in identifying a lesion that might progress to carcinoma. Similar findings have been reported by other investigators (12,13).

The mean duration of progression of hyperplasia without atypia to carcinoma is nearly 10 years, and it takes a mean of 4 years to progress from atypical hyperplasia to clinically evident carcinoma (4). All but one of the carcinomas that developed from atypical hyperplasia were well differentiated and minimally invasive. These findings and others suggest that carcinomas associated with hyperplasia are relatively innocuous compared with carcinomas not associated with it.

It has been shown that 17–25% of women with atypical hyperplasia in curettings will have a well-differentiated carcinoma in the uterus if a hysterectomy is performed within 1 month of the curettage (9,14). With long-term follow-up, only 11–23% of women with atypical hyperplasia develop carcinoma if a hysterectomy is not done (4,15). Thus, the lesion that is designated well-differentiated carcinoma would appear to remain stable for a long period of time. Since complex atypical hyperplasia is associated with a significant risk of persistence and progression to carcinoma, this lesion is regarded as a direct precursor of well differentiated endometrioid carcinoma of the endometrium.

Women with atypical hyperplasia on an endometrial biopsy who wish to preserve their fertility can be treated with progestin suppression. A conservative plan of management can be justified because the risk of progression to carcinoma in young women is relatively low and the carcinomas that do

Table 4 Risk of Hyperplasia Progressing to Carcinoma

Type of Hyperplasia	No. of Patients	Progressed to Carcinoma
Simple	93	1 (1%)
Complex	29	1 (3%)
Simple atypical	13	1 (8%)
Complex atypical	35	10 (29%)

(From Ref. 4.)

develop tend to be innocuous. Conservative management also can be considered for women diagnosed with well-differentiated carcinoma. If conservative management is elected, magnetic resonance imaging (MRI) must be performed to exclude deep myometrial invasion or the presence of a coexisting ovarian neoplasm.

Patients age 40–55 years with a diagnosis of atypical hyperplasia can be treated with progestins or a hysterectomy. In postmenopausal women over age 55, a biopsy diagnosis of hyperplasia or atypical hyperplasia should be evaluated with a curettage. Hysterectomy is the treatment of choice for a diagnosis of atypical hyperplasia based on a curettage.

Precursors of Type II Carcinomas

Serous carcinoma is frequently associated with a putative precursor lesion, termed "endometrial intraepithelial carcinoma" (EIC). EIC is characterized by markedly atypical nuclei, identical to those of invasive serous carcinomas, lining the surfaces and glands of the atrophic endometrium (16,17). The surface often demonstrates a slightly papillary contour and some cells display hobnail morphology and smudged, hyperchromatic nuclei (Fig. 6). This lesion also has been referred to as "carcinoma in situ" and "uterine surface carcinoma." We prefer the term EIC to carcinoma in situ (CIS) because EIC can be associated with metastatic disease (discussed later), whereas the term CIS implies a lesion that does not have metastatic potential. Additional evidence that EIC is a precursor of serous carcinoma is the observation that EIC can be found in uteri without evidence of an invasive serous carcinoma, frequently on the surface of a polyp in an atrophic endometrium. Molecular genetic evidence that supports the concept that EIC is a precursor lesion of serous carcinoma includes the demonstration of immunohistochemical overexpression of p53 protein, loss of heterozygosity of chromosome 17p, and corresponding p53 gene mutations in a high proportion of serous carcinomas and EIC. Moreover, in cases containing concomitant EIC and serous carcinoma, the identical p53 mutation was present in both lesions.

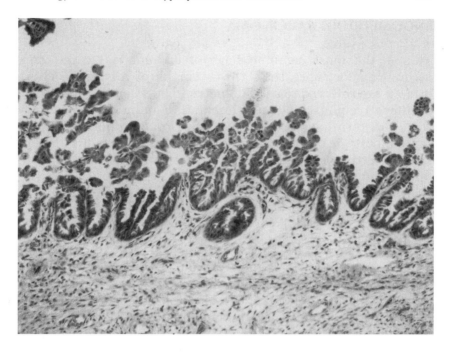

Figure 6 Endometrial intraepithelial carcinoma: The endometrial surface displays marked stratification with micropapillae and marked cytologic atypia. There is no invasion of the underlying endometrial stroma.

There are limited data on the behavior of pure EIC. A recent study found that patients with pure EIC and those with minimal uterine serous carcinoma (less than 1 cm of carcinoma in the endometrium) lacking myometrial or vascular invasion and no evidence of extrauterine disease, had an overall survival of 100% after a mean follow-up of 27 months. All but one of the patients in this group had not received chemotherapy. In contrast, patients with either EIC or minimal serous carcinoma and evidence of extrauterine disease (even microscopic disease) all died of disease despite intensive chemotherapy (18). Accordingly, patients with a diagnosis of EIC in an endometrial biopsy or curettage specimen should undergo careful surgical staging at the time of hysterectomy.

ENDOMETRIOID CARCINOMA

This is the most common form of endometrial carcinoma, accounting for more than three-fourths of all cases. These tumors are referred to as endometrioid because they resemble proliferative phase endometrium and to maintain consistency with the terminology used for describing tumors with the same histological appearance in the cervix, ovary, or fallopian tube. The tumors in this category, by definition, do not contain areas showing more than 10% of serous, mucinous, or clear cell differentiation. Such foci are common in endometrioid carcinoma and are designated as mixed.

Gross Findings

The gross appearance of endometrioid carcinoma is similar to the various other types of endometrial carcinoma with the possible exception of serous carcinoma (see the discussion following on serous carcinoma). The endometrial surface is shaggy, glistening, and tan, and may be focally hemorrhagic. Endometrioid carcinoma is almost uniformly exophytic even when deeply invasive. The neoplasm may be focal or diffuse. At times the tumor may appear to be composed of separate polypoid masses. Myometrial invasion by carcinoma may result in enlargement of the uterus, but a small atrophic uterus may harbor carcinoma diffusely invading the myometrium. Myometrial invasion often appears as well-demarcated, firm, gray-white tissue with linear extensions beneath an exophytic mass, or as multiple, white nodules with yellow areas of necrosis within the uterine wall. Extension into the lower uterine segment is common, and involvement of the cervix occurs in approximately 20% of cases.

Microscopic Findings

The microscopic appearance of endometrioid carcinoma is determined by the grade of the tumor. Grading is based on the architectural pattern and nuclear features. The architectural grade is determined by the extent to which the tumor is composed of solid masses of cells as compared with well-defined glands. In endometrioid carcinomas with squamous differentiation it is important to exclude masses of squamous epithelium in determining the amount of solid growth (see the following). The nuclear grade is determined by the variation in nuclear size and shape, chromatin distribution, and size of the nucleoli. Grade 1 nuclei are oval, mildly enlarged, and have evenly dispersed chromatin; grade 3 nuclei are markedly enlarged and pleomorphic, with irregular, coarse chromatin and prominent eosinophilic nucleoli; and grade 2 nuclei have features intermediate to grades 1 and 3. Mitotic activity is generally increased with increasing nuclear grade, as are abnormal mitotic figures.

The most recent revision of the FIGO Staging System and the WHO Histopathologic Classification of uterine carcinoma recommends that tumors be graded using both architectural and nuclear criteria (3,19). The grade of tumors that are architecturally grade 1 or 2 should be increased by one grade in the presence of "notable" nuclear atypia, defined as grade 3 nuclei. For example, a tumor that is grade 2 by architecture but in which there is marked nuclear atypia (nuclear grade 3) should be upgraded to grade 3. Thus, tumors are graded primarily by their architecture with the overall grade modified by the nuclear grade when there is discordance. Marked discordance between nuclear and architectural grade is unusual in endometrioid carcinoma and should raise suspicion that the tumor is a serous carcinoma (see the discussion on serous carcinoma).

Marked differences in architectural grade can be seen within a tumor. It is not unusual to see well-formed glandular elements immediately adjacent to solid masses of cells. When a tumor displays this type of heterogeneity the architectural grade should be based on the overall appearance. The heterogeneity in differentiation accounts for the differences in grade that can be observed between the endometrial curettings and the hysterectomy specimen. Discordance between the curettage and hysterectomy specimens occurs in 15–25% of cases.

Differential Diagnosis

The main problem in the differential diagnosis of low-grade endometrioid carcinoma is the distinction from atypical hyperplasia (see atypical hyperplasia, discussed earlier). Another problem in differential diagnosis is the distinction of an endometrial from an endocervical primary. Both endometrioid and mucinous carcinomas can arise in either location. The presence of associated endometrial hyperplasia favors a primary site in the endometrium whereas the presence of adenocarcinoma in situ favors endocervical origin. Immunohistochemical stains for carcinoembryonic antigen and vimentin can be of value in this distinction, as can testing for human papillomavirus DNA which is nearly always present in cervical carcinomas and absent in endometrial carcinomas.

Prognostic Factors

Based largely on a series of GOG studies it has been shown that the risk factors for endometrial carcinoma can be divided into uterine and extrauterine factors (20). Uterine factors include histological type, grade, depth of myometrial invasion, cervical involvement, vascular invasion, presence of atypical endometrial hyperplasia, and hormone receptor status. Extrauterine factors include adnexal involvement, intraperitoneal metastasis, positive peritoneal cytology, and pelvic and para-aortic lymph node metastasis. Patients with no evidence of extrauterine disease, no cervical involvement, and no evidence of vascular invasion are at a low overall risk of recurrence. For these patients the grade and depth of invasion are important prognostic factors. In contrast to this low-risk group of patients, women with evidence of extrauterine disease, cervical involvement, or vascular invasion constitute a high-risk group. If one of these three factors is positive, the frequency of recurrence is 20% and increases to 43% for two positive factors and to 63% for three factors (20).

Histologic grading has been discussed. Numerous studies have confirmed the value of grading. In a study of more than 600 women with clinical stage I or occult stage II endometrioid adenocarcinoma the 5-year relative survival was as follows: grade 1: 94%; grade 2: 84%; grade 3: 72% (21). According to a population-based study from the Norwegian Radium Hospital involving nearly 2000 patients, the 5- and 10-year survival rates for patients with grade 1 tumors was 88% and 80%, respectively; with grade 2 tumors, 77% and 62%; and with grade 3 tumors, 60% and 49% (22). Histologic grade is highly correlated with other prognostic factors such as age, stage, and depth of myometrial invasion, so its prognostic utility must also be examined in multivariate analyses. In such studies, the significance of histologic grade in the prediction of survival or recurrence is diminished after adjustment for the other factors, suggesting that grade primarily provides information about the probability of local or disseminated spread of tumor (22). Nevertheless, even for patients with metastatic (stage III) tumor, the histologic grade is significant in predicting outcome after multivariate analysis (23).

Recently, a two-tiered system for assessing uterine tumor grade was proposed and yielded a higher degree of interobserver agreement than the three-tiered FIGO system (24). This system uses three features: proportion of solid tumor growth, pattern of invasion (infiltrative versus expansile), and presence of tumor cell necrosis. There are several advantages of the binary system over the FIGO system. The assessment of solid growth does not require distinction of squamous from non-squamous growth, small amounts of solid growth (around 5%) need not be recognized, and nuclear grading is not necessary. This study found that patients with low grade advanced stage tumors had a 5-year survival of about 75%, similar to high grade tumors confined to the uterus. This system should be tested in other studies to verify its utility.

In the past, depth of myometrial invasion has been reported as the proportion of the uterine wall invaded by tumor and expressed in thirds. More recently, the revised FIGO staging of endometrial carcinoma limited to the uterine corpus (stage I) incorporates depth of myometrial invasion expressed as inner or outer half. Tumors confined to the endometrium are stage IA, those involving the inner half of the myometrium are stage IB, and those involving more than half the uterine wall thickness are stage IC. In addition, we recommend measuring the maximum depth of invasion in millimeters and expressing this as a percentage of the myometrial thickness.

Carcinoma may be confined to the endometrium and involve pre-existing endometrial glands that are beyond the basalis and are in the myometrium. It is important to remember that the endomyometrial junction is typically irregular and it is not unusual for endometrial glands to appear to be in the superficial myometrium. Tumors that involve these superficial glands should be reported as being confined to the endometrium. It may be difficult to distinguish myometrial invasion from extension of the carcinoma into adenomyosis. The distinction, however, is important because the presence of carcinoma in adenomyosis deeper than the maximum depth of true tumor invasion does not worsen the prognosis.

Myometrial invasion, independent of tumor grade, is an important predictor of prognosis. In fact, it probably is the single most important predictor of behavior in stages I and II disease and has been shown to be an independent predictor of outcome for women with early stage endometrial carcinoma (20,21). For example, in the GOG experience, recurrence developed in only 1 of 99 (1%) patients with no myometrial invasion compared with 15 of 196 (7.7%) with inner-third, 8 of 55 (14.5%) with middle-third, and 6 of 40 (15%) with outer-third invasion when grade was not taken into account (20). In another GOG study it was shown that the 5-year relative survival for endometrioid carcinoma confined to the endometrium was 94%, involving the inner third 91%, the middle third 84%, and the outer third 59% (21). The frequency of lymph node metastasis also is related to the depth of myometrial invasion. In clinical stage I endometrial carcinoma, inner-third myometrial invasion is associated with lymph node metastasis in 5% of cases, middle-third invasion with metastasis in 23%, and outer-third invasion with metastasis in 33%. When grade and myometrial invasion are analyzed together, grade 1 tumors invading the inner third of the myometrium do not have pelvic node metastasis, but with outer-third invasion, pelvic node metastasis occurs in 25%. A similar trend occurs with higher-grade tumors.

Cervical involvement also has been incorporated into the new FIGO staging system. Tumors confined to the uterus but involving the cervix are stage II. These neoplasms are then staged as IIA if tumor is confined to the surface epithelium or glands and stage IIB if the tumor invades the adjacent cervical stroma. Cervical stromal involvement is characterized by carcinoma that is not confined to the surface epithelium or pre-existing endocervical glands and typically elicits a stromal reaction. Cervical involvement is associated with a somewhat elevated risk of recurrence, with an overall relapse rate of 16% in the absence of extra-uterine disease (20). Generally, cervical involvement is associated with increasing grade, depth of invasion, and tumor volume so the higher recurrence rate is not surprising.

Between 5% and 15% of patients have positive peritoneal cytology as their only manifestation of extra-uterine spread of tumor. The presence of malignant cells identified cytologically in a peritoneal fluid sample is the basis for classification of a patient as stage IIIA. Positive peritoneal cytology has been associated with other risk factors for recurrence, such as high grade, deep myometrial invasion, or extra-uterine spread (25). Although some studies are conflicting, the weight of evidence in large studies with multivariate analysis supports the presence of malignant cells in peritoneal washings as a significant indicator of poor prognosis.

Vascular invasion is relatively uncommon in endometrioid adenocarcinoma of the uterus, but the frequency increases with deeper myometrial invasion, aggressive cell types, and decreasing histologic differentiation (26). The presence of perivascular lymphocytic infiltrates in the myometrium, but not lymphocytic infiltrate at the tumor-myometrial junction, is frequently associated with vascular invasion and hence is a useful marker of vascular invasion. Some studies have revealed a significant correlation between vascular invasion and tumor recurrence independent of differentiation and depth of myometrial invasion. In an analysis of stage I grade 1 endometrioid adenocarcinomas with a poor outcome, vascular invasion in addition to myometrial invasion, mitotic index, and absence of progesterone receptors were significant factors that predicted aggressive behavior (27). In another study aimed at comparing the significance of various pathologic risk factors in stage I endometrioid carcinoma, univariate analysis showed that vascular invasion was more important than grade and depth of myometrial invasion in predicting outcome. Some evidence suggests that lymphatic invasion may help to identify patients likely to have spread to lymph nodes or distant sites, but that its importance is diminished for those in whom thorough sampling of nodes has failed to identify metastases. Others have also found that vascular invasion was a significant prognosticator by univariate analysis, but less important after adjusting for other variables.

Among the extra-uterine risk factors, the presence of positive aortic lymph nodes is most important in predicting outcome (20). Only 36% of patients with positive aortic nodes were free of tumor at 5 years compared with 85% with negative aortic nodes. The highest correlation of positive para-aortic lymph nodes is with pelvic lymph nodes. Nearly one-third of patients with positive pelvic lymph nodes have positive para-aortic lymph nodes. Other features that correlate with positive aortic nodes are vascular invasion (19%), deep myometrial invasion (17%), positive peritoneal cytology (16%), cervical involvement (12%), and grade 3 tumors (8%).

Endometrioid carcinomas frequently express estrogen receptor and progesterone receptor, whereas serous and clear cell carcinomas are almost always negative. Although in most studies the presence and quantity of steroid receptors have been correlated with histologic differentiation, FIGO stage, and survival, several studies have reported variable results regarding the correlation of hormone receptor expression and prognosis. Given the disparity in results and the relationship with other strong risk factors, hormone receptor expression is best considered a prognostic indicator of uncertain utility.

In an analysis of 819 women with clinical stage I and occult stage II adenocarcinoma of the endometrium entered on a GOG protocol, multivariate analysis demonstrated that age, cell type, architectural grade, depth of myometrial invasion, vascular space involvement, and peritoneal cytology were independent risk factors for recurrence and death from tumor (29). From these data it appears possible to create a model for assignment of the relative risk of death from tumor for individual patients based solely on information gathered by pathological examination of the hysterectomy specimen. For example, a woman with grade 1 endometrioid carcinoma, with tumor confined to the endometrium and no vascular invasion, is arbitrarily assigned a risk of 1. Relative to this baseline risk, a woman with a grade 2 endometrioid carcinoma that invades superficial myometrium and lacks vascular space involvement has a relative risk of 2.6. Similarly, a woman with a grade 3 endometrioid carcinoma, with middle third myometrial invasion and positive vascular space involvement, has a relative risk of 10. The probability of disease-free survival at 5 years for these three women would be approximately 95%, 90%, and 65%, respectively. Knowledge of the specific risk for each patient would allow better prognostication and, potentially, individually tailored therapy.

Patterns of Spread

Endometrioid adenocarcinoma spreads by lymphatic and vascular dissemination, direct extension to contiguous organs, and transperitoneal and transtubal seeding. Lymphatic metastasis is more common than hematogenous spread, but involvement of the lungs without metastasis to mediastinal lymph nodes suggests that hematogenous spread may occur early in the course of disease. Endometrial carcinoma tends to spread to the pelvic lymph nodes before involving para-aortic lymph nodes.

Variants of Endometrioid Carcinoma

Villoglandular Adenocarcinoma

Villoglandular adenocarcinoma is a variant of endometrioid carcinoma that displays a papillary architecture in which the papillary fronds are composed of a delicate fibrovascular core covered by columnar cells that generally contain bland nuclei (30). The median age is 61 years, similar to that of women with typical endometrioid carcinoma. In all other respects, women with these tumors are similar to patients with low-grade endometrioid carcinoma.

The microscopic appearance of villoglandular adenocarcinoma is characterized by thin, delicate fronds covered by strat-

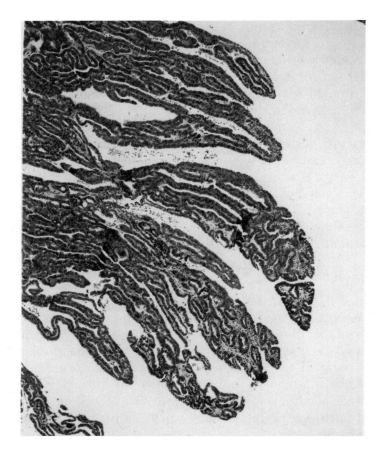

Figure 7 Endometrioid adenocarcinoma, villoglandular type:
Elongated and thin papillary processes have a complex branching
pattern.

ified columnar epithelial cells with oval nuclei that generally
display mild to moderate (grade 1 or 2) atypia (Figs. 7 and 8).
Occasionally more atypical (grade 3) nuclei may be observed.
Mitotic activity is variable, and abnormal mitotic figures are
rare (30). Myometrial invasion usually is superficial.

The main consideration in the differential diagnosis is
serous carcinoma because both villoglandular and serous

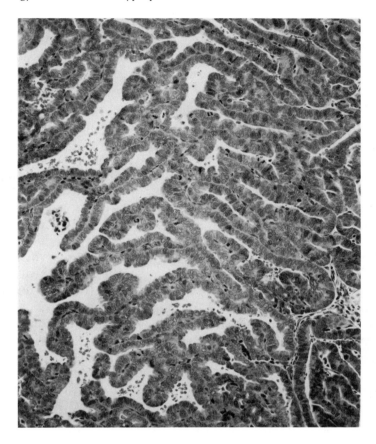

Figure 8   Endometrioid adenocarcinoma, villoglandular type: The papillary branches anastomose with one another, and the cytologic atypia is low grade.

carcinomas have a prominent papillary pattern (31). In contrast to serous carcinomas, villoglandular carcinomas have long delicate papillary fronds and are covered by columnar cells with only mild to moderate nuclear atypia. The cells look distinctly endometrioid with a smooth, luminal border. To have significance as a distinctive entity, the diagnosis is reserved for tumors in which most of the neoplasm has a villoglandular appearance. In contrast to villoglandular carcinomas, serous carcinomas tend to have shorter, thick, densely fibrotic papillary fronds. The most important distinguishing feature is the cytological appearance. The cells of serous carcinoma tend to be rounder, forming small papillary clusters that are detached from the papillary fronds, a finding that is often referred to as papillary tufts. As a consequence, the luminal border has a scalloped appearance. The nuclei of serous carcinomas are highly pleomorphic and atypical (grade 3). Macronucleoli typically are present. Many of the cells have a hobnail appearance, often with smudged, hyperchromatic nuclei. It should be noted that considerable nuclear heterogeneity can be observed (see the discussion on serous carcinoma).

Villoglandular carcinomas are generally grade 1 or 2, and when stratified by stage are not significantly different from endometrioid carcinoma with respect to depth of invasion or frequency of nodal metastases (30). In addition, villoglandular carcinomas are frequently admixed with typical endometrioid carcinoma. In view of the frequent admixture of the two patterns and similar prognosis, villoglandular carcinoma is considered a variant of endometrioid carcinoma.

Endometrioid Carcinoma with Squamous Differentiation

Many endometrioid adenocarcinomas contain squamous epithelium, but the amount of squamous epithelium can vary widely. In a well-sampled neoplasm, the squamous element should constitute at least 10% of a tumor to qualify as an adenocarcinoma with squamous differentiation. Adenocarcinomas with squamous elements were formerly divided into those with benign-appearing squamous elements and favorable prognosis, designated adenoacanthoma (AA), and those with malignant-appearing squamous epithelium and a worse prognosis, termed adenosquamous carcinoma (AS). Recent studies indicate that the difference in behavior between AA and AS mainly reflects the difference in the grade of these respective neoplasms (21,32). Thus, categorization of carcinomas with squamous epithelium according to the depth of myometrial invasion and the grade of the glandular component provides more useful prognostic information than the division into AA or AS because the grade of the glandular component generally parallels that of the squamous element (21). This had led to the view that AA and AS reflect a continuum in the degree of differentiation of the squamous epithelium that parallels the differentiation of the glandular component. Accordingly, it is recommended that endometrioid carcinomas with squamous epithelium be classified simply as endometrioid carcinoma with squamous differentiation, and graded based on the glandular component as well, moderately, or poorly differentiated (grade 1, 2, or 3, respectively).

There are no differences in the clinical features of adenocarcinoma containing squamous epithelium and endometrioid adenocarcinoma. Thus, there are no differences in the frequency of obesity, hypertension, diabetes, and nulliparity among the large series in which this has been analyzed (32).

Gross and Microscopic Findings

These tumors have no distinctive gross findings. Low grade tumors (grade 1) are composed of glandular and squamous elements but generally the glandular component predominates; the nests of squamous epithelium are confined to gland lumens (Fig. 9). The squamous epithelium resembles metaplastic squamous cells of the cervical transformation zone. Frequently, nests of cells with a prominent oval-to-spindle cell appearance, referred to as morules, are observed. Intercellular bridges can be identified within the squamous epithelium, and keratin formation is common. The nuclei of the squamous cells are bland, uniform, and lack prominent nucleoli. Mitotic figures are rare. In higher-grade tumors the squamous element is cytologically more atypical and is not confined to gland lumens but often extends out from the glands. Keratinization and pearl formation occur to varying degrees. Generally, the glandular component predominates, but masses of undifferentiated cells that may represent poorly differentiated glandular or squamous cells lie between glands. This undifferentiated epithelium should be considered glandular unless intercel-

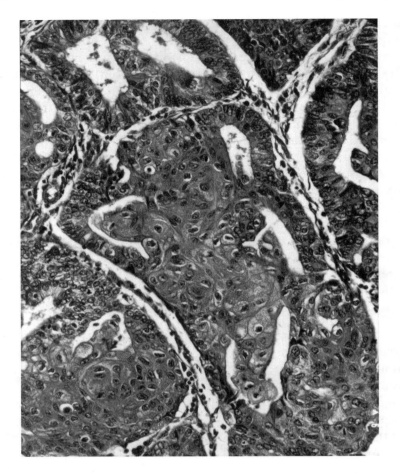

Figure 9 Endometrioid adenocarcinoma with squamous differentiation: The glands in the center of the field are solidified by squamous epithelium, which displays prominent cell borders and a pavement-like appearance.

lular bridges are demonstrated or the cells have prominent eosinophilic cytoplasm, well-defined cytoplasmic borders, and a sheet-like proliferation without evidence of gland formation. Both the glandular and squamous components display grade 2 or 3 nuclear atypia, an increased nuclear cytoplasmic ratio, and increased mitotic activity. The glandular architecture usually is poorly differentiated. Tumors of intermediate differentiation are common. These neoplasms contain glandular and solid areas in which the squamous cells display a moderate degree of nuclear atypia, defying the historical separation into a "benign" and "malignant" category.

A rare finding in patients with adenocarcinoma with squamous differentiation is the presence of keratin granulomas that may involve a wide variety of sites in the peritoneal cavity including the ovaries, tubes, omentum, and serosa of the uterus and bowel (33). Microscopically, these lesions consist of a central mass of keratin and necrotic squamous cells surrounded by a foreign body granulomatous reaction. The granulomas probably result from exfoliation of necrotic cells from the tumor, followed by transtubal spread and implantation on peritoneal surfaces. It is important to distinguish pure keratin granulomas from lesions with both viable-appearing tumor cells and keratin accompanied by a foreign body-type giant cell reaction because the former lesions have not been associated with an unfavorable prognosis.

Differential Diagnosis

The most common problem in the differential diagnosis of the low-grade tumors is with atypical hyperplasia showing squamous metaplasia. To distinguish between the two, the criteria for identifying endometrial stromal invasion (discussed earlier) should be employed. At times, a low-grade tumor may be confused with a high-grade carcinoma because the masses of squamous epithelium are misconstrued as a solid proliferation of neoplastic cells. The nuclear grade is high in poorly differentiated carcinoma, however. For high-grade adenocarcinomas with squamous epithelium the major problem in differential diagnosis in curettings is distinguishing a primary carcinoma of the endometrium from an adenosquamous carcinoma arising in the endocervix. In the cervix, the squamous component usually predominates, whereas in the endometrium the glandular component predominates. A profusion of cell types, especially mucinous or signet ring cells, is more characteristic of an endocervical neoplasm.

Behavior

As described previously, when stratified according to stage, grade, and depth of myometrial invasion, there are no notable differences in the behavior of carcinomas with squamous epithelium compared with endometrioid carcinomas without squamous epithelium (21,32). As occurs with endometrioid carcinomas, the low-grade carcinomas with squamous epithelium tend to be only superficially invasive and seldom invade vascular channels. In contrast, high-grade tumors have a high frequency of deep myometrial invasion, vascular space involvement, and pelvic and para-aortic lymph node metastasis. Metastasis of high-grade tumors occurs widely throughout the pelvis and abdomen, involving bowel, mesentery, liver, kidney, spleen, and lymph nodes. Distant metastasis may involve the lungs, heart, skin, and bones. Nearly two-thirds of metastases contain both glandular and squamous elements, but pure adenocarcinoma or squamous carcinoma is encountered in 20% and 8%, respectively. Often it is the squamous component that is identified in vascular channels. Accordingly, the treatment for carcinomas with squamous differentiation is the same as that for endometrioid carcinomas of comparable stage.

Mucinous Carcinoma

This uncommon type of endometrial carcinoma has an appearance similar to mucinous carcinoma of the endocervix (34). It represents the dominant cellular population in only 1–9% of endometrial carcinomas. To qualify as a mucinous carcinoma, more than one-half the cell population of the tumor must contain intracytoplasmic mucin (Fig. 10). Judging from the few published cases, the clinical features of patients with mucinous carcinoma of the endometrium do not differ from those with endometrioid carcinoma. Patients range in age from 47 to 89 years and typically present with vaginal bleeding. In one study more than 40% had a history

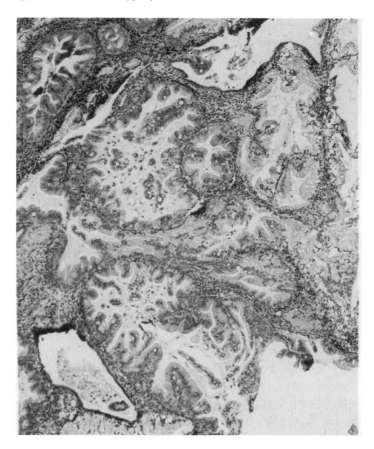

Figure 10 Mucinous adenocarcinoma: Glands are lined by mucinous epithelium, which displays low grade atypia and pale cytoplasm that contains mucin. The epithelium has papillary infoldings and the lumens are filled with extracellular mucin.

of receiving exogenous estrogens. The vast majority of patients present with stage I disease.

Endocervical epithelium merges with the endometrium in the lower uterine segment, so it is not surprising that the distinction of primary endocervical from endometrial mucinous carcinoma in curettings can be difficult. Rarely a low grade mucinous carcinoma or a mixed mucinous and endometrioid carcinoma may contain areas that simulate microglandular hyperplasia of the cervix. Such foci are characterized by cells showing mucinous change with microcystic spaces containing acute inflammatory cells. The patients are in their 50s and 60s, which is in contrast to women with microglandular hyperplasia who are young. The complexity of the glandular pattern distinguish this type of carcinoma from microglandular hyperplasia.

When stratified by stage, grade, and depth of myometrial invasion, mucinous tumors behave the same as endometrioid carcinomas (35). Mucinous carcinomas, however, tend to be low grade and minimally invasive, and therefore as a group have an excellent prognosis. Treatment is the same as for endometrioid carcinoma.

Rare variants of endometrioid carcinoma include ciliated and secretory carcinoma and are discussed in more specialized texts.

SEROUS CARCINOMA

Although papillary architecture is a common finding in serous carcinoma, most other types of endometrial carcinoma can display papillary architecture but are usually not highly aggressive tumors. What distinguishes serous carcinoma from these other types is the uniformly marked cytologic atypia. Thus, the designation "serous carcinoma" rather than "papillary serous carcinoma" is preferred so that cell type rather than architecture is emphasized, and so that confusion with the villoglandular type of endometrioid adenocarcinoma is reduced.

Gross Findings

On gross examination, uteri containing these tumors often are small and atrophic. Generally the tumor is exophytic and has a papillary appearance. Depth of invasion is difficult to assess on macroscopic examination. It is not unusual to find a benign-appearing polyp containing the carcinoma in the hysterectomy specimen after a diagnosis of serous carcinoma or endometrial intraepithelial carcinoma has been made on a curetting because these tumors frequently develop within a polyp.

Microscopic Findings

Although a papillary pattern typically predominates, glandular and solid patterns also occur (17,36). Serous carcinoma originally was described as having thick, short papillae but subsequent studies have shown that thin papillae may be present in more than half. The cytological features of these tumors also are quite varied. Polygonal cells with eosinophilic or clear cytoplasm often are seen but hobnail cells are among the most frequently observed cells. Marked nuclear atypia is always present and is required for a tumor to qualify as serous carcinoma. Thus, serous carcinoma is defined by the discordance between its architecture, which appears well differentiated (papillary or glandular pattern), and its nuclear morphology, which is high-grade (grade 3 nuclei) (37). Focal areas containing clear cells are commonly seen and do not preclude the diagnosis of serous carcinoma.

Microscopically, the exophytic component of a serous carcinoma typically has a complex papillary architecture resembling serous carcinoma of the ovary (Figs. 11 and 12). The papillary fronds may be either short and densely fibrotic or thin and delicate. The cells covering the papillae and lining the glands form small papillary tufts, many of which are detached and float freely in spaces between the papillae and in gland lumens (Figs. 11 and 12). The cells are cuboidal or hobnail-shaped (Fig. 11) and contain abundant granular eosinophilic or clear cytoplasm. There may be considerable cytological variability throughout the tumor, as many cells tend to show marked cytological atypia manifested by nuclear pleomorphism, hyperchromasia, and macronucleoli (Figs. 13 and 14), whereas others are small and not as ominous in appearance. Multinucleated cells, giant nuclei, and bizarre forms occur in half the tumors (Fig. 13). Mitotic activity usually is high and abnormal mitotic figures are easily identified (Fig. 14). Psammoma bodies are encountered in one-third of cases. The myoinvasive component of the neoplasm can show

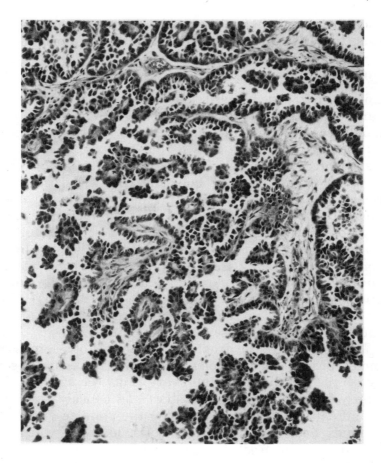

Figure 11 Serous carcinoma: A complex papillary pattern with a hobnail architecture creates a scalloped appearance. Detachment of cell clusters is prominent.

contiguous down-growth of papillary processes, or solid masses or glands, the latter often have a gaping appearance. Nests of cells within vascular spaces are commonly found.

The adjacent endometrium in hysterectomy specimens with serous carcinoma is atrophic in almost all cases. Hyperplasia, generally without atypia, is present in less than 10% of cases (17,36). In nearly 90% of cases the surface endometrium adjacent to the carcinoma or at other sites away

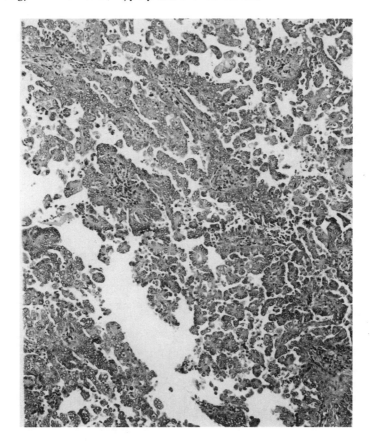

Figure 12 Serous carcinoma: The papillae vary in size and have minimal fibrovascular support. Detachment of cell clusters is present.

from the neoplasm is replaced by one or several layers of highly atypical cells that overlie atrophic endometrium and extend into normal glands. These cells are identical to those of the invasive carcinoma and at times form micropapillary processes. This lesion has been designated "endometrial intraepithelial carcinoma" (EIC) (see earlier discussion and Fig. 6) (16). The intraepithelial carcinoma can extensively replace the surface endometrium and underlying glands with-

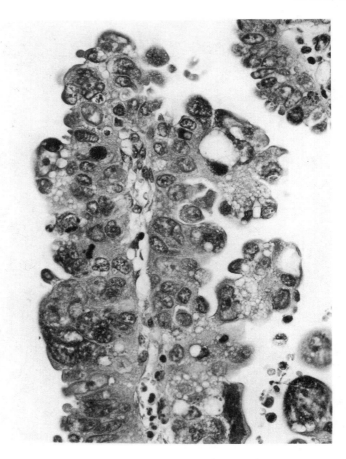

Figure 13 Serous carcinoma: Nuclear atypia is marked with hyperchromasia, pleomorphism, and occasional large, bizarre nuclear forms.

out stromal invasion. It is important to recognize that patients whose uteri demonstrate only EIC, without evidence of invasive serous carcinoma in the completely sampled endometrium, can have metastatic serous carcinoma in the ovary, peritoneum, and/or omentum, presumably as a result of exfoliation and implantation of the loosely cohesive tumor cells (17,36).

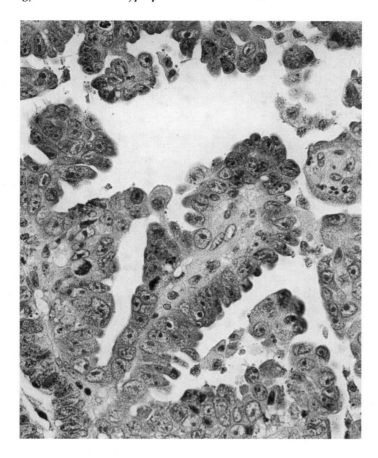

Figure 14 Serous carcinoma: Enlarged, prominent nucleoli and mitotic figures are commonly present.

Differential Diagnosis

Serous carcinoma must be distinguished from villoglandular carcinoma, which also has papillary architecture. The cells of villoglandular carcinoma are columnar, resembling cells in endometrioid carcinoma, and lack high-grade nuclear atypia. Endometrioid carcinomas with grade 3 nuclei are almost always solid, not glandular. In contrast, the glands in a serous carcinoma are lined by cells with high-grade nuclei, some of which are hobnail-shaped, thus imparting a scalloped luminal border to the glands (Fig. 11). In addition, in most cases papillary tufts project or lie detached in the gland lumens. Several studies have demonstrated a very high frequency of strong, diffuse positivity for p53 in serous carcinomas and this pattern of staining is correlated with the presence of mutations in the p53 gene (38). In a small proportion of cases, a missense mutation results in a truncated protein and p53 immunostaining will be completely negative. Strong, diffuse immunohistochemical expression of p53 is confined to a subset of grade 3 endometrioid carcinomas and is not encountered in lower grade endometrioid carcinomas. In addition, most serous carcinomas demonstrate a lack of expression of estrogen and progesterone receptors and very high proliferation indices as measured by immunohistochemical expression of Ki-67. In contrast, endometrioid carcinomas (particularly grade 1 and 2 tumors) frequently express hormone receptors and have lower proliferation indices. Hence, glandular carcinomas with high-grade cytology for which the differential diagnosis includes grade 2 endometrioid carcinoma and serous carcinoma can be distinguished by immunohistochemistry for p53, Ki-67, and hormone receptors.

Behavior

Serous carcinoma has a propensity for myometrial and lymphatic invasion. The hysterectomy specimen often discloses tumor in lymphatics extensively within the myometrium, cervix, broad ligament, fallopian tube, and ovarian hilum. In addition, intraepithelial carcinoma similar to that involving the endometrium has been reported on the surfaces of the ovaries, peritoneum, and mucosa of the endocervix and fallopian tube in the absence of gross disease in these sites (17,36). Involvement of peritoneal surfaces in the pelvis and abdomen, as in ovarian serous carcinoma, occurs early in the course of disease. Not surprisingly, most studies report that uterine serous carcinoma is clinically understaged in approximately 40% of cases. In addition to intraperitoneal spread, serous carcinoma can metastasize to the liver, brain, and skin.

CLEAR CELL CARCINOMA

The prevalence of clear cell carcinoma ranges from 1% to 6% in most series. Almost all studies report that those with clear cell carcinoma are older than women with endometrioid carcinoma (mean age in late 60s) (39). Some studies have reported a higher likelihood of abnormal cytology, a lower frequency of some of the associated constitutional symptoms, such as obesity and diabetes mellitus, and a lack of association of estrogen replacement therapy compared with endometrioid carcinomas, but this has not been confirmed by other studies.

These tumors do not have distinctive gross features. Clear cell carcinoma may exhibit solid, papillary, tubular, and cystic patterns (Figs. 15 and 16). The solid pattern is composed of masses of clear cells intermixed with eosinophilic cells, whereas papillary, tubular, and cystic patterns are composed predominantly of hobnail-shaped cells with interspersed clear and eosinophilic cells (Fig. 15). Cystic spaces frequently are lined by flattened cells. Psammoma bodies can be found in association with papillary areas. The cells typically are large, with clear or lightly stained eosinophilic cytoplasm. The clear cytoplasm is due to the presence of glycogen, demonstrated with a PAS stain and diastase digestion. Cells that have discharged their glycogen and lost most of their cytoplasm are characterized by a naked nucleus, the hobnail cell. Nuclear atypia is nearly always marked, at least focally, and is manifested by pleomorphic, often large, multiple nuclei with prominent nucleoli. Mitotic activity is high, and abnormal mitoses are readily seen. PAS-positive, diastase-resistant intracellular and extracellular hyaline bodies, similar to those in endodermal sinus tumors, can be found in nearly two-thirds of clear cell carcinomas and serve as a useful identifying feature.

Clear cell carcinoma tends to be high grade, deeply invasive, and presents in an advanced stage. Similar to serous carcinoma, clear cell carcinomas are more frequently associated with deep myometrial invasion, high nuclear grade, lymph-vascular space invasion, and pelvic lymph node metas-

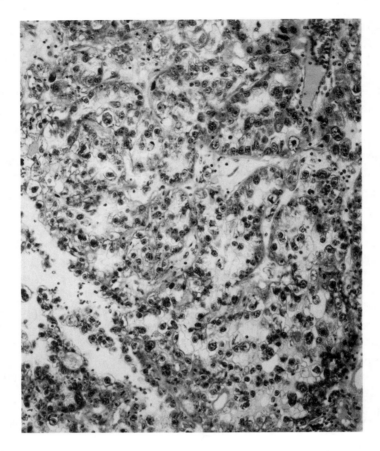

Figure 15   Clear cell carcinoma: Clear cytoplasm, prominent cell borders, and high grade nuclear atypia characterize this variant of endometrial adenocarcinoma. Both glands and solid areas are present.

tasis compared to endometrioid carcinomas (40). Occasionally they are confined to a polyp. The reported survival of patients with clear cell carcinoma differs considerably as reported in various series, ranging from 21% to 75%. The wide range in survival suggests that different investigators may be applying different criteria for the diagnosis of clear cell carcinoma, resulting in a heterogeneous group of cases being studied.

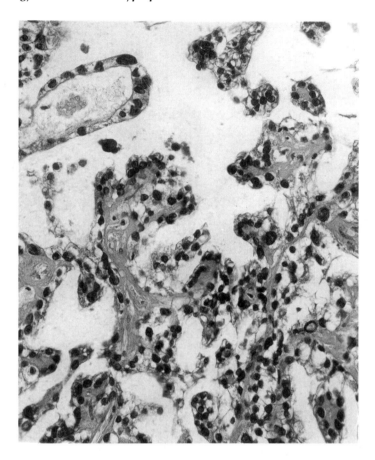

Figure 16 Clear cell carcinoma: A papillary architecture with a dense collagenized stroma is present.

MIXED TYPES OF CARCINOMA

An endometrial carcinoma may show combinations of two or more of the pure types. By convention, a mixed carcinoma has at least one other component comprising at least 10% of the tumor. There are very little data that can be used as a basis for making valid recommendations concerning what proportion of an additional component that justifies being separately classified. Mixed serous and endometrioid carcinomas containing as little as 25% of a serous component behave as pure serous carcinomas (17). Except for serous and possibly clear cell components, it is likely that the combination of other tumor types has little, if any, clinical significance.

MALIGNANT MESODERMAL MIXED TUMOR (MMMT)/CARCINOSARCOMA

These tumors represent less than 5% of malignant neoplasms of the uterine corpus. By definition, they are composed of malignant epithelial and mesenchymal components as recognized by light microscopy. Because of the biphasic appearance of MMMTs, there has been considerable controversy about their histopathogenesis. Recent clinicopathologic, immunohistochemical, and molecular genetic studies have provided compelling evidence that MMMTs should be classified as variants of carcinoma. One study demonstrated that both patients with MMMTs and those with endometrial carcinomas have similar risk factor profiles, consistent with the concept that the pathogenesis of the two tumor types is similar (41). These factors include body weight, exogenous estrogen use, and nulliparity, all of which are associated with increased risk of developing either tumor type, as well as oral contraceptive use and current smoking, which are associated with decreased risk. It has also been observed that MMMTs respond better to cisplatin-based chemotherapy, which is used for the treatment of carcinomas and thus targets the carcinomatous component, than to regimens directed at the sarcomatous component (42). These observations support the view that MMMTs are high-grade variants of carcinoma. Several immunohistochemical studies have demonstrated that the mesenchymal components of MMMTs express cytokeratins and epithelial membrane antigen in the majority of cases, supporting the view that these portions of the tumor arise from the carcinomatous areas via divergent differentiation (43).

There have been a small number of molecular studies that have suggested that the majority of MMMTs show common molecular alterations in both components, supporting a monoclonal origin. In sum, most molecular studies support a monoclonal origin of MMMTs with subsequent divergent differentiation. In conjunction with the observations that the behavior of these tumors is dictated by the carcinomatous component and immunohistochemical stains commonly demonstrate keratin expression in the mesenchymal components, it has been proposed that MMMTs be classified as aggressive variants of carcinoma rather than as sarcomas.

MMMTs are frequently polypoid and usually fill the entire endometrial cavity. Many invade the myometrium but some are confined to polyps. Because they are often polypoid, the tumors often protrude through the cervical os, simulating a cervical neoplasm. The protruding tip of the mass is often necrotic, making diagnosis based on biopsy of this portion of the tumor difficult. In approximately one-fourth of the cases the uterine tumor extends into the endocervix. The tumors are variably soft to firm and tan with areas of necrosis and hemorrhage.

MMMTs are composed of an intimate admixture of histologically malignant epithelial and mesenchymal components (44). The most common type of epithelial component is endometrioid carcinoma, which is often accompanied by squamous differentiation. Serous, clear cell, mucinous, squamous, and undifferentiated carcinoma also can be found as the epithelial component. Approximately one-half of the cases demonstrate a homologous type of stromal component, which is endometrial stromal sarcoma or fibrosarcoma in most and only occasionally leiomyosarcoma. When heterologous elements are present, rhabdomyosarcoma and chondrosarcoma are the most common types encountered (44,45). Rhabdomyosarcoma can be identified by finding round or elongated cells with granular or fibrillar eosinophilic cytoplasm. On occasion, striated rhabdomyoblasts can be found.

MMMTs metastasize to pelvic and para-aortic lymph nodes, pelvic soft tissues, the vagina, peritoneal surfaces of the upper abdomen, and the lungs. The histologic appearance of metastases is variable. Three studies on metastases of MMMTs have demonstrated that invasive foci in lymphatic or vascular spaces are always pure carcinoma and metastatic lesions are most commonly purely carcinoma; occasionally, mixtures of carcinoma and sarcoma are found and only rarely is pure sarcoma encountered (46). Another study, however, found biphasic metastases to be the most common type.

UNDIFFERENTIATED CARCINOMA

Tumors that fail to show evidence of either glandular or squamous differentiation are regarded as undifferentiated carcinomas. The prevalence is 1–2%. The mean age of patients with undifferentiated carcinoma is 64 years. The clinical features of women with undifferentiated carcinoma insofar as age, parity, hypertension, and diabetes are similar to those of endometrioid carcinoma.

In a study of 31 undifferentiated carcinomas, these tumors were divided into large cell and small cell/intermediate types (47). Some small cell carcinomas display a trabecular pattern simulating a carcinoid tumor. It is not infrequent to find these tumors admixed with adenocarcinoma, adenocarcinoma with squamous differentiation, or malignant mesodermal mixed tumor. The small cell carcinomas are positive for neuroendocrine markers such as neuron-specific enolase, synaptophysin, chromogranin, or leu-7. The survival difference of the large cell compared with the small/intermediate cell carcinomas was not statistically significant (54% vs. 64%, respectively, at 5 years) (47). As a group, the survival rates for patients with undifferentiated carcinoma at 5 and 10 years were 58% and 48%, respectively, which was similar to grade 3 endometrioid carcinoma. Recent studies have confirmed the aggressive behavior of small cell carcinoma of the endometrium.

MOLECULAR GENETICS OF ENDOMETRIAL CANCER

As discussed, endometrial carcinoma can be broadly divided into two types based on clinical, epidemiological, immunohistochemical, and molecular genetic features. In addition to confirming this subdivision, the molecular studies have provided insights into the genetic events involved in the development and progression of endometrial carcinoma. Since the initial clinical observation of endometrial carcinoma as two broad disease entities, it has been recognized by pathologists that there is a general correlation of the clinical type with the morphologic features of the endometrial tumor. For the most part, Type I tumors are associated with endometrioid features and arise in the setting of hyperplasia, whereas Type II tumors are often of serous type and present in a background of endometrial atrophy. Although somewhat oversimplified, this histologic distinction is important to the understanding of endometrial carcinoma at the molecular level. For this reason, the two tumor types are discussed separately, recognizing that many molecular studies have not clearly classified the tumors by morphologic type.

Endometrioid Carcinoma

Over the past decade a number of cancer causing genes (oncogenes and tumor suppressor genes) have been analyzed in endometrial carcinoma. Recently, several studies have shown that the most frequently altered gene in endometrioid carcinoma is the PTEN tumor suppressor gene, which is mutated in 30–50% of cases (51). PTEN is located on chromosome 10q23.3 and encodes a phosphatase. The primary target is the lipid molecule phosphatidylinositol 3,4,5-triphosphate (PIP3) that is involved in a signal transduction pathway that regulates cell growth and apoptosis. The frequency of mutation of the gene is similar in all three grades of endometrioid carcinoma and it is also mutated in approximately 20% of atypical and non-atypical hyperplasias (52). These findings suggest that inactivation of this gene is important early in the pathogenesis of endometrioid carcinoma. In addition, an immunohistochemical study found that the majority of endometrioid carcinomas show loss of PTEN expression, indicating that it may play a central role in the development of this tumor type. Furthermore, this study found loss of PTEN expression was found in clusters of otherwise benign appearing endometrial glands, suggesting that PTEN inactivation may occur before the development of a recognizable histopathological lesion.

Clearly, understanding PTEN and its role in the development of endometrioid carcinomas may provide novel markers for detecting endometrial glands predisposed to progress to malignancy and provide targets for therapeutic intervention prior to the development of malignant disease.

The p53 tumor suppressor gene, like in other tumors, has been extensively studied in endometrial cancer. p53 encodes a DNA-binding phosphoprotein that is involved in cell-cycle control and apoptosis. Mutations in p53 are found in approximately 10% of all endometrioid carcinomas, with the vast majority occurring in grade 3, and occasionally in grade 2, tumors. Overall, p53 mutations occur in 40–50% of grade 3 tumors and they have not been identified in grade 1 tumors or endometrial hyperplasia (38). This finding is consistent with a role for p53 in the progression, but not initiation, of endometrioid carcinoma.

Another molecular alteration in endometrioid carcinomas that has received substantial attention is the molecular phenotype called microsatellite instability. Microsatellite instability is defined as alterations in the length of short, repetitive DNA sequences, called microsatellites, in tumors when compared to DNA prepared from the same patient's normal tissue. This molecular phenotype is detected in tumors that lack an intact DNA mismatch repair system, a fundamental cellular mechanism for preventing DNA alterations that are created largely during DNA replication. In tumors that display microsatellite instability the DNA mismatch repair system has been inactivated either through mutation or "silencing" by promoter hypermethylation of one of the DNA mismatch repair genes (53). The consequence of inactivating the DNA mismatch repair system is an increase in the rate at which mutations occur, a factor that clearly contributes to tumorigenesis. Microsatellite instability is found in tumors from patients affected by hereditary nonpolyposis colorectal carcinoma (HNPCC), a syndrome in which endometrial carcinoma is the most common non-colorectal malignancy. Microsatellite instability also is present in approximately 20% of sporadic endometrial cancers and can be found in complex atypical hyperplasias that are associated with cancers that demonstrate instability. It has not, however, been found in lesser degrees of hyperplasia. It remains unclear exactly when in the development of endometrial neoplasia the DNA mismatch repair system becomes inactivated (54). Further studies of endometrial hyperplasia are warranted to address this important biological and potentially clinically relevant question.

Over the past decade several oncogenes have been studied in endometrial carcinomas, but only a few are altered in a significant number of cases. Mutations in the K-ras proto-oncogene have been identified consistently in 10–30% of endometrial cancers in several studies (55). The mutations have been found in all grades of endometrioid carcinoma and have been reported in complex atypical hyperplasia, suggesting a relatively early role for K-ras mutations in this tumor type. K-ras encodes a guanine nucleotide binding protein of 21kd that plays a role in the regulation of cell growth and differentiation by transducing signals from activated transmembrane receptors. In the mutant form, K-ras is constitutively "on" even in the absence of an activated receptor. Other oncogenes that have been found to be overexpressed or amplified are c-myc, HER-2/neu, bcl-2 and c-fms. More recently, mutations in the β-catenin gene have been found in approximately 15–20% of endometrioid carcinomas (56).

bcl-2 is a proto-oncogene that inhibits programmed cell death, which is manifest morphologically as apoptosis. In the endometrium, bcl-2 expression assessed by immunohistochemistry varies during the menstrual cycle, and is highly expressed in the proliferative phase, with down regulation during the secretory phase. In general, available data support the concept that bcl-2 protein expression persists at high levels in simple hyperplasia, but progressively diminishes in atypical hyperplasia and with decreasing differentiation in invasive endometrial adenocarcinoma (48,49). Apoptotic cells and apoptotic bodies are also increased in poorly differentiated endometrioid carcinomas, clear cell carcinomas, and serous carcinomas compared with well differentiated endometrioid adenocarcinomas. Loss of bcl-2 expression has also been associated with other features of poor prognosis including increasing depth of invasion, negative PR status, increasing FIGO stage, aggressive cell types, and lymph node metastasis (48,49).

HER-2/neu is a proto-oncogene, the product of which is a transmembrane growth factor receptor, p185erb-2, which shares some homology with the epidermal growth factor receptor. It is normally expressed at low levels in the cycling endometrium. Gene amplification and/or overexpression occur in about 20% to 40% of endometrial carcinomas. Overexpression of HER-2/neu protein has been associated with advanced stage, decreased differentiation, aggressive cell types particularly clear cell type, and increased depth of myometrial invasion (50). Reports of its utility as a predictor of survival have been mixed, with no apparent association of overexpression to outcome identified in several studies, but a statistically significant relationship in most others (50). At present, HER-2/neu overexpression is a prognostic factor of uncertain utility. Additional studies on these genes are needed to more definitively determine their role in endometrial cancer.

Serous Carcinoma

Compared to endometrioid carcinoma, relatively little is known about serous carcinoma at the molecular level. This is in part due to its relative infrequency and because this tumor type is not analyzed separately in many molecular studies. Although a number of candidate cancer genes have been analyzed in serous carcinoma, only the p53 tumor suppressor gene has been shown to be altered in a significant number, with mutations identified in almost 90% of cases (38). In fact, there are few other tumor types that demonstrate a mutation frequency in a single gene as high as that of p53 in serous endometrial carcinoma. Furthermore, approximately 75% of endometrial intraepithelial carcinomas, the putative precursor of serous carcinoma, have mutations in p53. In this setting, it has been shown that intense, diffuse immunohistochemical staining for p53 correlates well with p53 mutation. These findings suggest that in serous carcinoma p53 mutations occur relatively early and are central to the development of this tumor type. This is in contrast to endometrioid carcinoma in which p53 mutations are relatively uncommon and, when they do occur, they are largely confined to grade 3 tumors. Thus, it is possible that the mutation of p53 early in the pathogenesis of serous carcinoma is an important factor that accounts for its aggressive behavior. In addition, the fact that p53 mutations occur most commonly in grade 3 endometrioid and serous carcinomas most likely explains the finding that it is an independent indicator of tumors that behave aggressively (57).

In contrast to endometrioid carcinoma, mutations in K-ras and PTEN appear to be very uncommon in serous carcinoma and microsatellite instability has not definitively been described in this tumor type. Studies have suggested that there is amplification and overexpression of c-myc and HER-2/neu; however, it is not clear from the literature what percentage of serous carcinomas demonstrate these alterations.

As is clear from this discussion there is relatively little known about the molecular pathogenesis of the two major types of endometrial carcinoma. However, it is evident from the described studies above that endometrioid and serous carcinoma of the endometrium are distinct biological entities. As in other tumor systems, the molecular studies of endometrial cancer support the notion that epithelial-derived tumors often develop from preinvasive precursors that accumulate a combination of genetic alterations, thus providing the cell with the attributes necessary for unregulated growth. In endometrioid carcinoma it appears that PTEN alterations may be central to the initiation of proliferative lesions that then acquire mutations in other cancer causing genes (e.g., DNA mismatch repair genes, K-ras, p53) in the progression to malignancy. On the other hand, p53 mutations appear to be important in the conversion of relatively quiescent, atrophic endometrium to an intraepithelial form of serous carcinoma that then sets the stage for the accumulation of alterations in yet unidentified cancer-causing genes.

REFERENCES

1. Bokhman JV. Two pathogenetic types of endometrial carcinoma. *Gynecol Oncol* 1983; 15:10–17.

2. Sherman ME, Sturgeon S, Brinton LA, Potischman N, Kurman RJ, Berman ML, et al. Risk factors and hormone levels in patients with serous and endometrioid uterine carcinomas. *Mod Pathol* 1997; 10:963–968.

3. Scully RE, Bonfiglio TA, Kurman RJ, Silverberg SG, Wilkinson EJ. Histologic typing of female genital tract tumours (international histological classification of tumours). 2nd ed. Berlin: Springer-Verlag, 1994.

4. Kurman RJ, Kaminski PF, Norris HJ. The behavior of endometrial hyperplasia. A long-term study of "untreated" hyperplasia in 170 patients. *Cancer* 1985; 56:403–412.

5. Iozzo RV. Proteoglycans and neoplastic—mesenchymal cell interactions. *Hum Pathol* 1984; 15:2–10.

6. Liotta LA, Rao CN, Barsky SH. Tumor invasion and the extracellular matrix. *Lab Invest* 1983; 49:636–649.

7. Kurman RJ, Norris HJ. Evaluation of criteria for distinguishing atypical endometrial hyperplasia from well-differentiated carcinoma. *Cancer* 1982; 49:2547–2559.

8. Norris HJ, Tavassoli FA, Kurman RJ. Endometrial hyperplasia and carcinoma. Diagnostic considerations. *Am J Surg Pathol* 1983; 7:839–847.

9. King A, Seraj IM, Wagner RJ. Stromal invasion in endometrial adenocarcinoma. *Am J Obstet Gynecol* 1984; 149:10–14.

10. Janicek MF, Rosenshein NB. Invasive endometrial cancer in uteri resected for atypical endometrial hyperplasia. *Gynecol Oncol* 1994; 52:373–378.

11. Widra EA, Dunton CJ, McHugh M, Palazzo JP. Endometrial hyperplasia and the risk of carcinoma. *Int J Gynecol Cancer* 1995; 5:233–235.

12. Baak JP, Wisse-Brekelmans EC, Fleege JC, van der Putten HW, Bezemer PD. Assessment of the risk on endometrial cancer in hyperplasia, by means of morphological and morphometrical features. *Pathol Res Pract* 1992; 188:856–859.

13. Ferenczy A, Gelfand M. The biologic significance of cytologic atypia in progestogen-treated endometrial hyperplasia. *Am J Obstet Gynecol* 1989; 160:126–131.

14. Tavassoli FA, Kraus FT. Endometrial lesions in uteri resected for atypical endometrial hyperplasia. *Am J Clin Pathol* 1978; 70:770–779.

15. Gusberg SB, Kaplan AL. Precursors of corpus cancer. IV. Adenomatous hyperplasia as Stage 0 carcinoma of the endometrium. *Am J Obstet Gynecol* 1963; 87:662–678.

16. Ambros RA, Sherman ME, Zahn CM, Bitterman P, Kurman RJ. Endometrial intraepithelial carcinoma: a distinctive lesion specifically associated with tumors displaying serous differentiation. *Hum Pathol* 1995; 26:1260–1267.

17. Sherman ME, Bitterman P, Rosenshein NB, Delgado G, Kurman RJ. Uterine serous carcinoma. A morphologically diverse neoplasm with unifying clinicopathologic features. *Am J Surg Pathol* 1992; 16:600–610.

18. Wheeler DT, Bell KA, Kurman RJ, Sherman ME. Minimal uterine serous carcinoma: diagnosis and clicopathologic correlation. *Am J Surg Pathol* 2000; 24:797–806.

19. Creasman WT. Announcement. FIGO Stages—1988 Revision. *Gynecol Oncol* 1989; 35:125–127.

20. Morrow CP, Bundy BN, Kurman RJ, Creasman WT, Heller P, Homesley HD, et al. Relationship between surgical-pathological risk factors and outcome in clinical stage I and II carcinoma of the endometrium: a Gynecologic Oncology Group study. *Gynecol Oncol* 1991; 40:55–65.

21. Zaino RJ, Kurman R, Herbold D, Gliedman J, Bundy BN, Voet R, et al. The significance of squamous differentiation in endometrial carcinoma. Data from a Gynecologic Oncology Group study. *Cancer* 1991; 68:2293–2302.

22. Abeler VM, Kjordstad K, Berle E. Carcinoma of the endometrium in Norway: a histopathological and prognostic survey of a total population. *Int J Gynecol Cancer* 1992; 9–22.

23. Greven KM, Lanciano RM, Corn B, Case D, Randall ME. Pathologic stage III endometrial carcinoma. Prognostic factors and patterns of recurrence. *Cancer* 1993; 71:3697–3702.

24. Lax SF, Kurman RJ, Pizer ES, Wu L, Ronnett BM. A binary architectural grading system for uterine endometrial endometrioid carcinoma has superior reproducibility compared with FIGO grading and identifies subsets of advance-stage tumors with favorable and unfavorable prognosis. *Am J Surg Pathol* 2000; 24:1201–1208.

25. Grimshaw RN, Tupper WC, Fraser RC, Tompkins MG, Jeffrey JF. Prognostic value of peritoneal cytology in endometrial carcinoma. *Gynecol Oncol* 1990; 36:97–100.

26. Sivridis E, Buckley CH, Fox H. The prognostic significance of lymphatic vascular space invasion in endometrial adenocarcinoma. *Br J Obstet Gynaecol* 1987; 94:991–994.

27. Tornos C, Silva EG, el-Naggar A, Burke TW. Aggressive stage I grade 1 endometrial carcinoma. *Cancer* 1992; 70:790–798.

28. Ambros RA, Kurman RJ. Combined assessment of vascular and myometrial invasion as a model to predict prognosis in stage I endometrioid adenocarcinoma of the uterine corpus. *Cancer* 1992; 69:1424–1431.

29. Zaino RJ, Kurman RJ, Diana KL, Morrow CP. Pathologic models to predict outcome for women with endometrial adenocarcinoma: the importance of the distinction between surgical stage and clinical stage—a Gynecologic Oncology Group study [published erratum appears in *Cancer* 1997 Jan 15; 79(2):422]. *Cancer* 1996; 77:1115–1121.

30. Zaino RJ, Kurman RJ, Brunetto VL, Morrow CP, Bentley RC, Cappellari JO, et al. Villoglandular adenocarcinoma of the endometrium: a clinicopathologic study of 61 cases. A Gynecologic Oncology Group study. *Am J Surg Pathol* 1998; 22:1379–1385.

31. Hendrickson MR, Ross J, Eifel P, Martinez A, Kempson R. Uterine papillary serous carcinoma: a highly malignant form of endometrial adenocarcinoma. *Am J Surg Pathol* 1982; 6:93–108.

32. Zaino RJ, Kurman RJ. Squamous differentiation in carcinoma of the endometrium: a critical appraisal of adenoacanthoma and adenosquamous carcinoma. *Semin Diagn Pathol* 1988; 5:154–171.

33. Kim KR, Scully RE. Peritoneal keratin granulomas with carcinomas of endometrium and ovary and atypical polypoid adenomyoma of endometrium. A clinicopathological analysis of 22 cases. *Am J Surg Pathol* 1990; 14:925–932.

34. Tiltman AJ. Mucinous carcinoma of the endometrium. *Obstet Gynecol* 1980; 55:244–247.

35. Ross JC, Eifel PJ, Cox RS, Kempson RL, Hendrickson MR. Primary mucinous adenocarcinoma of the endometrium. A clinicopathologic and histochemical study. *Am J Surg Pathol* 1983; 7:715–729.

36. Carcangiu ML, Chambers JT. Uterine papillary serous carcinoma: a study on 108 cases with emphasis on the prognostic significance of associated endometrioid carcinoma, absence of invasion, and concomitant ovarian carcinoma. *Gynecol Oncol* 1992; 47:298–305.

37. Demopoulos RI, Genega E, Vamvakas E, Carlson E, Mittal K. Papillary carcinoma of the endometrium: morphometric predictors of survival. *Int J Gynecol Pathol* 1996; 15:110–118.

38. Lax SF, Kendall B, Tashiro H, Slebos RJ, Hedrick L. The frequency of p53, K-ras mutations, and microsatellite instability differs in uterine endometrioid and serous carcinoma: evidence of distinct molecular genetic pathways. *Cancer* 2000; 88:814–824.

39. Abeler VM, Kjorstad KE. Clear cell carcinoma of the endometrium: a histopathological and clinical study of 97 cases. *Gynecol Oncol* 1991; 40:207–217.

40. Sakuragi N, Hareyama H, Todo Y, Yamada H, Yamamoto R, Fujino T, et al. Prognostic significance of serous and clear cell adenocarcinoma in surgically staged endometrial carcinoma. *Acta Obstet Gynecol* Scand 2000; 79:311–316.

41. Zelmanowicz A, Hildesheim A, Sherman ME, Sturgeon SR, Kurman RJ, Barrett RJ, et al. Evidence for a common etiology for endometrial carcinomas and malignant mixed müllerian tumors. *Gynecol Oncol* 1998; 69:253–257.

42. Van Rijswijk REN, Tognon G, Burger CW, Baak JP, Kenemans P, Vermorken JB. The effect of chemotherapy on the different components of advanced carcinomas (malignant mixed meso-

dermal tumors) of the female genital tract. *Int J Gynecol Cancer* 1994; 4:52–60.

43. Bitterman P, Chun B, Kurman RJ. The significance of epithelial differentiation in mixed mesodermal tumors of the uterus. A clinicopathologic and immunohistochemical study. *Am J Surg Pathol* 1990; 14:317–328.

44. Barwick KW, LiVolsi VA. Malignant mixed müllerian tumors of the uterus. A clinicopathologic assessment of 34 cases. *Am J Surg Pathol* 1979; 3:125–135.

45. Dinh TV, Slavin RE, Bhagavan BS, Hannigan EV, Tiamson EM, Yandell RB. Mixed müllerian tumors of the uterus: a clinicopathologic study. *Obstet Gynecol* 1989; 74:388–392.

46. Sreenan JJ, Hart WR. Carcinosarcomas of the female genital tract. A pathologic study of 29 metastatic tumors: further evidence for the dominant role of the epithelial component and the conversion theory of histogenesis. *Am J Surg Pathol* 1995; 19:666–674.

47. Abeler VM, Kjorstad KE, Nesland JM. Undifferentiated carcinoma of the endometrium. A histopathologic and clinical study of 31 cases. *Cancer* 1991; 68:98–105.

48. Sakuragi N, Ohkouchi T, Hareyama H, Ikeda K, Watari H, Fujimoto T, et al. Bcl-2 expression and prognosis of patients with endometrial carcinoma. *Int J Cancer* 1998; 79:153–158.

49. Geisler JP, Geisler HE, Wiemann MC, Zhou Z, Miller GA, Crabtree W. Lack of bcl-2 persistence: an independent prognostic indicator of poor prognosis in endometrial carcinoma. *Gynecol Oncol* 1998; 71:305–307.

50. Rolitsky CD, Theil KS, McGaughy VR, Copeland LJ, Niemann TH. HER-2/neu amplification and overexpression in endometrial carcinoma. *Int J Gynecol Pathol* 1999; 18:138–143.

51. Risinger JI, Hayes AK, Berchuck A, Barrett JC. PTEN/MMAC1 mutations in endometrial cancers. *Cancer Res* 1997; 57:4736–4738.

52. Levine RL, Cargile CB, Blazes MS, van Rees B, Kurman RJ, Ellenson LH. PTEN mutations and microsatellite instability in complex atypical hyperplasia, a precursor lesion to uterine endometrioid carcinoma. *Cancer Res* 1998; 58:3254–3258.

53. Esteller M, Levine R, Baylin SB, Ellenson LH, Herman JG. MLH1 promoter hypermethylation is associated with the microsatellite instability phenotype in sporadic endometrial carcinomas. *Oncogene* 1998; 17:2413–2417.

54. Esteller M, Catasus L, Matias-Guiu X, Mutter GL, Prat J, Baylin SB, et al. hMLH1 promoter hypermethylation is an early event in human endometrial tumorigenesis. Am J Pathol 1999; 155:1767–1772.

55. Enomoto T, Fujita M, Inoue M, Rice JM, Nakajima R, Tanizawa O, et al. Alterations of the p53 tumor suppressor gene and its association with activation of the c-K-ras-2 protooncogene in premalignant and malignant lesions of the human uterine endometrium. *Cancer Res* 1993; 53:1883–1888.

56. Fukuchi T, Sakamoto M, Tsuda H, Maruyama K, Nozawa S, Hirohashi S. Beta-catenin mutation in carcinoma of the uterine endometrium. *Cancer Res* 1998; 58:3526–3528.

57. Soong R, Knowles S, Williams KE, Hammond IG, Wysocki SJ, Iacopetta BJ. Overexpression of p53 protein is an independent prognostic indicator in human endometrial carcinoma. *Br J Cancer* 1996; 74:562–567.

58 Ronnett BM, Zaino RJ, Ellenson LH, Kurman RJ. Endometrial carcinoma. In: Kurman RJ, ed. *Blaustein's Pathology of the Female Genital Tract*, 5th ed. New York: Springer-Verlag, 2002.

6

Pathology of Uterine Sarcomas

MICHAEL R. HENDRICKSON, TERI A. LONGACRE, AND RICHARD L. KEMPSON

Stanford University Medical Center,
Stanford, California, U.S.A.

CLASSIFICATION OF UTERINE MESENCHYMAL, AND MIXED MESENCHYMAL/EPITHELIAL NEOPLASMS

The uterine sarcomas comprise a heterogeny of pure mesenchymal and mixed epithelial-mesenchymal neoplasms whose clinical profiles range from relatively indolent neoplasms that characteristically present at low clinical stage and are cured by removal, to very aggressive neoplasms that routinely present at a high stage, spread locally, disseminate both regionally and distantly, and are, over the course of one to several years, characteristically fatal.

The classification of these neoplasms is relatively complex. The primary division is between pure mesenchymal and mixed epithelial/mesenchymal neoplasms. The former is further subdivided into those neoplasms that exhibit differentiation normally encountered in the uterus (homologous; i.e., endometrial stromal or smooth muscle), neoplasms exhibiting differentation not normally present in the uterus (heterologous; e.g., skeletal muscle, cartilage, bone) and neoplasms that are undifferentiated. Of course, the vast majority of neoplasms in this pure mesenchymal group are ordinary leiomyomas. A much smaller percentage of smooth muscle neoplasms are leiomyosarcomas. Most neoplasms exhibiting endometrial stromal differentiation are low-grade sarcomas (endometrial stromal sarcoma); less than 10% are benign (stromal nodules). Heterologous differentiation is usually encountered in mixed neoplasms but, rarely, may be the only differentiated type present; these are almost always malignant.

Any of the malignant mesenchymal patterns of differentiation may be combined with benign or malignant glandular elements to yield, respectively, adenofibroma/adenosarcoma or carcinosarcoma (a.k.a. malignant mixed müllerian tumor). These mixed neoplasms may be further subdivided into "homologous" or "heterologous" depending upon the type of mesenchymal differentiation present.

The classification of mesenchymal and mixed epithelial/mesenchymal neoplasms becomes greatly simplified when clinical behavior is used as the organizing principle. We distinguish four patterns of clinical behavior (Table 1).

This chapter will concern itself chiefly with clinical diseases III and IV. These considerations include a clinicopathologic cross-classification.

Leiomyosarcomas and carcinosarcomas (also known as malignant mixed müllerian tumors) comprise the majority of uterine sarcomas. Most of the remainder are accounted for by low-grade endometrial sarcoma and adenosarcoma.

ENDOMETRIAL STROMAL SARCOMA (ESS) (1–3)

Neoplasms in the endometrial stromal group resemble, in their differentiated features, the stroma of normal prolifera-

Table 1 Patterns of Clinical Behavior

Clinical Disease I (ClinD-1) "Benign"	Local excision is usually curative; at most, local recurrence in uterus after incomplete local excision
Clinical Disease II (ClinD-2) "Benign, but. . . ."	Usually clinically benign but infrequently presents at high stage or recurs after initial presentation at low stage; indolent clinical course with recurrence; only rarely fatal (e.g., intravenous leiomyomatosis with cardiac involvement)
Clinical Disease III (ClinD-3) "Low Grade Malignancy"	Sometimes presents at high stage; recurrence not unusual; disease is indolent
Clinical Disease IV (ClinD-4) "Highly Malignant"	Often presents at high stage; local, regional and distant failures; rapid evolution

tive phase endometrium. A diagnostically problematic feature (see the following) of this group of neoplasms is that the histologic features of both the benign and malignant member groups are identical—they betray their clinical potential by their relationship to surrounding normal structures, not by subtle features of their morphology. By morphologic definition, the malignant tumor in this group, endometrial stromal sarcoma (ESS), infiltrates the myometrium and/or invades the uterine vasculature. Its much less common benign counterpart, endometrial stromal nodule (ESN), lacks both of these features. ESS is a clinically indolent neoplasm (ClinD-3) (Table 1) that at the time of clinical presentation is usually confined to the uterus but, even when it presents with extrauterine disease or recurs after hysterectomy, is compatible with long term survival. It has been traditional to grade ESS based upon an assessment of mitotic index using 10 mf/10 hpf as the threshold dividing "low grade" from "high grade" sarcoma. The utility of this classification has been drawn into question in recent years. ESS must be distinguished from "undifferentiated sarcoma"—a clinically highly aggressive neoplasm (ClinD-4), which shares with ESS a generally undifferentiated appearance but is distinguished by its greater degree of anaplasia and the absence of the arborizing vasculature so characteristic of endometrial stromal neoplasms.

Clinical Features

ESS occurs almost exclusively in adults and has a peak incidence in the fifth decade; over three-fourths of women are premenopausal (4–11). There is no association with prior irradiation, nor do patients share the risk profile of patients with endometrial carcinoma. A few cases have been reported in patients receiving tamoxifen (12,13). Patients usually come to clinical attention because of a mass that may be associated with abdominal pain or uterine bleeding. Not infrequently, ESS is an unexpected or incidental finding. Difficult management problems are created when this occurs in an endometrial sampling or a myomectomy specimen in a patient for whom uterine conservation is an issue (3).

Gross Pathology

When advanced, ESS has a characteristic gross appearance: The uterus is asymmetrically enlarged by a typically yellowish tumor mass that infiltrates the surrounding normal myometrium and often extends as a polypoid growth into the endometrial cavity. Intravascular plugs of tumor may sometimes be appreciated grossly, both within the uterus and extending outside the uterus into the adnexa.

Microscopic Pathology (Figs. 1 and 2)

ESS is a neoplasm that in its differentiated features most resembles proliferative endometrial stroma. That is, it is composed of a monomorphous population of rounded-to-oblong-to-spindled cells possessing scanty cytoplasm and small, bland, uniform nuclei with evenly distributed chromatin. These cells are embedded in an abundant reticulin framework which contains a highly characteristic, delicate, arborizing vasculature. ESS, by definition, exhibits myoinvasion and/or intravascular intrusion by plugs of tumor. Myoinvasive ESS has a distinctive pattern featuring irregularly shaped "tongues" or islands of tumor cells splaying apart bundles of smooth muscle. Occasionally, a decidual-like reaction or foam cells may be seen. In most cases of ESS, mitotic figures are difficult to find, but occasional tumors have been

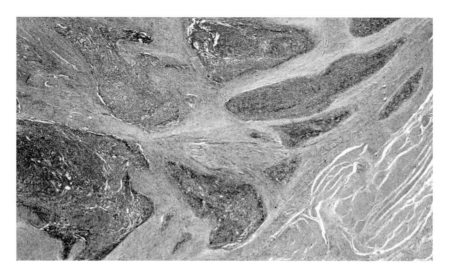

Figure 1   Endometrial stromal sarcoma. Tongues of tumor infiltrate the myometrium. Intravascular tumor is present.

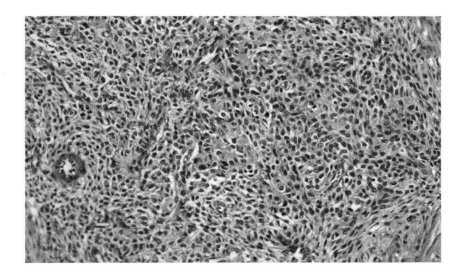

Figure 2   Endometrial stromal sarcoma. Blunt, spindled cells with scanty cytoplasm are arranged in a tuft-and-weave pattern.

found in excess of 10 mf/10 hpf. Uncommonly, foci of glands and/or tubules may be encountered; more rarely these structures can be uniformly distributed throughout the tumor (14,15), a pattern that blends imperceptibly into adenosarcoma (see the following). Alternatively, rare neoplasms in this class contain epithelial-like structures resembling sex-cord stromal tumors (see the section entitled "Uterine Neoplasms with Sex Cord-like Elements").

While most endometrial stromal proliferations are easily separated from the vastly more common uterine smooth muscle neoplasms, there is a range over which clear distinction is not possible using conventional light microscopy. This ambiguity, unfortunately, is propagated to all levels of more refined examination, including immunohistochemistry. Initially, it was reseasonably supposed that a variety of smooth muscle markers (desmin, muscle specific actin, etc.) would be demonstrable in smooth muscle neoplasms and would be absent in endometrial stromal neoplasms. Unfortunately, these hopes have not been realized; there is a substantial cross reactivity between these two phenotypes (16–20). Indeed, both stromal and smooth muscle neoplasms may occasionally be positive for the epithelial marker, keratin (19). There has been recent interest in the antibody CD 10 as a reliable marker for endometrial stroma (21–23). With the acquisition of more experience, the specificity of this stain has dropped considerably (20). Thus, currently the utility of immunohistochemistry in assigning problematic cases to one or the other group is limited. However, *strong*, diffuse desmin and caldesmon positivity is practically never seen in otherwise characteristic endometrial stromal tumors (20,24,25). When immunohistochemical signals remain ambiguous and when the probability of an endometrial stromal proliferation is high on other grounds, the case should be assigned to the endometrial stromal group for management purposes.

The glandular and epithelioid cells in endometrial stromal proliferations are sometimes keratin positive, or, at other times, may have the immunophenotype of smooth muscle cells (20,26–30).

Clinicopathologic Correlation

The prognosis of ESS depends chiefly on the extent of disease at the time of diagnosis and the adequacy of surgical therapy. The importance of grading is less established. The first modern clinicopathologic study of endometrial stromal neoplasms was that of Norris and Taylor (31). These workers divided endometrial stromal sarcomas into low- and high-grade types on the basis of mitotic index. After excluding anaplastic undifferentiated sarcomas (ClinD-4) (Table 1), they drew the line between low- and high-grade stromal sarcomas at 10 mitotic figures per 10 hpf. Subsequently, Evans revised the Norris and Taylor primary division between "undifferentiated endometrial sarcoma" and "endometrial stromal sarcoma" but, based upon an analysis of 11 cases, questioned the value of stratifying the latter into "low-grade" and "high-grade" groups based upon mitotic index (32). Those endometrial stromal neoplasms composed of relatively bland monomorphous, oblong-to-spindle cells resembling proliferative-phase endometrial stromal cells independent of the mitotic counts are considered by Evans to be "endometrial stromal sarcomas," while those composed of pleomorphic or anaplastic cells he places in the undifferentiated endometrial sarcoma group. The latter typically contain large numbers of mitotic figures, some of which may be abnormal. The main difference between the two points of view is that Norris and Taylor concluded that stratifying neoplasms (that both they and Evans would agree are endometrial stromal sarcomas) by mitotic index is useful while Evans's data did not support this approach. A study of 93 stromal sarcomas at Stanford supports Evans's conclusions, so we do not stratify endometrial stromal sarcomas into high-grade and low-grade types (5). However, we continue to use the term "low grade" to modify the diagnosis of ESS (independent of its mitotic index) in order to emphasize its ClinD-3 (Table 1) behavior and to avoid confusion with the ClinD-4 disease, undifferential endometrial sarcoma.

Low-grade endometrial stromal sarcomas, including those few with a characteristic histologic pattern but with significantly increased (normal) mitotic figures, are indolent, slowly progressing neoplasms that occur at all ages. In the Stanford series, 45% percent of clinical stage I patients who had both rare mitotic figures and minimal atypia had one or more relapses and of these, 2 (13%) died of disease at 85 and 360 months, respectively. There was no significant difference in relapse rate or survival between patients on either side of the MI = 10 mf/10 hpf line (5). Patients with high-stage disease fare significantly worse than those with disease confined to the uterus; high-stage patients tend to have higher mitotic indices and, within the high-stage group, patients with an MI ≥ 10 mf/10 hpf fare worse than those with an MI <10. Thus the single most important prognostic factor would appear to be the stage at presentation while bland histology and low mitotic indices are no guarantees that recurrence will not occur. The course of this disease is protracted and recurrences and metastases are observed 20 to 30 years after the primary tumor has been removed (33,34). The cells composing endometrial stromal sarcomas possess estrogen and progesterone receptors and metastatic neoplasms frequently respond to progestational therapy; the role of progesterones in an adjuvant setting is not settled (35,36).

Managerially Relevant Differential Diagnostic Issues

Clinical Disease I (Benign) Conditions with which ESS May Be Confused

The distinction between stromal nodule and ESS can usually be made only with the entire uterus in hand and is based on the presence of infiltrating margins and/or vascular invasion in the former but not in the latter. Endometrial samples that do not allow for the evaluation of the interface between normal structure and the cellular process in question pose a difficult problem in the patient for whom uterine conservation is relevant. Methods short of "diagnostic hysterectomy" can be used in an attempt to clarify the situation including imaging studies, hysteroscopy, and further sampling. Highly cellular leiomyoma may mimic endometrial stromal proliferations, particularly in an endometrial sampling. Strategies useful in identifying a smooth muscle tumor include close attention to the architecture of the process (fascicles of blunt-ended spin-dled cells, thick-walled vessels, lack of arborizing vascula-ture) and, in some instances, immunohistochemical studies provided a panel approach is utilized (desmin, caldesmon, and CD 10) (37). Less commonly, ESS may be mimicked in a sampling by florid endometritis, or in a hysterectomy speci-men by adenomyosis with sparse or absent glands (38) or menstrual endometrium within vessels (39).

Clinical Disease II Conditions with which ESS May Be Confused

ESS shares with intravascular leiomyomatosis (IVL) intravascular tumor growth. The two conditions differ in the phenotype of the neoplastic cell: smooth muscle in IVL and endometrial stromal in ESS. In most cases the two are easily distinguished. The clinical stakes are between a ClinD-2 (IVL) and a ClinD-3 (ESS) (Table1). Frustratingly, but not surprisingly, the two phenotypes may either blend or coexist in an individual case (40). In our experience the mixed and blended cases behave more like ESS than IVL, and we indi-cate this in our diagnostic comment.

Other Clinical Disease II Conditions with which ESS May Be Confused

Mixed müllerian proliferations that feature a prominent endometrial stromal component and benign glands pose diffi-cult taxonomic problems but no serious managerial problems as long as the stroma is not high grade. The usual confusion is between an epithelium-poor adenosarcoma with an endome-trial stromal sarcoma mesenchymal component, and ESS with a prominent glandular component—both of which are ClinD-3. There is currently no non-arbitrary way of distinguishing these two conditions over this range of appearance.

Clinical Disease IV Conditions with which ESS May Be Confused

Even though it is composed of cells with bland nuclei, ESS is a relatively undifferentiated neoplasm and it is not surprising that it figures in the uterine version of one of the major differential diagnosis set pieces of diagnostic pathology: the "undifferentiated neoplasm." When the few minimally distinctive features that ESS does posess are muted, the differential diagnostic possibilities are numerous. These include lymphoma, leukemia, and poorly differentiated carcinomas— both primary endometrial and metastatic, particularly lobular carcinoma of the breast metastatic to the uterus. Strategies for distinguishing among these are beyond the scope of this chapter; however, most of these conditions lack the arborizing vasculature of ESS and feature a higher degree of cytologic atypia and higher mitotic index than is customary for ESS.

UTERINE NEOPLASMS WITH SEX CORD-LIKE ELEMENTS (26,29,30,41–43)

The neoplstic cells that give this tumor its name are arranged, at least focally, in cords, hollow tubules, trabeculae, and/or sheets resembling epithelial cells, and they most often have scant cytoplasm, indistinct cell margins, and round nuclei, imparting a sex cord-like appearance (Fig. 3). In some tumors the constituent cells may have abundant eosinophilic or clear cytoplasm. The stroma between the epithelioid structures varies from paucicellular and fibroblastic to an appearance similar to normal proliferative endometrial stroma. Hyaline matrix may be prominent. Many of these tumors contain only focal sex cord-like differentiation and are otherwise identical to one or another form of ESS. Vascular intrusion and infiltrative margins may be present in such tumors and pelvic recurrences have been reported; for this reason we include this group in the endometrial stromal category. We use the same criteria to distinguish benign from malignant endometrial stromal neoplasms with sex cord-like differentiation as we do to distinguish stromal nodules from low-grade ESS; i.e., only tumors with circumscribed borders and uniform cells are considered to be benign.

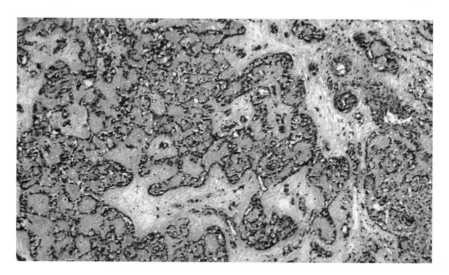

Figure 3 Endometrial stromal sarcoma. Sex cord-like areas (medium power).

However, there is another group of uterine tumors composed predominantly or exclusively of sex cord elements without an obvious stromal component. The cells composing the sex cord-like areas in these tumors are often inhibin positive and may express keratin, and thus appear to more closely simulate sex cord elements than their ESS counterparts (30). Most of these latter neoplsms are benign (ClinD-1) (Table 2) and may be treated with a less aggressive surgical procedure than the usual ESS. Because of the apparently benign clinical course and the distinctly unusual appearance of these tumors, we prefer to regard them as distinct entities and reserve the designation "uterine tumor resembling ovarian sex cord tumor" for those neoplasms that are composed almost exclusively of sex cord-like differentiation.

Table 2 Classification of Uterine Mesenchymal, Mixed Mesenchymal, and Epithelial Elements

	Clincial Disease I Behavior	Clinical Disease II Behavior	Clinical Disease III Behavior	Clincial Disease IV Behavior
PHENOTYPE	Clinically benign	Clincially benign with very few exceptions. If there is dissemination beyond the uterus, the tempo of disease is slow and compatible with long term survival	Clincially malignancy of low aggressiveness: local, reginal and distant recurrence; slow tempo of disease; fatal in a minority of cases	Clinically aggessive malignancy from outset; local, regional, distant spread
Endometrial stromal differentiation	• Stromal nodule: Without sex cord elements or glands With sex cord elements or gland		• Endometrial stromal sarcoma: Without sex cord elements or glands With sex cord elements or glands	
Smooth muscle differentiation	• Leiomyoma and variants	• Intravenous leiomyomatosis (IVL) • Atypical leiomyoma with low risk of recurrence • Benign metastazing leiomyomas (BML) • Leiomyomatosis peri-otonealis disseminata (LPD)		• Leiomyosarcoma Usual Epithelioid Myxoid

Pure heterologous differentiation	• Metaplastic bone or cartilage	• Osteosarcoma • Chondrosarcoma • Liposarcoma • Rhabdomyosarcoma
Undifferentiated pleomorphic spindled cells		• Angiosarcoma • Undifferentiated sarcoma
Mixed müllerian differentiation	• Adenofibroma • Atypical polypoid adenomyoma (APA)	Carcinosarcoma (malignant mixed müllerian tumor)
	Atypical polypoid adeno-myoma of LMP	Adenosarcoma with morphologic malignant stromal overgrowth
	Adenosarcoma Adenosarcoma with bland sarcomatous overgrowth	

LEIOMYOSARCOMA (1,3)

A deceptively simple definition of leiomyosarcoma is "a malignant neoplasm differentiated as smooth muscle." This leaves us with the dual problems of, first, distinguishing smooth muscle differentiation from other phenotypes (e.g., endometrial stromal) and, second, specifying morphologic criteria for separating clinically benign from clinically malignant smooth muscle neoplasms. This effort has extended over the past several decades and as a result, the morphologic definition of leiomysarcoma has undergone substantial changes.

What counts as smooth muscle differentiation? The smooth muscle phenotype has been expanded over recent years to include neoplasms with either epithelioid differentiation or myxoid differentiation. These subcategories are important to recognize because the criteria for malignancy within these differentiated groups differ from those used for neoplasms exhibiting the more common "standard" smooth muscle differentiation. Over a certain range of appearance, cellular smooth muscle and endometrial stromal proliferations resemble one another. Distinguishing the two can sometimes have important management consequences, discussed earlier in connection with ESS.

What features of a smooth muscle neoplasm predict for a malignant clinical course? Taxonomic efforts to separate benign from malignant neoplasms exhibiting standard smooth muscle differentiation have focused on two general areas. First, at the benign end of the morphologic spectrum, progress has been made in separating clinically malignant uterine smooth muscle neoplasms (i.e., leiomyosarcoma) from clinically benign uterine smooth muscle neoplasms that feature one or more of the following: 1) alternative differentiation (e.g., myxoid or epithelioid); 2) increased cellularity; 3) marked cytological atypia; and 4) necrosis. Second, a number of benign or, at most clinically indolent, smooth muscle proliferations have been recognized that involve extrauterine sites that are often incidental findings; while they may produce morbidity, they only rarely lead to patient death. In short, these proliferations exhibit clinical disease II behavior. These include intravenous leiomyomatosis (44,45), benign metastasizing leiomyoma (46,47), and disseminated peritoneal leiomyomatosis (48,49).

Clinical Features

Leiomyosarcoma represents about 1–2% of uterine malignancies and about one-third of uterine sarcomas. Approximately 1 of every 800 smooth muscle tumors of the uterus is a leiomyosarcoma, but less than 1% of women thought clinically to have leiomyoma prove to have leiomyosarcoma (50). The average age of women with leiomyosarcoma is 52, nearly a decade older than women with leiomyoma although the disease is well known to occur in women in the third decade of life (51–56). There is no consistent racial predisposition, nor is there a relationship with gravidity or parity. The clinical presentation is nonspecific. The main symptoms are abnormal vaginal bleeding, lower abdominal pain, or a pelvic or abdominal mass (51,53,54,57,58). The average duration of symptoms before diagnosis is 5 months (58). There appears to be little support for the clinical dictum that a rapidly enlarging uterine smooth muscle neoplasm is indicative of leiomyosarcoma. In a recent study, only 1 of 371 women operated with this indication harbored a leiomyosarcoma (59). Unlike carcinosarcoma, leiomyosarcoma is seldom associated with a history of pelvic radiation (60).

Gross Pathology

Most leiomyosarcomas are intramural and 50–75% are solitary masses (55,60–62). A higher proportion involves the cervix than is the case with leiomyoma. Leiomyosarcoma averages 6–9 cm in diameter and is soft or fleshy with poorly defined margins (63). Relative to leiomyomas, leiomyosarcomas tend to be larger and softer, to have irregular margins, and are more likely to be hemorrhagic and necrotic.

Rarely, leiomyosarcoma may completely mimic leiomyoma, hence the need to grossly serial section and histologically sample all large, peculiar leiomyomas. Myxoid
leiomyosarcomas in particular may appear extensively gelatinous and deceptively circumscribed (64–67). On the other
hand, leiomyomas may mimic leiomyosarcoma by virtue of a
large number of "degenerations." These are, by and large, consequences of ischemia that produce changes ranging from
acute hemorrhagic necrosis to patterns of scarring that result
in a peculiar gross appearance.

Microscopic Appearance (Figs. 4 and 5; Table 3)

The typical leiomyosarcoma is composed of fascicles of spindle cells possessing abundant eosinophilic cytoplasm with
longitudinal cytoplasmic fibrils. The nuclei are fusiform,

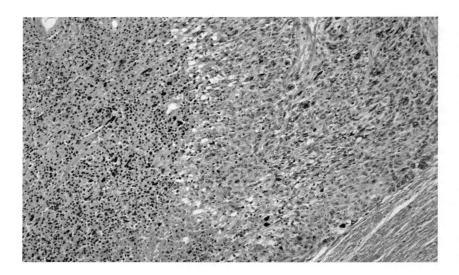

Figure 4   Leiomyosarcoma. A cellular smooth muscle neoplasm
featuring nuclear pleomorphism, abnormal mitotic figures, and
tumor cell necrosis.

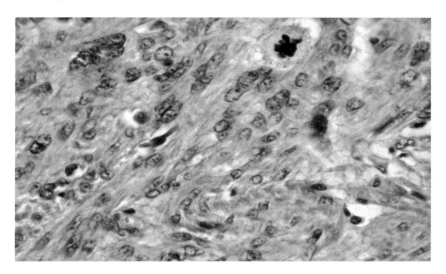

Figure 5   Leiomyosarcoma. A higher-power view showing marked nuclear pleomorphism in cells with abundant eosinophilic cytoplasm. An abnormal mitotic figure is present at the top of the field.

usually have blunt ends, and are hyperchromatic, with coarse chromatin and prominent nucleoli. Cellular pleomorphism is marked in poorly differentiated neoplasms. Multinucleated tumor cells are found in 50% of leiomyosarcomas and osteoclast-like giant cells may rarely be present (62,68–70). Many leiomyosarcomas invade the surrounding myometrium, but a leiomyosarcoma with a circumscribed margin can give rise to metastases. Vascular invasion is identified in 10–20% of leiomyosarcomas (62,71–73). Tumor cell necrosis is typically prominent but need not be present. In a recent series the mitotic index was in excess of 15 mf/10 hpf in 80% of 59 cases (71).

Problems arise in identifying clinically malignant smooth muscle neoplasms that lack tumor cell necrosis but have some other feature that suggests malignancy. For example, it has been known for some time that clinically benign uterine smooth muscle cells may exhibit striking nuclear pleomorphism and atypia. Again, although historically the finding of a mitotic index in excess of 10 mf/10 hpf was sufficient to warrant a diagnosis of leiomyosarcoma, in recent years it has become apparent that absent significant nuclear atypia and tumor cell necrosis, mitotic indices as high as 20 mf/10 hpf may be encountered in clinically benign smooth muscle neoplasms. Criteria reflecting these observations are given in Table 3 (56,74,75).

Myxoid leiomyosarcoma is a large, gelatinous neoplasm that usually appears to be circumscribed on gross examination (64–67). Microscopically, the smooth muscle cells are usually widely separated by myxoid material. The characteristic low cellularity partly accounts for the presence of only a few mf/10 hpf in most myxoid leiomyosarcomas. Sometimes, however, the mitotic index is high and most often there is a substantial degree of cytological atypia (76,77). In the absence of significant numbers of mitotic figures, other microscopic features are helpful in identifying a myxoid uterine tumor as a leiomyosarcoma. Some may invade blood vessels. Despite the low mitotic counts, myxoid leiomyosarcoma has the same unfavorable prognosis as typical leiomysarcomas; therefore, myxoid smooth muscle tumors of the uterus must be regarded with suspicion. It is critical to distinguish the myxoid differentiation found in myxoid leiomyosarcomas from the vastly more prevalent myxoid and hydropic changes seen in "degenerating" leiomyomas (78). In myxoid leiomyosarcomas, not only is the stroma myxoid but the cells are enlarged with hyperchromatic nuclei and pleomorphism is usually obvious. The usual case of myxoid leiomyosarcoma bears a striking resemblance to soft tissue myxoid malignant fibrous histiocytoma.

Epithelioid leiomyosarcomas exhibit one of the patterns of epithelioid differentiation in addition to the usual features of malignancy seen in the more conventional leiomyosarcoma: cytologic atypia, tumor cell necrosis, and a high mitotic index (79–85).

Clinicopathologic Correlation

Most leiomyosarcoma are clinically confined to the uterus on presentation; when extrauterine disease is present, it is likely to involve the lung (91). Leiomyosarcoma spreads intraperitoneally to regional lymph nodes, and hematogenously, particularly to the lungs, liver, brain, kidney, and bone. Recurrences in a recent large series of stage I and II leiomyosarcomas were hematogenous in 57% and pelvic in 20%. The incidence of lymph node metastasis varies from series to series. In the Gyneocologic Oncology Group (GOG) study (71) 83% of 59 clincial stage I and II leiomyosarcoma patients were surgical stage I; 2 of 59 (3%) had lymph node involvement, 2 had adnexal involvement, and 1 had positive peritoneal cytology. Because patients in this series underwent lymph node sampling rather than lymph node dissection, these figures probably somewhat underestimate the true incidence of lymph node involvement. Lymph node involvement is higher in series reporting advanced stage leiomyosarcoma, with figures as high as 44% reported in autopsy series (91–93). Goff et al. (91) found in their series of 15 surgically staged patients that lymph nodes were involved only when there was peritoneal disease. Moreover, a high percentage of lymph node negative patients failed (91). In view of this, there would appear to be little role for lymph node sampling in this disease.

Leiomyosarcoma diagnosed using current morphologic criteria is a highly malignant neoplasm; survival is worse with this disease than with carcinosarcoma (71,94). The prognosis of leiomyosarcoma depends chiefly upon stage (72,89,95–99). For stage I tumors, some investigators have found the size of the neoplasm to be an important prognostic factor (62,72). In Evans's series, all patients with tumors larger than 5 cm died of disease while only 3 of 8 patients with tumors smaller than 5 cm died of disease (62). In another series of metastasizing leiomyosarcomas, only 20% were less than 5 cm (82). Premenopausal women have a more favorable outcome in some series (58,60,73,96–98) but not in others (51,63). Several recent series, including the large GOG study of early stage leiomyosarcoma, have found the mitotic index to be of prognostic significance (58,71,98) while others have not (62). A modification of the classification of Bell et al. (56) has been employed as a grading scheme and found to provide independent prognostic information (89). A grading scheme designed for soft tissue neoplasms has been applied to uterine sarcomas but was not of prognostic significance (100).

What should be incorporated in the pathology report in the face of these conflicting claims about prognostically relevant features? We do not grade leiomyosarcomas since no universally agreed upon grading scheme exists, but we do comment on the features listed above: maximum diameter of tumor, mitotic index, the presence or absence of necrosis and its extent if present, and the presence or absence of vascular space involvement.

Managerially Relevant Differential Diagnostic Issues

Clinical Disease I (Table 3) with which Leiomyosarcoma May Be Confused

Grossly, "degenerating" leiomyomas may simulate malignancy; microscopically, after adequate sampling for histologic examination, these lack the criteria for leiomyosarcoma given in Table 3. Infarcted leiomyomas have areas of necrosis and in this way simulate malignancy microscopically. The gross appearance (e.g., submucous leiomyomas with torsion) and the lack of anything other than necrosis to recommend a diagnosis of malignancy usually are sufficient to arrive at the correct diagnosis.

Clinical Disease II (Table 3) with which Leiomyosarcoma May Be Confused

A variety of smooth muscle proliferations simulate leiomyosarcoma in virtue of the distribution of disease. These include intravenous leiomyomatosis (44,45), benign metastasizing leiomyoma (46,47), and disseminated peritoneal leiomyomatosis (48,49). None of these entities meets the morphologic criteria for leiomyosarcoma set out in Table 3. "Atypical leiomyoma with low incidence of recurrence" falls into this category (56).

Table 3   Criteria for the Diagnosis of Leiomyosarcoma

Morphologic features to be evaluated
- Degree of cytologic atypia: none to mild *or* moderate to marked
- Presence or absence of coagulative tumor cells necrosis
- Mitotic index

Smooth muscle tumors with usual differentiation
- Mitotic index (MI) ≤ 20 mf/10 hpf, *no* coagulative necrosis, *no* atypia or *no more* than *mild cytologic atypia* (i.e., bland cytology) = leiomyoma
- MI > 20 mf/20 hpf, *no* coagulative necrosis, *no* atypia or *no* more than *mild cytologic* atypia (i.e, the cytology must be bland) = leiomyoma with increased MI but experience limited
- MI < 10 mf/10 hpf, *no* coagulative necrosis but with *diffuse moderate* to *severe* cytologic atypia = atypical leiomyoma with low risk of recurrence
- MI > 10 mf/10 hpf, *no* coagulative necrosis but with *diffuse moderate* to *severe* cytologic atypia = leiomyosarcoma
- MI ≤ 10 mf/10 hpf, *no* coagulative necrosis but with *focal* moderate to severe cytologic atypia = leiomyoma with atypia but limited experience
- Any MI and any degree of cytologic atypia with coagulative necrosis = leiomyosarcoma *Note:* Most often there will be significant atypia and/or elevated mitotic counts in leiomyosarcoma in addition to the coagulative tumor cell necrosis. Be careful of the case that does not have these additional morphologic features

Smooth muscle tumors with myxoid stroma
- MI < 5 mf/10 hpf, *no* or mild cytologic atypia, no coagulative necrosis = myxoid leiomyoma
- Any MI, moderate to marked atypia with or without coagulative necrosis = myxoid leiomyosarcoma

Smooth muscle tumor with epithelioid differentiation
- MI < 5 mf/10 hpf, *no* coagulative necrosis, *no* atypia or *no more* than mild cytologic atypia = epithelioid leiomyoma (limited experience)
- MI ≥ 5 mf/10 hpf, *no* coagulative necrosis, none or any degree of atypia = epithelioid leiomyosarcoma (limited experience)
- Any MI and any degree of cytologic atypia *with coagulative necrosis* = epithelioid leiomyosarcoma (limited experience)

Clinical Disease III (Table 3) with which Leiomyosarcoma May Be Confused

ESS features myoinvasion and/or intravascular growth and accordingly may raise the possibility of leiomyosarcoma. The diagnosis can usually be established by attention to the differentiated features of the constituent cells (smooth muscle vs. endometrial stromal), and by noting that ESS is cytologically bland while angio-invasive leiomyosarcoma almost always features a high degree of cytologic atypia.

Clinical Disease IV (Table 3) with which Leiomyosarcoma May Be Confused

These include carcinosarcoma with inconspicuous glandular elements, undifferentiated sarcoma, and poorly differentiated endometrial carcinomas. This is usually only a problem when examining limited or very necrotic samplings; most often the situation is clarified by examination of the hysterectomy specimen.

UNDIFFERENTIATED UTERINE SARCOMA (31,32,101)

Undifferentiated uterine sarcoma is much less common than ESS once one has carefully excluded, with suitable studies, other large-cell undifferentiated neoplasms: leukemia, lymphoma, high grade carcinoma, carcinosarcoma, and differentiated pure sarcomas (see earlier discussion). Undifferentiated uterine sarcomas are easily recognized as cytologically malignant and are composed of pleomorphic, undifferentiated rounded-to-spindled cells with a high mitotic index. They lack the bland, uniform cells, arborizing vasculature, and areas of hyalinization characteristic of low-grade ESS, and the constituent cells do not resemble smooth muscle cells and are not arranged in fascicles. Most resemble the undifferentiated malignant stroma often encountered in carcinosarcomas (32). All pure undifferentiated sarcomas of the uterus, including the giant cell variety, can for convenience be placed in this category. Pure sarcomas containing cells differentiating along recognizable mesenchymal lines are named in a way that reflects their differentiation, i.e., leiomyosarcoma, osteosarcoma, rhabdomyosarcoma, etc. Undifferentiated uterine sarcomas, in sharp contrast to endometrial stromal sarcomas, exhibit ClinD-4 behavior and, in this respect, resemble carcinosarcomas, leiomyosarcomas, or pure heterologous sarcomas.

MISCELLANEOUS PURE SARCOMAS

A variety of pure sarcomas has been reported in the uterus but they are all very rare. These include osteosarcoma (102–104), chondrosarcoma (105,106), rhabdomyosarcoma (107–111), liposarcoma (112), and angiosarcoma (113). The chief differential diagnostic consideration in all of these exotic types is a carcinosarcoma with an inconspicuous epithelial component. Since all of these neoplasms are high grade, the distinction, currently, is not of great importance. This might change if it becomes apparent that carcinosarcomas respond to treatment more like carcinomas than sarcomas. Finally, primitive neuroectodermal tumor (PNET) has been reported in the uterus (114–116).

MIXED MÜLLERIAN NEOPLASMS

Mixed müllerian neoplasms are biphasic epithelial mesenchymal proliferations that exhibit a range of clinical behaviors from benign (adenofibroma, adenomyoma, and atypical polypoid adenomyoma) to highly malignant (carcinosarcoma).

The classification of mixed müllerian neoplasms is based upon an assessment of both the epithelial and mesenchymal components; assignment of each of these to a morphologically "benign" or morphologically "malignant" category results in a fourfold classification.

Table 4 Mixed Müllerian Neoplasms

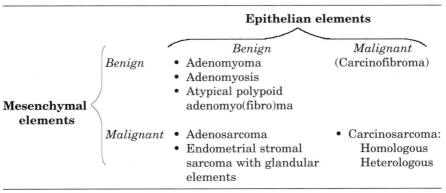

Mesenchymal elements		Epithelian elements	
		Benign	*Malignant*
	Benign	• Adenomyoma • Adenomyosis • Atypical polypoid adenomyo(fibro)ma	(Carcinofibroma)

	Malignant	• Adenosarcoma
		• Endometrial stromal sarcoma with glandular elements
			• Carcinosarcoma:
			  Homologous
			  Heterologous

The terms "adenofibroma," "adenomyoma," and "atypical polypoid adenomyoma" are used for neoplasms with benign epithelium and benign proliferating stroma; the term "adenosarcoma" is used for neoplasms with benign epithelium and mitotically active or sarcomatous stroma; and the term carcinosarcoma (malignant mixed müllerian tumor) is used for neoplasms composed of malignant epithelium and malignant stroma. It is usual to classify all tumors containing malignant epithelium with benign stroma as "carcinomas." The term "carcinofibroma" has been proposed for tumors in which the stroma is deemed to be "neoplastic" rather than reactive; however, this terminology is rarely used because determining whether a stroma is reactive or a benign neoplastic proliferation is problematic at best (117,118).

ADENOSARCOMA (1,119–125)

Adenosarcoma is a neoplasm composed of benign glands distributed throughout a cellular, mitotically active, or overtly malignant stroma.

Clinical Features

Patients with adenosarcoma are usually postmenopausal, although this neoplasm may occur during the reproductive years. Most patients present with abnormal bleeding. An association with tamoxifen has been reported (126–129).

Gross Pathology

Grossly, adenosarcoma is a fleshy polypoid neoplasm that grows into the uterine cavity and enlarges the uterus. The cut surface is punctuated by microcysts. 5–10% of adenosarcomas arise primarily in the uterine cervix (125,130).

Microscopic Pathology

Two microscopic patterns are encountered. The majority of cases feature irregular, often dilated, glandular elements uniformly distributed throughout a cytologically bland but, at least focally, cellular stroma producing a pattern similar to that seen in its benign counterpart, adenofibroma (Fig. 6). The stroma is characteristically more cellular immediately adjacent to the glands and produces a distinctive "cambium layer" or "collar." Asymmetric growth of stroma compresses the epithelial component to produce irregular stellate glandular configurations; sometimes, when this asymmetry is extreme, polypoid invaginations are produced. The glands are formed by non-stratified cytologically bland cells exhibiting a variety of müllerian differentiated types. Occasionally, the epithelium is hyperplastic but, by definition, it is rarely morphologically malignant. On occasion there are regions of stroma devoid of glands—so-called stromal overgrowth. To qualify as stromal overgrowth these areas without glands must comprise 25% or more of the tumor. A second pattern of adenosar-

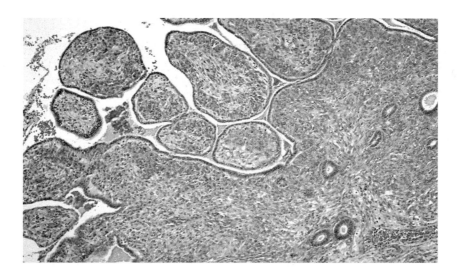

Figure 6 Adenosarcoma. Cytologically bland epithelium lines glands and papillary structures. The stroma is cellular and condenses below the epithelium.

174   *Hendrickson, Longacre, and Kempson*

coma is characterized by a more conspicuously malignant stroma in which there is pleomorphism and usually a high mitotic index (122). Rarely, the stromal cells in an adenosarcoma may arrange themselves in cord-like patterns reminiscent of the structures seen in the uterine tumors resembling ovarian sex cord tumors and endometrial stromal tumors with epithelial elements (121).

Clinicopathologic Correlation

Approximately one-fourth of adenosarcomas are myoinvasive and vascular invasion may be present. Interestingly, myoinvasive foci, intravascular tumors, and extrauterine tumors tend to be purely mesenchymal. In the absence of overtly malignant stromal overgrowth, a 15–25% recurrence rate is seen; in the presence of this finding, a recurrence rate of 45–70% is the rule, thus warranting a ClinD-3 designation for the former and ClinD-4 for the latter.

Most patients with adenosarcoma are cured by hysterectomy. Patients at higher risk to develop recurrent disease are those with high-stage tumor at the time of diagnosis, deep (>30% of the uterine wall) myoinvasion, a high-grade sarcomatous component, and stromal overgrowth, particularly if the stroma is high grade. Recurrent disease typically appears in the pelvis; distant metastasis from low-grade tumors is unusual but may occur many years after pelvic recurrence. Death from adenosarcoma is reported to occur in 10–25% of cases and more often the patients who died had a primary tumor that featured stromal overgrowth; death may be delayed until many years after the initial diagnosis, particularly if the stroma is low grade.

Managerially Relevant Differential Diagnostic Issues

Clinical Disease (Table 3) Considerations

Adenosarcomas without stromal overgrowth may have the typical low-power appearance of benign uterine adenofibroma but differ from that lesion in that the stroma is more cellular (particularly the cambium layer-like cuff immediately adjacent to the epithelium) and is mitotically active. Authorities differ on the appropriate mitotic index conventions for distinguishing adenofibroma from adenosarcoma. Clement and Scully (119) advocate a threshold of 2 mitotic figures (mf) per 10 high-power fields (hpf) while Zaloudek and Norris suggest a dividing line in the neighborhood of 4 mf per 10 hpf. We use the 4 mf/10 hpf criterion to make a diagnosis of adenosarcoma, but we consider tumors with particularly cellular stroma and/or borderline mitotic counts as being of uncertain malignant potential, particularly if subepithelial condensation is present. Other benign proliferations that feature a mixture of glands and stroma include endometrial polyps and polypoid adenomyoma (both typical and atypical). These lack the characteristic peri-glandular cuffing and the polypoid invaginations seen in adenosarcoma (131).

Clinical Disease III (Table 3) Considerations

The differential diagnosis of adenosarcoma in addition to adenofibroma includes ESS with a prominent glandular component. Over a certain range of appearance, there is no crisp distinction between the two. Features favoring adenosarcoma include dilated, irregularly shaped glands with intraluminal polypoid protrusions, a variety of müllerian epithelial types, and periglandular stromal condensation. The absence of these features combined with endometrial-type, regularly contoured glands favor ESS. Fortunately, as long as the stromal component is as bland as that seen in ESS, the tumor under either assumption will exhibit Clinical Disease III behavior.

Clinical Disease IV (Table 3) Considerations

Adenosarcoma with stromal overgrowth feature areas with "pure" stromal proliferation (greater than 25% of the tumor) alternating with stroma containing scattered, enlarged, dilated, morphologically benign glandular elements. The stroma in the areas of "overgrowth" is usually obviously sarcomatous. Heterologous sarcoma (particularly rhabdomyosarcoma) is seen in one-fourth of adenosarcomas with stromal overgrowth. The mitotic counts in tumors with stromal overgrowth are almost always well over 4 per 10 hpf. When the stroma is cytologically malignant, distinction of adenosarcoma from a pure uterine sarcoma or carcinosarcoma depends on identifying neoplastic glands in some part of the tumor—benign in adenosarcoma and malignant in the case of carcinosarcoma. Again, in all of these cases, Clinical Disease IV behavior is to be anticipated.

CARCINOSARCOMA (43,132–136)

The terminology for mixed neoplasms composed of carcinoma and sarcoma is in flux. Malignant mixed müllerian tumor (MMMT) has the advantage of long entrenchment and, consequently, is the term clinicians are most likely to recognize. This observation notwithstanding, the Nomenclature Committee of International Society of Gynecologic Pathologists and the World Health Organization has recommended that the term be replaced by "carcinosarcoma" and, for a variety of reasons, we think this practice should be adopted.

The claim advanced by advocates for changing this nomenclature is that carcinosarcoma is not a "true" sarcoma but a carcinoma with metaplastic sarcomatous elements. This histogenetic claim, then, is that the targeted stem in the development of carcinosarcoma is not a normal mesenchymal cell (for example, a normal myocyte in the case of leiomyosarcoma) but an epithelial cell of the sort that is responsible for the development of endometrial carcinoma. The production of a sarcomatous component is, then, a developmental afterthought, hence the "metaplasia" designation. Support for this taxonomic claim comes from several quarters. The epidemiologic profile of patients with carcinosarcoma is similar to patients with endometrial adenocarcinoma (137), the sarcomatous component often marks with keratins as do the cells in endometrial adenocarcinoma (133,135,139–144), and molecular studies support both the similarity of the two components and their monclonality (145–148). Whether this taxonomic insight has any implications for therapy, as some suggest, remains to be confirmed (152).

Clinical Features

Carcinosarcoma, with rare exceptions, is a disease of elderly menopausal women; most patients present with uterine bleeding. Uterine enlargement is common. There is an association between carcinosarcoma and prior pelvic radiation (53,134,153–159).

Gross Pathology

Carcinosarcomas are almost invariably fleshy, necrotic, hemorrhagic, polypoid growths that fill the uterine cavity and commonly extend through the cervical os. Cervical and extrauterine involvement at the time of hysterectomy is common. Gross sectioning of the uterus typically reveals extensive myometrial invasion. A small minority of cases are incidental findings in uteri removed for other reasons. Despite their small size, disseminated disease in these cases has been reported

Microscopic Pathology (Figs. 7 and 8)

Almost all carcinosarcoma are easily recognized as high-grade malignant neoplasms, whether the tumor is initially encountered in an endometrial sampling or a hysterectomy specimen. Both the high-grade nuclear features and the biphasic pattern of this neoplasm are obvious in the typical case. However, in many instances, one or the other component predominates and differential diagnostic problems arise when this biphasic pattern is inconspicuous, particularly in endometrial samplings. The most common problem is trying to determine whether an anaplastic carcinoma also contains sarcoma. The epithelial component of a carcinosarcoma may be any type of müllerian carcinoma—mucinous, squamous, endometrioid, serous, clear cell, undifferentiated, or mixtures of these—although endometrioid is the most common. It is traditional to divide the stromal components into "homologous" (leiomyosarcoma, stromal sarcoma, "fibrosarcoma") and "heterologous" (chondrosarcoma, rhabdomyosarcoma, osteosarcoma, liposarcoma) types, although there is little evidence that this ritual is clinically useful. On the other hand, identification of heterolo-

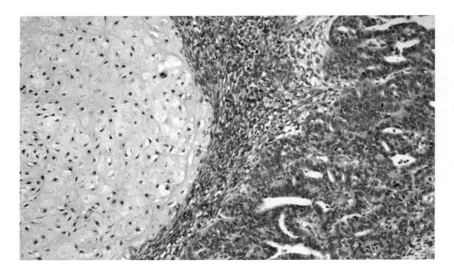

Figure 7 Carcinosarcoma. Malignant glands and malignant stroma are the defining characteristics of this neoplasm.

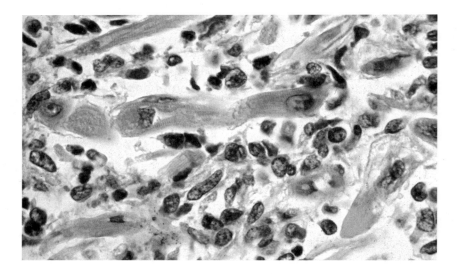

Figure 8 Carcinosarcoma. A focus of rhabdomyosarcoma is present as indicated by several rhabdomyoblasts.

gous sarcoma is often diagnostically useful in identifying the tumor as a carcinosarcoma rather than pure carcinoma. An unusual occurrence is the carcinosarcoma in which the carcinoma and sarcoma are both low grade. Although very few cases have been studied, these appear to have low-grade behavior similar to that of low-grade adenosarcoma and therefore this feature should be documented.

The clinical course of patients with carcinosarcoma is that of a high-grade aggressive malignant neoplasm with a prognosis that is significantly worse than high grade endometrial carcinoma including serous and clear cell variants (143). One-third of the patients present with clinical evidence of extrauterine spread and, in some series, as high as 40–50% of patients thought to have stage I disease clinically are upstaged after surgical staging. The most important prognostic features are the stage, size of the tumor, and the depth of myometrial invasion. For practical purposes, the only patients to achieve long-term survival are those with small tumors that are most minimally myoinvasive. However, the converse does not hold; even tumors that, after extensive sectioning of the uterus, are apparently confined to the endometrium (or to an endometrial polyp) can metastasize. The type(s) of sarcoma, level of mitotic counts, and grade of the sarcoma have not been shown to be significantly related to survival in large clinicopathologic series. There are conflicting reports about the significance of vascular invasion, cervical involvement, and the subtype of carcinoma. The GOG has reported that the subtype (especially, serous and clear cell) and grade of the carcinomatous element are significant predictors of survival (132).

The pathology report of a carcinosarcoma should specify the size and location of the tumor, the extent of myometrial invasion if any, the status of the cervix, the presence or absence of vascular invasion, the type of carcinoma, and the status of the resection margins.

Managerially Relevant Differential Diagnostic Issues

Carcinosarcoma is almost invariably easily identified as a highly malignant proliferation. As indicated formerly, there are infrequent problems of separating carcinosarcoma from adenosarcoma with high-grade stromal overgrowth; this is a managerial non-problem as both are Clinical Disease IV. More commonly, it is not obvious from an endometrial sampling whether the malignancy is carcinosarcoma, high-grade endometrial carcinoma, or a pure, high-grade sarcoma. Again, in the usual situation, hysterectomy is the next move and complete examination resolves the problem. Much less commonly, the possibility of a hemotolymphoid malignancy is raised by the sampling; again, the usual immunohistochemical strategies suffice to clarify the situation.

REFERENCES

1. Zaloudek C, Hendrickson MR. Mesenchymal tumors of the uterus. In: Kurman RJ, ed. *Blaustein's Pathology of the Female Genital Tract*. New York: Springer-Verlag, 2002, 561–616.

2. Oliva E, Clement PB, Young RH. Endometrial stromal tumors: an update on a group of tumors with a protean phenotype. *Adv Anat Pathol* 2000; 7:257–281.

3. Kempson RL, Hendrickson MR. Smooth muscle, endometrial, stromal, and mixed müllerian tumors of the uterus. *Mod Pathol* 2000; 13:328–342.

4. Berchuck A, Rubin S, Hoskins W, Saigo P, Pierce V, Lewis JJ. Treatment of endometrial stromal tumors. *Gynecol Oncol* 1990; 36:60–65.

5. Chang K, Crabtree G, Lim-Tam S, Kempson R, Hendrickson M. Primary uterine endometrial stromal neoplasms. A clinicopathologic study of 117 cases. *Am J Surg Pathol* 1990; 14:415–438.

6. Chauveine L, Deniaud E, Plancher C, et al. Uterine sarcomas: the Curie Institut experience. Prognosis factors and adjuvant treatments. *Gynecol Oncol* 1999; 72:232–237.

7. el-Naggar AK, Abdul-Karim FW, Silva EG, McLemore D, Garnsey L. Uterine stromal neoplasms: a clinicopathologic and DNA flow cytometric correlation. *Hum Pathol* 1991; 22:897–903.

8. Gadducci A, Sartori E, Landoni F, et al. Endometrial stromal sarcoma: analysis of treatment failures and survival. *Gynecol Oncol* 1996; 63:247–253.

9. Hart W, Yoonessi M. Endometrial stromatosis of the uterus.*Obstet Gynecol* 1977; 49:393–403.

10. Mansi J, Ramachandra S, Wiltshaw E, Fisher C. Endometrial stromal sarcomas. *Gynecol Oncol* 1990; 36:113–118.

11. Piver M, Rutledge F, Copeland L, Webster K, Blumenson L, Suh O. Uterine endolymphatic stromal myosis: a collaborative study. *Obstet Gynecol* 1984; 64:173–178.

12. Eddy GL, Mazur MT. Endolymphatic stromal myosis associated with tamoxifen use. *Gynecol Oncol* 1997; 64:262–264.

13. Pang LC. Endometrial stromal sarcoma with sex cord-like differentiation associated with tamoxifen therapy. *South Med J* 1998; 91:592–594.

14. Clement P, Scully R. Endometrial stromal sarcomas of the uterus with extensive endometrioid glandular differentiation: a report of three cases that caused problems in differential diagnosis. *Int J Gynecol Path* 1992; 11:163–173.

15. Oliva E, Clement PB, Young RH. Epithelioid endometrial and endometrioid stromal tumors: a report of four cases emhasizing their distinction from epithelioid smooth muscle tumors and other oxyphilic uterine and extrauterine tumors. *Int J Gynecol Pathol* 2002; 21:48–55.

16. Franquemont DW, Frierson HF Jr, Mills SE. An immunohistochemical study of normal endometrial stroma and endometrial stromal neoplasms. Evidence for smooth muscle differentiation. *Am J Surg Pathol* 1991; 15:861–870.

17. Farhood AI, Abrams J. Immunohistochemistry of endometrial stromal sarcoma. *Hum Pathol* 1991; 22:224–230.

18. Devaney K, Tavassoli FA. Immunohistochemistry as a diagnostic aid in the interpretation of unusual mesenchymal tumors of the uterus. *Mod Pathol* 1991; 4:225–231.

19. Binder SW, Nieberg RK, Cheng L, al-Jitawi S. Histologic and immunohistochemical analysis of nine endometrial stromal

tumors: an unexpected high frequency of keratin protein positivity. *Int J Gynecol Pathol* 1991; 10:191–197.

20. Oliva E, Young RH, Amin MB, Clement PB. An immunohistochemical analysis of endometrial stromal and smooth muscle tumors of the uterus: a study of 54 cases emphasizing the importance of using a panel because of overlap in immunoreactivity for individual antibodies. *Am J Surg Pathol* 2002; 26:403–412.

21. Agoff SN, Grieco VS, Garcia R, Gown AM. Immunohistochemical distinction of endometrial stromal sarcoma and cellular leiomyoma. *Appl Immunohistochem Mol Morphol* 2001; 9:164–169.

22. Chu PG, Arber DA, Weiss LM, Chang KL. Utility of CD 10 in distinguishing between endometrial stromal sarcoma and uterine smooth muscle tumors: an immunohistochemical comparison of 34 cases. *Mod Pathol* 2001; 14:465–471.

23. McCluggage WG, Sumathy VP, Maxwell P. CD 10 is a sensitive and diagnostically useful immunohistochemical marker of normal endometrial stroma and of endometrial stromal neoplasms. *Histopathology* 2001; 39:273–278.

24. Nucci MR, O'Connell JT, Huettner PC, Cviko A, Sun D, Quade BJ. h-Caldesmon expression effectively distinguishes endometrial stromal tumors from uterine smooth muscle tumors. *Am J Surg Pathol* 2001; 25:455–463.

25. Rush DS, Tan J, Baergen RN, Soslow RA. h-Caldesmon, a novel smooth muscle-specific antibody, distinguishes between cellular leiomyoma and endometrial stromal sarcoma. *Am J Surg Pathol* 2001; 25:253–258.

26. Fekete PS, Vellios F, Patterson BD. Uterine tumor resembling an ovarian sex-cord tumor: report of a case of an endometrial stromal tumor with foam cells and ultrastructural evidence of epithelial differentiation. *Int J Gynecol Pathol* 1985; 4:378–387.

27. Sullinger J, Scully R. Uterine tumors resembling ovarian sex-cord tumors. A clinicopathologic and immunohistochemical study [abstract]. *Mod Pathol* 1989; 2:93A.

28. Lillemoe T, Perrone T, Norris H, Dehner L. Myogenous phenotype of epithelial-like areas in endometrial stromal sarco-

mas. *Lab Investigations* [abstract]; 1990 (unpublished manuscript).

29. Fukunaga M, Miyazawa Y, Ushigome S. Endometrial low-grade stromal sarcoma with ovarian sex-cord-like differentiation: report of two cases with an immunohistochemical and flow cytometric study. *Pathol Int* 1997; 47:412–415.

30. Baker RJ, Hildebrandt RH, Rouse RV, Hendrickson MR, Longacre TA. Inhibin and CD99 (MIC2) expression in uterine stromal neoplasms with sex cord-like elements. *Mod Pathology* 1998; 11:100A.

31. Norris H, Taylor H. Mesenchymal tumors of the uterus. I. A clinical and pathological study of 53 endometrial stromal tumors. *Cancer* 1966; 19:755–766.

32. Evans H. Endometrial stromal sarcoma and poorly differentiated endometrial sarcoma. *Cancer* 1982; 50:2170–2182.

33. Aubry MC, Myers JL, Colby TV, Leslie KO, Tazelaar HD. Endometrial stromal sarcoma metastatic to the lung: a detailed analysis of 16 patients. *Am J Surg Pathol* 2002; 26:440–449.

34. Gloor E, Schnyder P, Cikes M, et al. Endolymphatic stromal myosis. Surgical and hormonal treatment of extensive abdominal recurrence 20 years after hysterectomy. *Cancer* 1982; 50:1888–1893.

35. Sabini G, Chumas JC, Mann WJ. Steroid hormone receptors in endometrial stromal sarcomas. A biochemical and immuno-histochemical study. *Am J Clin Pathol* 1992; 97:381–386.

36. Reich O, Regauer S, Urdl W, Lahousen M, Winter R. Expression of oestrogen and progesterone receptors in low-grade endometrial stromal sarcomas. *Br J Cancer* 2000; 82:1030–1034.

37. Oliva E, Young RH, Clement PB, Bhan AK, Scully RE. Cellular benign mesenchymal tumors of the uterus. A comparative morphologic and immunohistochemical analysis of 33 highly cellular leiomyomas and six endometrial stromal nodules, two frequently confused tumors. *Am J Surg Pathol* 1995; 19:757–768.

38. Goldblum JR, Clement PB, Hart WR. Adenomyosis with sparse glands. A potential mimic of low-grade endometrial stromal sarcoma. *Am J Clin Pathol* 1995; 103:218–223.

39. Banks ER, Mills SE, Frierson HF Jr. Uterine intravascular menstrual endometrium simulating malignancy. *Am J Surg Pathol* 1991; 15:407–412.

40. Oliva E, Clement PB, Young RH, Scully RE. Mixed endometrial stromal and smooth muscle tumors of the uterus: a clinicopathologic study of 15 cases. *Am J Surg Pathol* 1998; 22:997–1005.

41. Clement P, Scully R. Uterine tumors resembling ovarian sex-cord tumors. A clinicopathologic analysis of fourteen cases. *Am J Clin Pathol* 1976; 66:512–525.

42. Kantelip B, Cloup N, Dechelotte P. Uterine tumor resembling ovarian sex cord tumors: report of a case with ultrastructural study. *Hum Pathol* 1986; 17:91–94.

43. Clement P, Scully R. Uterine tumors with mixed epithelial and mesenchymal elements. *Semin Diagn Pathol* 1988; 5:199–222.

44. Norris H, Parmley T. Mesenchymal tumors of the uterus. V. Intravenous leiomyomatosis. A clinical and pathologic study of 14 cases. *Cancer* 1975; 36:2164.

45. Clement P, Young R, Scully R. Intravenous leiomyomatosis of the uterus. A clinicopathological analysis of 16 cases with unusual histologic features. *Am J Surg Pathol* 1988; 12:932–459.

46. Esteban JM, Allen WM, Schaerf RH. Benign metastasizing leiomyoma of the uterus: histologic and immunohistochemical characterization of primary and metastatic lesions. *Arch Pathol Lab Med* 1999; 123:960–962.

47. Tietze L, Gunther K, Horbe A, et al. Benign metastasizing leiomyoma: a cytogenetically balanced but clonal disease. *Hum Pathol* 2000; 31:126–128.

48. Hales HA, Peterson CM, Jones KP, Quinn JD. Leiomyomatosis peritonealis disseminata treated with a gonadotropin-releasing hormone agonist. A case report [published erratum appears in *Am J Obstet Gynecol* 1993 Aug; 169(2Pt 1):439]. *Am J Obstet Gynecol* 1992; 167:515–516.

49. Tavassoli F, Norris H. Peritoneal leiomyomatosis (leiomyomatosis peritonealis disseminata): a clinicopathologic study

of 20 cases with ultrastructural observations. *Int J Gynecol Pathol* 1982; 1:59–74.

50. Leibsohn S, d'Ablaing G, Mishell DR Jr, Schlaerth JB. Leiomyosarcoma in a series of hysterectomies performed for presumed uterine leiomyomas. *Am J Obstet Gynecol* 1990; 162:968–974; discussion 974–976.

51. Hart W, Billman JJ. An reassessment of uterine neoplasms originally diagnosed as leiomyosarcomas. *Cancer* 1978; 41:1902–1910.

52. Barter J, Smith E, Szpak C, Hinshaw W, Clarke-Pearson D, Creasman W. Leiomyosarcoma of the uterus: clinicopathologic study of 21 cases. *Gynecol Oncol* 1985; 21:220–227.

53. Wheelock JB, Krebs HB, Schneider V, Goplerud DR. Uterine sarcoma: analysis of prognostic variables in 71 cases. *Am J Obstet Gynecol* 1985; 151:1016–1022.

54. Covens AL, Nisker JA, Chapman WB, Allen HH. Uterine sarcoma: an analysis of 74 cases. *Am J Obstet Gynecol* 1987; 156:370–374.

55. Schwartz LB, Diamond MP, Schwartz PE. Leiomyosarcomas: clinical presentation. *Am J Obstet Gynecol* 1993.

56. Bell SW, Kempson RL, Hendrickson MR. Problematic uterine smooth muscle neoplasms. A clinicopathologic study of 213 cases. *Am J Surg Pathol* 1994; 18:535–558.

57. Sakala EP, Gaio KL. Fundal uterine leiomyoma obscuring first-trimester transabdominal sonographic diagnosis of fetal holoprosencephaly. A case report. *J Reprod Med* 1993; 38:400–402.

58. Larson B, Silfversward C, Nilsson B, Pettersson F. Prognostic factors in uterine leiomyosarcoma. A clinical and histopathological study of 143 cases. The Radiumhemmet series 1936–1981. *Acta Oncol* 1990; 29:185–191.

59. Parker WH, Fu YS, Berek JS. Uterine sarcoma in patients operated on for presumed leiomyoma and rapidly growing leiomyoma. *Obstet Gynecol* 1994; 83:414–418.

60. Vardi J, Tovelli H. Leiomyosarcoma of the uterus: clinicopathologic study. *Obstet Gynecol* 1980; 56:428–434.

61. Burns B, Curry R, Bell M. Morphologic features of prognostic significance in uterine smooth muscle tumors: a review of eighty-four cases. *Am J Obstet Gynecol* 1979; 135:109–114.

62, Evans HL, Chawla SP, Simpson C, Finn KP. Smooth muscle neoplasms of the uterus other than ordinary leiomyoma. A study of 446 cases, with emphasis on diagnostic criteria and prognostic factors. *Cancer* 1988; 62:2239–2247.

63. Barter JF, Smith EB, Szpak CA, Hinshaw W, Clarke-Pearson DL, Creasman WT. Leiomyosarcoma of the uterus: clinicopathologic study of 21 cases. *Gynecol Oncol* 1985; 21:220–227.

64. King M, Dickersin G, Scully R. Myxoid leiomyosarcoma of the uterus. A report of six cases. *Am J Surg Pathol* 1982; 6:589–598.

65. Chen K. Myxoid leiomyosarcoma of the uterus. *Int J Gynecol Pathol* 1984; 3:389–392.

66. Peacock G, Archer S. Myxoid leiomysarcoma of the uterus: case report and review of the literature. *Am J Obstet Gynecol* 1989; 160:1515–1518; discussion 1518–1519.

67. Atkins K. Bell S, Kempson RL, Hendrickson MR. Myxoid smooth muscle neoplasms of the uterus. 2000 (forthcoming).

68. Darby A, Papadaki L, Beilby J. An unusual leiomyosarcoma of the uterus containing osteoclast-like giant cells. *Cancer* 1975; 36:495–504.

69. Marshall RJ, Braye SG, Jones DB. Leiomyosarcoma of the uterus with giant cells resembling osteoclasts. *Int J Gynecol Pathol* 1986; 5:260–268.

70. Watanabe K, Hiraki H, Ohishi M, Mashiko K, Saginoya H, Suzuki T. Uterine leiomyosarcoma with osteoclast-like giant cells: histopathological and cytological observations. *Pathol Int* 1996; 46:656–660.

71. Major FJ, Blessing JA, Silverberg SG, et al. Prognostic factors in early-stage uterine sarcoma. A Gynecologic Oncology Group study. *Cancer* 1993.

72. Nordal RR, Kristensen GB, Kaern J, Stenwig AE, Pettersen EO, Trope CG. The prognostic significance of stage, tumor size, cellular atypia and DNA ploidy in uterine leiomyosarcoma. *Acta Oncol* 1995; 34:797–802.

73. Mayerhofer K, Obermair A, Windbichler G, et al. Leiomyosarcoma of the uterus: a clinicopathologic multicenter study of 71 cases. *Gynecol Oncol* 1999; 74:196–201.

74. Downes KA, Hart WR. Bizarre leiomyomas of the uterus: a comprehensive pathologic study of 24 cases with long-term follow-up. *Am J Surg Pathol* 1997; 21:1261–1270.

75. Prayson RA, Hart WR. Mitotically active leiomyomas of the uterus. *Am J Clin Pathol* 1992; 97:14–20.

76. Kunzel KE, Mills NZ, Muderspach LI, d'Ablaing G III. Myxoid leiomyosarcoma of the uterus. *Gynecol Oncol* 1993; 48:277–282.

77. Schneider D, Halperin R, Segal M, Maymon R, Bukovsky I. Myxoid leiomyosarcoma of the uterus with unusual malignant histologic pattern—a case report. *Gynecol Oncol* 1995; 59A:156–158.

78. Clement P, Young R, Scully R. Diffuse, perinodular, and other patterns of hydropic degeneration within and adjacent to uterine leiomyomas. Problems in differential diagnosis. *Am J Surg Pathol* 1992; 16:26–32.

79. Oliva E, Nielsen PG, Clement PB, Young RH, Scully RE. Epithelioid smooth muscle tumors of the uterus: a clinicopathologic study of 80 cases [abstract]. *Mod Pathol* 1997; 10:107A.

80. Prayson RA, Goldblum JR, Hart WR. Epithelioid smooth-muscle tumors of the uterus: a clinicopathologic study of 18 patients. *Am J Surg Pathol* 1997; 21:383–391.

81. Atkins K, Bell S, Kempson RL, Hendrickson MR. Epithelioid smooth muscle neoplasms of the uterus. 2000 (forthcoming).

82. Jones MW, Norris HJ. Clinicopathologic study of 28 uterine leiomyosarcomas with metastasis. *Int J Gynecol Pathol* 1995; 14:243–249.

83. Clement PB. The pathology of uterine smooth muscle tumors and mixed endometrial stromal-smooth muscle tumors: a selective review with emphasis on recent advances. *Int J Gynecol Pathol* 2000; 19:39–55.

84. Kurman R, Norris H. Mesenchymal tumors of the uterus. VI. Epithelioid smooth muscle tumors including leiomyoblas-

toma and clear-cell leiomyoma: a clinical and pathologic analysis of 26 cases. *Cancer* 1976; 37:1853–1865.

85. Karpuz V, Joris F, Letovanec N, Branchmanski F, Kapanci Y. Metastizing lowgrade clear cell leiomyosarcoma of the uterus. *Pathol Int* 1998; 48:82–85.

86. Malmstrom H, Schmidt H, Perrson PG, Carstensen J, Nordenskjold B, Simonsen E. Flow cytometric analysis of uterine sarcoma: ploidy and S-phase rate as prognostic indicators. *Gynecol Oncol* 1992; 44:172–177.

87. Peters WA III,Howard DR, Andersen WA, Figge DC. Deoxyribonucleic acid analysis by flow cytometry of uterine leiomyosarcomas and smooth muscle tumors of uncertain malignant potential. *Am J Obstet Gynecol* 1992; 166:1646–1653; discussion 1653–1654.

88. Layfield LJ, Liu K, Dodge R, Barsky SH. Uterine smooth muscle tumors: utility of classification by proliferation, plordy, and prognostic markers versus traditional histopathology. *Arc Pathol Lab Med* 2000; 124:221–227.

89. Bloom R, Guerrieri C, Stal O, Malmstrom H, Simonsen E. Leiomyosarcoma of the uterus: a clinicopathologic, DNA flow cytometric, p53, and mdm-2–analysis of 49 cases. *Gynecol Oncol* 1998; 68:54–61.

90. Jeffers MD, Oakes SJ, Richmond JA, Macaulay EM. Proliferation, ploidy and prognosis in uterine smooth muscle tumours. *Histopathology* 1996; 29:217–223.

91. Goff BA, Rice LW, Fleischhacker D, et al. Uterine leiomyosarcoma and endometrial stromal sarcoma: lymph node metastases and sites of recurrence. *Gynecol Oncol* 1993; 50:105–109.

92. Fleming W, Peters W III, Kumar N, Morley G. Autopsy findings in patients with uterine sarcoma. *Gynecol Oncol* 1984; 19:168–172.

93. Rose PG, Piver MS, Tsukada Y, Lau T. Patterns of metastasis in uterine sarcoma. An autopsy study. *Cancer* 1989; 63:935–938.

94. Olah KS, Dunn JA, Gee H. Leiomyosarcomas have a poorer prognosis than mixed mesodermal tumours when adjusting for known prognostic factors: the result of a retrospective

study of 423 cases of uterine sarcoma. *Br J Obstet Gynaecol* 1992; 590–594.

95. Marchese M, Liskow A, Crum C, McCaffrey R, Frick H II. Uterine sarcomas: a clinicopathologic study, 1965–1981. *Gynecol Oncol* 1984; 18:299–312.

96. Kahanpaa K, Wahlstrom T, Grohn P, Heinonen E, Nieminen U, Widholm O. Sarcomas of the uterus: a clinicopathologic study of 119 patients. *Obstet Gynecol* 1986; 67:417–424.

97. Wolfson AH, Wolfson DJ, Sittler SY, et al. A multivariate analysis of clinicopathologic factors for predicting outcome in uterine sarcomas. *Gynecol Oncol* 1994; 52:56–62.

98. Gadducci A, Landoni F, Sartori E, et al. Uterine leiomyosarcoma: analysis of treatment failures and survival. *Gynecol Oncol* 1996; 62:25–32.

99. Nola M, Babic D, Ilic J, et al. Prognostic parameters for survival of patients with malignant mesenchymal tumors of the uterus. *Cancer* 1996; 78:2543–2550.

100. Pautier P, Genestic C, Rey A, et al. Analysis of clinicopathologic prognostic factors for 157 uterine sarcomas and evaluation of a grading score validated for soft tissue sarcoma. *Cancer* 2000; 88:1425–1431.

101. Yoonessi M, Hart W. Endometrial stromal sarcomas. *Cancer* 1977; 40:898–906.

102. De Young B, Bitterman P, Lack EE. Primary osteosarcoma of the uterus: report of a case with immunohistochemical study. *Mod Pathol* 1992; 5:212–215.

103. Emoto M, Iwasaki H, Kawarabayashi T, et al. Primary osteosarcoma of the uterus: report of a case with immunohistochemical analysis. *Gynecol Oncol* 1994; 54:385–388.

104. Hardisson D, Simon RS, Burgos E. Primary osteosarcoma of the uterine corpus: report of a case with immunohistochemical and ultrastructural study. *Gynecol Oncol* 2001; 82:181–186.

105. Kofinas A, Suarez J, Calame R, Chipeco Z. Chondrosarcoma of the uterus. *Gynecol Oncol* 1984; 19:231–237.

106. Clement P. Chondrosarcoma of the uterus: report of a case and review of the literature. *Hum Pathol* 1978; 9:726–732.

107. McCluggage WG, Lioe TF, McClelland HR, Lamki H. Rhabdomyosarcoma of the uterus: report of two cases, including one of the spindle cell variant. *Int J Gynecol Cancer* 2002; 12:128–132.

108. Takano M, Kikuchi Y, Aida S, Sato K, Nagata I. Embryonal rhabdomyosarcoma of the uterine corpus in a 76-year-old patient. *Gynecol Oncol* 1999; 75:490–494.

109. Chiarle R, Godio L, Fusi D, Soldati T, Palestro G. Pure alveolar rhabdomyosarcoma of the corpus uteri: description of a case with increased serum level of CA 125. *Gynecol Oncol* 1997; 66:320–332.

110. Holcomb K, Francis M, Ruiz J, Abulafia O, Matthews RP, Lee YC. Pleomorphic rhabdomyosarcoma of the uterus in a postmenopausal woman with elevated serum CA 125. *Gynecol Oncol* 1999; 74:499–501.

111. Ordi J, Stamatakos MD, Tavassoli FA. Pure pleomorphic rhabdomysarcomas of the uterus. *Int J Gynecol Pathol* 1997; 16:369–377.

112. Bapat K, Brustein S. Uterine sarcoma with liposarcomatous differentiation: report of a case and review of the literature. *Int J Gynecol Obstet* 1989; 28:71–75.

113. Schammel DP, Tavassoli FA. Uterine angiosarcomas: a morphologic and immunohistochemical study of four cases. *Am J Surg Pathol* 1998; 22:246–250.

114. Hendrickson M, Scheithauer B. Primitive neuroectodermal tumor of the endometrium: report of two cases, one with electron microscopic observations. *Int J Gynecol Pathol* 1986; 5:249–259.

115. Daya D, Lukka H, Clement P. Primitive neuroectodermal tumors of the uterus: a report of four cases. *Hum Pathol* 1992; 23:1120–1129.

116. Fraggetta F, Magro G, Vasquez E. Primitive neuroectodermal tumour of the uterus with focal cartilaginous differentiation. *Histopathology* 1997; 309:483–485.

117. Chen K, Vergon J. Carcinomesenchymoma of the uterus. *Am J Clin Pathol* 1981; 75:746–748.

118. Engdhal E, Wolfhagen U. Carcinofibroma—a rare variant of mixed müllerian tumor. *Acta Obstet Gynecol Scand* 1988; 67:85–88.

119. Clement P, Scully R. Müllerian adenosarcoma of the uterus: a clinicopathologic analysis of 100 cases with a review of the literature. *Hum Pathol* 1990; 21:363–383.

120. Zaloudek C, Norris H. Adenofibroma and adenosarcoma of the uterus: a clinicopathologic study of 35 cases. *Cancer* 1981; 48:354–366.

121. Clement P, Scully R. Müllerian adenosarcomas of the uterus with sex cord-like elements. A clinicopatholgic analysis of eight cases. *Am J Clin Pathol* 1989; 91:664–672.

122. Clement P. Müllerian adenosarcomas of the uterus with sarcomatous overgrowth. A clinicopathological analysis of 10 cases. *Am J Surg Pathol* 1989; 13:28–38.

123. Czernobilsky B, Hohlweg-Majert P, Dallenbach-Hellweg G. Uterine adenosarcoma: a clinicopathologic study of 11 cases with a reevaluation of histologic criteria. *Arch Gynecol* 1983; 233:281–294.

124. Hirschfield L, Kahn L, Chen S, Winkler B, Rosenberg S. Müllerian adenosarcoma with ovarian sex cord-like differentiation. A light and electron-microscopic study. *Cancer* 1986; 57:1197–1200.

125. Kaku T, Silverberg S, Major F, Miller A, Fetter B, Brady M. Adenosarcoma of the uterus: a Gynecologic Oncology Group Clinicopathologic study of 31 cases. *Int J Gynecol* 1992; 11:75–88.

126. Clement PB, Oliva E, Young RH. Müllerian adenosarcoma of the uterine corpus associated with tamoxifen therapy: a report of six cases and a review of tamoxifen-associated endometrial lesions. *Int J Gynecol Pathol* 1996; 15:222–229.

127. Jessop FA, Roberts PF. Müllerian adenosarcoma of the uterus in association with tamoxifen therapy. *Histopathology* 2000; 36:91–129.

128. Carvalho FM, Carvalho JP, Motta EV, Souen J. Müllerian adenosarcoma of the uterus with sarcomatous overgrowth

following tamoxifen treatment for breast cancer. *Rev Hosp Clin Fac Med Sao Paulo* 2000; 55:17–20.

129. Jagavkar RS, Shakespeare TP, Stevens MJ. Endometrial adenosarcoma with adjuvant tamoxifen therapy for primary breast carcinoma. *Australas Radiol* 1998; 42:157–158.

130. Jones MW, Lefkowitz M. Adenosarcoma of the uterine cervix: a clinicopathological study of 12 cases. *Int J Gynecol Pathol* 1995; 14:223–229.

131. Longacre TA, Chung MH, Rouse RV, Hendrickson MR. Atypical polypoid adenomyofibromas (atypical polypoid adenomyomas) of the uterus. A clinicopathologic study of 55 cases. *Am J Surg Pathol* 1996; 20:1–20.

132. Silverberg S, Major F, Blessing J, et al. Carcinosarcoma (malignant mixed mesodermal tumor) of the uterus. A Gynecologic Oncology Group pathologic study of 203 cases. *Int J Gynecol Pathol* 1990; 9:1–19.

133. Geisinger K, Dabbs D, Marshall R. Malignant mixed müllerian tumors. An ultrastructural and immunohistochemical analysis with histogenetic considerations. *Cancer* 1987; 59:1781–1790.

134. Gagne E, Tetu B, Blondeau L, Raymond PE, Blais R. Morphologic prognostic factors of malignant mixed Müllerian tumor of the uterus: a cllinicopathologic study of 58 cases. *Mod Pathol* 1989; 2:433–438.

135. Meiss JM, Lawrence WD. The immunohistochemical profile of malignant mixed müllerian tumor. Overlap with endometrial adenocarcinoma. *Am J Clin Pathol* 1990; 94:1–7.

136. Ronnett BM, Zaino RJ, Ellenson LH, Kurman RJ. Endometrial carcinomas. In: Kurman RJ, ed. *Blaustein's Pathology of the Female Genital Tract*. New York: Springer-Verlag, 2002. 501–560.

137. Zelmanowicz A, Hildesheim A, Sherman ME, et al. Evidence for a common etiology for endometrial carcinomas and malignant mixed müllerian tumors. *Gynecol Oncol* 1998; 69–253–257.

138. Yoshida Y, Kurokawa T, Fukano N, Nishikawa Y, Kamitani N, Kotsuji F. Markers of apoptosis and angiogenesis indicate that carcinomatous components play an important role in the

malignant behavior of uterine carcinosarcoma. *Hum Pathol* 2000; 31:1448–1454.

139. Auerbach H, LiVolsi V, Merino M. Malignant mixed müllerian tumors of the uterus. An immunohistochemical study. *Int J Gynecol Pathol* 1988; 7:123–131.

140. Bitterman P, Chun B, Kurman R. The significance of epithelial differentiation in mixed mesodermal tumors of the uterus. A clinicopathologic and immunohistochemical study. *Am J Surg Pathol* 1990; 14:317–328.

141. Costa MJ, Khan R, Judd R. Carcinoma [malignant mixed müllerian (mesodermal) tumor] of the uterus and ovary. Correlation of clinical, pathologic, and immunohistochemical features in 29 cases. *Arch Pathol Lab Med* 1991; 115:583–590.

142. de Brito PA, Silverberg SG, Orenstein JM. Carcinosarcoma [malignant mixed müllerian (mesodermal) tumor] of the female genital tract: immunohistochemical and ultrastructural analysis of 28 cases. *Human Pathol* 1993; 24:132–142.

143. George E, Lillemoe TJ, Twiggs LB, Perrone T. Malignant mixed müllerian tumor versus high-grade endometrial carcinoma and aggressive variants of endometrial carcinoma: a comparative analysis of survival. *Int J Gynecol Pathol* 1995; 14:39–44.

144. Ramadan M, Goudie RB. Epithelial antigens in malignant mixed müllerian tumors of endometrium. *J Pathol* 1986; 148:13–18.

145. Kounelis S, Jones MW, Papadaki H, Bakker A, Swalsky P, Finkelstein SD. Carcinosarcomas (malignant mixed müllerian tumors) of the female genital tract: comparative molecular analysis of epithellial and mesenchymal components. *Hum Pathol* 1998; 29:82–87.

146. Thompson L, Chang B, Barksy SH. Monoclonal origins of malignant mixed tumors (carcinosarcomas). Evidence for a divergent histogenesis. *Am J Surg Pathol* 1996; 20:277–285.

147. Wada H, Enomoto T, Fujita M, et al. Molecular evidence that most but not all carcinosarcomas of the uterus are combination tumors. *Cancer Res* 1997; 57:5379–5385.

148. Fujii H, Yoshida M, Gong ZX, et al. Frequent genetic heterogeneity in the clonal evolution of gynecological carcinosar-

coma and its influence on phenotypic diversity. *Cancer Res* 2000; 60:114–201.

149.   Emoto M, Iwasaki H, Kikuchi M, Shirakawa K. Characteristics of cloned cells of mixed müllerian tumor of the human uterus. Carcinoma cells showing myogenic differentiation in vitro. *Cancer* 1993; 71:3065–3075.

150.   Gorai I, Doi C, Minaguchi H. Establishment and characterization of carcinosarcoma cell line of the human uterus. *Cancer* 1993; 71:775–786.

151.   Gorai I, Yanagibashi T, Taki A, et al. Uterine carcinosarcoma is derived from a single stem cell: an in vitro study. *Int J Cancer* 1997; 72:821–827.

152.   van Rijswijk RE, Tognon G, Burger CW, Baak JP, Kenemans P, Vermorken JB. The effect of chemotherapy on the different components of advanced carcinosarcomas (malignant mixed mesodermal tumors) of the female genital tract. *Int J Gynecol Cancer* 1994; 4:52–60.

153.   Chuang JT, Van Velden DJ, Graham JB. Carcinosarcoma and mixed mesodermal tumor of the uterine corpus. Reivew of 49 cases. *Obstet Gynecol* 1970; 35:769–780.

154.   Meredith RF, Eisert DR, Kaka Z, Hodgson SE, Johnston GA Jr, Boutselis JG. An excess of uterine sarcomas after pelvic irradiation. *Cancer* 1986; 58:2003–2007.

155.   Norris H, Taylor H. Post irradiation sarcomas of the uterus. *Obstet Gynecol* 1965; 26:689–694.

156.   Perez CA, Askin F, Baglan RJ, et al. Effects of irradition on mixed müllerian tumors of the uterus. *Cancer* 1979; 43:1274–1284.

157.   Peters WA III, Kumar NB, Fleming WP, Morley GW. Prognostic features of sarcomas and mixed tumors of the endometrium. *Obstet Gynecol* 1984; 63:550–556.

158.   Shaw RW, Lynch PF, Wade-Evans T. Müllerian mixed tumor of the uterine corpus: a clinical histopathological review of 28 patients. *Br J Obstet Gynaecol* 1983; 90:562–569.

159.   Varela-Duran J, Nochomovitz LE, Prem KA, Dehner LP. Postirradiation mixed müllerian tumors of the uterus: a comparative clinicopathologic study. *Cancer* 1980; 45:1625–1631.

7

Clinical Evaluation of Abnormal Uterine Bleeding

JAY M. COOPER

University of Arizona School of Medicine, Phoenix, Arizona, U.S.A.

BARBARA J. STEGMANN

Phoenix Integrated Residency in Obstetrics and Gynecology, Phoenix, Arizona, U.S.A.

Abnormal uterine bleeding (AUB) is the presenting symptom in up to 33% of women referred to the gynecologist. Annually, more than 10 million women complain of AUB, and 6 million will seek treatment for symptoms, including bleeding, chronic anemia, pain, and cramping (1).

DEFINITION

The normal menstrual cycle varies from 21–45 days, with flow lasting between 3 and 7 days. Average blood loss ranges from 30–40 ml, but it is usually less than 80 ml. Bleeding in

195

excess of 80 ml and cycles occurring more frequently than 21 days or at intervals greater than 45 days constitute abnormal uterine bleeding (AUB). The following are common terms used when discussing AUB and the menstrual cycle.

- *Menorrhagia*: Blood loss in excess of 80 ml per cycle (increased volume).
- *Hypomenorrhea*: Decreased blood flow with menses (decreased volume).
- *Oligomenorrhea*: Decrease in the total number of menstrual bleeding episodes (greater than 45 days between cycles).
- *Polymenorrhea*: Increase in the number of bleeding episodes (less than 21 days between cycles).
- *Metrorrhagia:* Irregular bleeding episodes that occur at frequent intervals between menses.
- *Menometrorrhagia:* Prolonged bleeding at irregular intervals.
- *Intermenstrual bleeding*: Bleeding that occurs between normal cycles.
- *Menopause:* Spontaneous cessation of menses for >1 year due to loss of reproductive hormones or surgical castration.
- *Postmenopausal bleeding*: Bleeding occurring >1 year after the onset of menopause or at unanticipated times during hormone replacement therapy.
- *Dysmenorrhea:* Painful menses.

HISTORY AND PHYSICAL EXAMINATION

An evaluation of AUB begins with a complete history including a menstrual history, and complete physical examination including a pelvic exam. Recent weight gain/loss, use of medications, previous episodes of bleeding not related to menses, psychological and physical stress, and eating disorders provide salient clues in the history that are helpful in narrowing one's focus in determining the etiology of AUB. A menstrual history outlining the length of the cycle, number of days of flow, evidence of intermenstrual bleeding, dysmenorrhea, and the characteristics of the menstrual flow are essential. In assessing a patient who is having difficulty recalling the events of the menstrual cycle, a daily menstrual diary containing this information is helpful.

The physical exam includes a breast and pelvic exam. The breasts are evaluated for evidence of nipple discharge, tenderness, or breast masses. The vulva should be inspected for trauma and lacerations, and the vagina should be examined for evidence of foreign bodies (including a retained tampon), mucosal lesions, and signs of estrogen deficiency and atrophy. The cervix should be examined for evidence of erosion, inflammation, lesions, or polyps. Finally, the size and position of the uterus should be documented and the adnexa evaluated for masses, tenderness, and mobility.

Laboratory evaluation includes hematologic indices, coagulation panel, and hormonal evaluation including assessment of the thyroid and the pituitary, and androgen status. A pregnancy test should be included for all women of childbearing age. Liver function testing and a renal panel should be performed if there is a suggestion of liver or renal impairment.

ETIOLOGY

Complications of Pregnancy

Threatened, incomplete, or missed abortion, ectopic pregnancy, trophoblastic disease, placental polyps, subinvolution of the placental site, postabortion endometritis, and retained products of conception can present with abnormal uterine bleeding, and can vary from spotting to hemorrhage. Especially in the case of early spontaneous abortion, women may present with symptoms of AUB before the diagnosis of pregnancy has been confirmed. Patients should be questioned about recent or current pregnancies, and all women of childbearing age should have a pregnancy test performed as part of the baseline evaluation of AUB. If positive, pelvic ultrasound and serial B-HCG evaluations are indicated.

Infections

Infections of the genital tract present with a variety of symptoms, including spotting, discharge, and pain. When the cervix is visualized during the speculum exam, careful attention should be paid to the possibility of cervical lesions suggestive of cervicitis. Infections with organisms such as *Trichomonas vaginalis, Neisseria gonorrhea, Chlamydia trachomatis*, and *Condylomata* may be confirmed with appropriate genital cultures and a wet prep (2).

Endometrial infections such as acute pelvic inflammatory disease or chronic endometritis can cause AUB. Women with pelvic inflammatory disease experience characteristic pain, fever, and constitutional symptoms associated with abnormal bleeding. Findings on physical exam include tenderness, purulent discharge from the cervical os an adenexal mass, or tenderness. An elevated white count and an abnormal transvaginal ultrasound may suggest an adenexal mass or abnormal endometrial stripe. Overt sepsis, with associated platelet deficiencies and consumptive coagulopathies, should be considered in patients presenting with bleeding in conjunction with other severe illnesses. In the absence of overt symptoms of pelvic inflammatory disease, AUB may be the only symptom of chronic endometritis. An endometrial biopsy can provide important information.

Systemic Causes

Oligomenorrhea and/or menorrhagia may be the earliest symptoms of hypothyroidism. The presence of a goiter, heat/cold intolerance, recent weight gain or loss, and dry skin are all suggestive of thyroid disease. High prolactin levels, which can occur with hypothyroidism or as an independent event, suppress luteinizing hormone (LH) and follicle-stimulating hormone (FSH) production, leading to anovulation and amenorrhea. Some women will have galactorrhea along with menstrual abnormalities; therefore, a careful breast exam is indicated in all women.

Patients with liver disease may present with AUB as a result of two possible mechanisms. Cirrhosis impairs the metabolism of sex steroids, leading to high levels of free estrogen that, in turn, may cause endometrial overgrowth or hyperplasia associated with intermittent sloughing expressed as breakthrough bleeding. Severe liver disease also depletes vitamin K-dependent clotting factors that can lead to heavy bleeding in women with a functional endometrium due to an acquired coagulopathy (2).

Adrenal anomalies such as Cushing's disease and Addison disease lead to AUB based on fluctuations of endogenous glucocorticoids. Exogenous ingestion of glucocorticoids can lead to AUB on the same basis. Chronic renal failure is also an uncommon cause of AUB (2).

A history of easy bleeding (especially during dental procedures), easy bruising, bleeding from other orifices, excessive bleeding associated with minor trauma or surgery, and a family history of bleeding disorders are suggestive of a coagulation disorder (3). Coagulopathies are frequently first diagnosed at the time of heavy menstrual bleeding, especially in young women who present with heavy flow during their initial menstrual period. At times, the flow may be heavy enough to cause significant anemia requiring hospitalization and transfusion. von Willebrand's disease, a hereditary autosomic dominant defect of platelet activity, is the most common coagulopathy encountered affecting approximately 1% of the population (2,4). Heavy menstrual bleeding may also result from platelet deficiencies associated with disorders such as leukemia, severe sepsis, idiopathic thrombocytopenic purpura, aplastic anemia, and hypersplenism. Prothrombin deficiency, thalassemia major, Fanconi's anemia, and Ganzmann's disease, though uncommon, are additional causes of AUB.

Benign Lesions

Benign lesions of the reproductive tract may be responsible for symptoms of AUB. Cervical and vaginal lesions are usually identified during physical exam, while uterine anomalies require more extensive testing such as ultrasound, sonohysterography, or hysteroscopy.

Cervical polyps are most common in multiparous women in their fourth to sixth decades of life. They arise from either the endocervix or ectocervix, with the former being most common. Polyps vary in size from a few millimeters to 3 cm, are usually smooth or reddish, and are elongated or round (5). Removal can often be accomplished in the office. Although the majority are benign mucous lesions, all polyps should receive pathologic evaluation to rule out dysplasia. Whether removed in an office setting or in an ambulatory surgical setting, care should be taken to remove the lesion in its entirety. This often requires visualization of both the uterine cavity and endocervical canal, most easily accomplished by hysteroscopy.

Nonfunctional endometrial polyps are a common cause of menorrhagia, and their incidence also increases with advancing age. Endometrial polyps account for 6.8% of all cases of menometrorrhagia in women 20–40 years of age, and in postmenopausal women the incidence ranges as high as 3.6% to 23.8%. In a study by O'Connell et al. of 104 postmenopausal women with AUB, the prevalence of endometrial polyps was 32%, triple the anticipated rate (6). These polyps are generally larger, are more regular in shape, and often have a thick, surface endometrium (7). Degeneration of a polyp is occasionally encountered and can account for significant pelvic pain.

Malignant transformation of polyps is rare. However, there is an association between polyps and endometrial cancer. In one series, 10–34% of cases of endometrial cancer in postmenopausal women were associated with polyps (8). A higher prevalence of endometrial polyps has also been noted in women using tamoxifen, in women of advanced age, and in those undergoing hormonal replacement therapy (8).

Like cervical and uterine polyps, leiomyomata (or fibroids) are uncommon findings in the adolescent age group, but the incidence increases as the woman ages. Torrejon et al. found that 24.8% of premenopausal women with AUB had myomata (9). Both submucosal and intramural fibroids can cause excessive bleeding, which is typically cyclical in nature. Diagnosis requires evaluation of the endometrial cavity, either with ultrasound or a hysteroscope.

Adenomyosis is often associated with abnormal or excessive bleeding, and should be suspected when bluish or brown spots with a punctate appearance are seen on hysteroscopic examination of the endometrial cavity (7). Arteriovenous malformations are a rare cause of AUB, and when present can be diagnosed with Doppler ultrasound. Estrogen-producing ovarian tumors cause abnormal bleeding by increasing endogenous estrogen levels. Other estrogen-producing tumors include thecoma, Sertoli-Leydig cell tumors, and yolk sac tumors. Granulosa-cell tumors commonly present in the prepubertal years with AUB. Ultrasound evaluation is helpful in the diagnosis.

Dysfunctional Bleeding

Dysfunctional uterine bleeding (DUB), or abnormal endometrial bleeding without structural pathology, is a diagnosis of exclusion (2,10,11). DUB is associated with both anovulatory and ovulatory states. Anovulatory DUB, most commonly due to an immature pituitary ovarian axis, is often seen in young women and can continue for several years following the onset of menstruation (2,5). Likewise, the woman who is in her later reproductive years often becomes anovulatory as she approaches menopause and, as such, is at risk for DUB. Ovulatory DUB is less common than anovulatory DUB, and some experts do not consider this to be a pathologic state.

In cases of anovulation, estrogen is present, but because there is no LH surge to induce ovum release, no progesterone is produced. Unopposed estrogen levels cause a thick buildup of the endometrial lining, which often outgrows its nutritional support, leading to necrosis and slough. If the lining is shed in a dyssynchronous manner, menometrorrhagia is the presenting symptom. Anovulatory states can present with oligomenorrhea as well as menometrorrhagia, as seen with olycystic ovarian syndrome.

Ovulatory DUB should be considered in a patient with menorrhagia but regular cycles. Because appropriate levels of progesterone are present, the cycle is not disrupted (11). This diagnosis should be entertained only after the endometrial cavity has been shown to be free of pathology and all other systemic disease states, such as von Willebrand's disease, have been ruled out (12).

Malignancy

Cervical cancer is the third most common cancer of the female reproductive tract. In 2000, it was estimated that there would be 12,800 new cases and 4600 deaths from cervical cancer (13). All women with abnormal bleeding require a thorough speculum exam, including inspection of the vulva, vagina, and cervix, and a Pap smear. Any suspicious lesions should be biopsied and colposcopy should be performed as indicated. Colposcopy is mandatory in cases of abnormal cytology.

Sarcoma botryoides of the vagina generally presents in infancy, while the same tumor in the cervix presents in adolescence (5). Both tumors are rare and are a variant of embryonal rhabdomyosarcoma, which derives its name from its grape-like appearance. Daya and Scully reported an average age of 18 years in women with cervical sarcoma botryoides, with the most common presenting complaint being vaginal bleeding.

Prior to the 1970s, diethylstilbestrol (DES) was commonly prescribed for pregnant women with threatened abortions, and about 3–5 million women were exposed to this agent. In utero exposure to diethylstilbestrol predisposed female fetuses to the development of clear cell adenocarcinoma of the vagina with an incidence rate of 0.14 to 1.4 per 1000 women aged 7–29 years (14). Because DES use was discontinued in the early 1970s, the incidence of clear cell carcinoma of the vagina is decreasing.

Women with a history of anovulatory bleeding and endometrial hyperplasia are at increased risk for endometrial carcinoma (12). Indeed, some experts consider endometrial hyperplasia to be a precancerous state, and while cancer is not the most common cause of AUB, it is certainly the most important. The incidence of endometrial hyperplasia in premenopausal women is 2–10% and without treatment, up to 3–23% will progress to endometrial carcinoma (15). In the year 2000, 36,000 new cases of endometrial cancer were predicted with 6500 deaths resulting from this disease (16).

Ninety-eight percent of cases of endometrial adenocarcinomas are diagnosed in postmenopausal women (9). The most common presenting symptom of endometrial cancer is vaginal bleeding, but only 12.5% of women with postmenopausal bleeding will be found to have endometrial cancer (13). While endometrial carcinoma is rare in adolescence, the incidence is sufficiently high in women over the age of 35 to warrant evaluation.

Significant risk factors for endometrial cancer have been found in as many as 20% of women over 35 (17). Women of any age, with an intact uterus, who are under the influence of unopposed estrogen, whether endogenous or exogenous, should receive progesterone to decrease their risk of endometrial hyperplasia. As the length of time a woman is exposed to unopposed estrogen increases, so does the risk of endometrial cancer. Gelfand and Ferenczy reported only a 1% incidence of hyperplasia in women receiving both estrogen and progesterone in combination, indicating that progesterone is protective to the endometrium (6). Additional risk factors include hypertension, obesity (body weight over 90 kg), diabetes, estrogen-secreting tumors, nulliparity, family history of colon or endometrial carcinoma, and tamoxifen use (15). Hereditary nonpolyposis colorectal cancer or Lynch type II syndrome is the only clearly defined hereditary cancer syndrome associated with endometrial cancer (13).

The presence of endometrial polyps may be a risk factor for endometrial carcinoma. Although malignant transformation rates are low, a case control study from Sweden showed a two-fold increase in the risk of subsequent endometrial cancer when polyps are present (8).

Iatrogenic

Foreign Bodies

Foul-smelling, purulent, or blood-tinged vaginal discharge may indicate the presence of a foreign body in the vagina. The most common objects found in the vagina are tampons and toilet paper. Particularly in adolescents or postmenopausal women with narrow or stenotic vaginas, an exam under anesthesia may be necessary to remove the object and wash the vagina. If the object has penetrated the bladder or rectum, appropriate consultation is necessary. Patients should be questioned regarding sexual abuse when unusual objects are found in the vagina or if there is evidence of trauma to the vagina and perineum.

Medications

Women in their peri- and postmenopausal years frequently use hormone replacement therapy (HRT) to provide relief of vasomotor disturbances or estrogen deficient states. Because of the problems with unopposed estrogen exposure, progesterone is added to most HRT regimens and to oral contraceptives. However, when progesterone is withdrawn, the endometrium is shed and bleeding occurs. Women should be questioned about hormone use, as well as the use of oral contraceptives, which can also lead to AUB.

Other pharmacological causes of AUB include medications used in the treatment of hirsutism, dysmenorrhea, premenstrual syndrome, acne, and endometriosis. Anticoagulants, tranquilizers, antidepressants, corticosteroids, and psychotropic medications may cause AUB as a result of hormonal disruption. All patients should be questioned about medication use as part of their admission history.

Tamoxifen

Tamoxifen deserves special mention as a cause of AUB. This nonsteroidal estrogen is frequently used as adjuvant therapy for breast cancer, and as preventive therapy for women at risk for breast cancer (6). Since this is a selective estrogen receptor modulator (SERM), it acts as a mixed agonist/antagonistic and can cause endometrial hyperplasia by stimulating the endometrium (14). The endometrium generally has a bizarre, microcystic appearance that can be misleading and difficult to interpret (6,12). In up to two-thirds of the women taking tamoxifen, the endometrial stripe will have an altered appearance on tranvaginal ultrasound exam in the absence of significant disease. However, women on tamoxifen therapy are at increased risk for the development of endometrial cancer, and the risk may be up to two- to three-times greater than that of the general population (13). A high index of suspicion should be maintained in women using tamoxifen, and some have suggested routine screening in these patients (i.e., ultrasound, endometrial biopsy) (13).

Herbal Medicines

More than 500 plants contain phytoestrogen. An increasing number of women are forsaking traditional hormone medication and are making use of these preparations to help cope with menopausal symptoms. Because they often fail to equate herbs to prescription medications, up to 70% of women may fail to disclose the use of herbs to their physicians without specific questioning (14,18). The most commonly used estrogen-like herbs are dong quai, red clover, alfalfa, licorice *(Glycyrrhiza glabra)*, black cohosh *(Cimicifuga racemosa)*, squaw vine *(Mitchella repens)*, and soybeans. If used in sufficient quantities, these substances can lead to troublesome unopposed estrogen effects (18). Chaparral *(Larrea tridentata)* has been used as a contraceptive preparation because of its estrogenic properties, and can produce an unusual bleeding pattern (18).

Other herbal preparations are used to alter progesterone levels, treat fibroids, or as a diuretic. Herbs commonly used to "balance" progesterone levels include chaste tree, wild yam *(Dioscorea villosa)*, and lady's mantle *(Alchemilla vulgaris)*, and if these are abruptly discontinued, withdrawal bleeding may occur. Herbal remedies used to treat fibroids include ginseng or herbal combinations of rhubarb, cinnamon, and sargassum seaweed. While ginseng itself does not have estrogenic effects, it can interfere with the metabolism of estrogen, and patients should be cautioned about the use of any ginseng preparation, including face creams, while taking oral estrogen preparations (18). Saw palmetto is used because of its diuretic effects and to

"promote good urinary health." However, it may have additive effects with estrogen replacement therapy and oral contraceptives, so caution is advised in patients using these
agents (18).

Diet and Stress

Excessive dieting, stress, and strenuous exercise affect the
hypothalamic-pituitary-ovarian axis. Endurance-trained ath-
letes and dancers with a low percentage of body fat often
experience amenorrhea or oligomenorrhea related to their
exercise habits. Young women with eating disorders and
excessive weight loss present with amenorrhea because of
depleted nutritional stores. Women should be questioned
about exercise patterns and eating habits, and their body
weight and habitus should be noted (5).

DIAGNOSIS

Imaging and/or visualization of the uterine cavity along with
histologic sampling of the endometrium are the cornerstones
in the diagnosis of AUB. The current gold standard for diagnosis is either transvaginal sonography with saline infusion
sonography, or hysteroscopy with directed histologic sampling.

Imaging Techniques

A variety of techniques, including transvaginal sonography
(TVS), saline infusion sonography (SIS), hysterosalpingogram
(HSG), and magnetic resonance imaging (MRI) are used to
image the uterus.

Transvaginal Sonography

TVS can be used to image the endometrial stripe and
myometrium and evaluate the uterus for overall size and
deformity. According to Emanuel et al., an ultrasound finding
of a normal uterus was predictive of the absence of abnormalities, even when the observer had only moderate experi-

ence in interpreting ultrasound images (19). Endometrial stripe measurements of 4–5 mm have been reported to be highly associated with lack of significant disease. However, to make this a reliable assessment, the endometrial echo must be homogeneous, surrounded by an intact hypoechoic junctional zone, and the operator must constantly remember that the endometrial cavity is a three-dimensional structure.

A normal endometrial stripe can range from 1–15 mm, with thicker stripes seen in premenopausal women just before menses. Therefore, if TVS is to be used, it is best scheduled in the proliferative phase. Cutoff levels for abnormal endometrial stripe thickness have been proposed by various investigators, and range from 4–12 mm (20). However, controversy exists as to the appropriate cutoff for premenopausal women or women who are receiving hormone replacement therapy. In fact, if the unenhanced TVS clearly shows a distinct homogenous endometrium that is 5 mm or less in the early proliferative phase of the woman's cycle, some authors feel that further investigation, including undirected endometrial sampling, is unnecessary. In postmenopausal women, significant pathologic features may still be present with an endometrium measuring as little as 5 mm in thickness (21).

In Holbert's study group of 327 asymptomatic postmenopausal women (21), those receiving unopposed estrogen had an endometrial stripe ranging from 4–13 mm, those receiving estrogen and progesterone had a stripe ranging from 2–15 mm, and those women on no hormonal therapy had a stripe ranging from 2–29 mm. The mean was 6.0 mm. There did appear to be a small, statistically significant correlation between increasing estrogen dose and endometrial stripe thickness. One patient had adenocarcinoma with a stripe thickness of 5 mm, leading to Holbert's recommendation that 4 mm be used as the cutoff for normal endometrial stripe thickness in postmenopausal women (21). Dorum et al. also recommended 4 mm as a cutoff, stating that when used alone, TVS missed 6% of carcinomas when a cutoff for a normal value of 5 mm was used (22). Bradley reported a sensitivity of 94% and a specificity of 78% when > 5 mm was used as the cutoff, with a 6.1% probability of missing a pathologic diagnosis (33). Another study involving 1100 women found no cases of endometrial cancer with a stripe of 4 mm or less (13). O'Connell et al. reported a sensitivity of 79% and a specificity of 57% with an endometrial stripe thickness of 5 mm or greater (6). With a cutoff of 4 mm in postmenopausal women, the sensitivity improved to 96%, but the specificity for detecting any endometrial pathology remained low (68%) (6,12). When the cutoff is increased to 5 mm, the sensitivity drops to 79–94% with a specificity of 57–78%. Therefore, further procedures such as endometrial sampling or hysteroscopy are required for definitive diagnosis (6).

Saidi (23) showed results contrary to the studies listed above. He reported a sensitivity that was higher for TVS and SIS than hysteroscopy in the diagnosis of AUB (95.7%, 90.9%, 78.3%, respectively) and a specificity that was higher for SIS than TVS or hysteroscopy (83.8%, 63.6%, 65.2%, respectively) (23). Other investigators' results do not support these findings.

The value of TVS is further limited when fibroids or polyps distort the uterine cavity, leading to a high frequency of equivocal scans (24). Kamel et al. (25) reported a false positive rate of 25% and a false negative rate of 36.5% when TVS alone was used to visualize intracavitary abnormalities other than hyperplasia. For the detection of endometrial polyps, the sensitivity, when compared to hysteroscopy, was only 64.5% with a specificity of 75.5% (25). de Vries et al. (20) reported a sensitivity of only 60% in the diagnosis of intracavitary lesions, with a specificity of 93%. The sensitivity increased to 85% when the criteria were modified to include an endometrial stripe of > 5 mm in the diagnosis of abnormalities, but the specificity fell to only 21% (20). For this reason these investigators did not feel that TVS was a reasonable triage tool for women with AUB.

Bradley et al. (33) were unable to visualize lesions less than 2 cm with TVS, and reported that 22% of patients with fibroids had normal TVS report (22% false negative rate). Additionally, it was difficult to differentiate various intracavitary abnormalities; when the cavity was distorted, measurements of the stripe proved difficult. In this study, the sensitivity for the diagnosis of fibroids ranges from 88–96%.

Sonohysterography (SIS)

The sensitivity and specificity of TVS can be significantly increased with the addition of saline infusion. Arsons and Lense first described this simple technique in 1993 (26). As with TVS, it is best to schedule the procedure in the early or midproliferative phase. A narrow, flexible pediatric feeding tube is fed into the uterine cavity, and saline infusion is observed with TVS. Schwarzler et al. found that sensitivy rose from 67% to 87% and specificity improved from 89% to 91% when SIS was added to TVS (27).

Laughead and Stones (26) reported that saline infusion sonohysterography (SIS) afforded enhanced visualization of the endometrium in patients with leiomyomas. Evaluation of the size of myomas and degree of penetration into the endometrial cavity was possible with this technique, which they felt could be helpful in identifying patients who might benefit from hysteroscopic resection. SIS is highly sensitive for polyps and myomas, while providing a three-dimensional view of the uterine cavity. Therefore, some feel it is more objective in assessing polyp and myoma size than hysteroscopy, and that SIS is the most appropriate initial diagnostic procedure in the evaluation of AUB (26,28).

While SIS can suggest an abnormality such as simple hyperplasia, histologic diagnosis is necessary to confirm the diagnosis (26). Widrich et al. reported SIS was comparable with office hysteroscopy in the diagnosis of endometrial polyps, myomas, synechiae, hyperplasia, endometrial cancer, or normal uterine cavities (29). de Vries et al. reported a sensitivity of 88%, specificity of 95% when SIS was used to diagnose intracavitary abnormalities in premenopausal women and believed SIS could be a useful triage tool, minimizing the need for hysteroscopy (20).

Widrich et al. compared hysteroscopy with SIS in 113 patients. They found excellent sensitivity and specificity with SIS (96% and 88%, respectively), and found no statistically significant difference in the detection of endometrial polyps, myomas, synechiae, hyperplasia, and endometrial cancer, or normal uterine cavities (29). Positive correlation with fractional curettage-hysteroscopy had been reported to be as high as 92% (6).

Cooper and Brady reported a good sensitivity but low specificity (80%) for SIS because of difficulty interpreting the images, stating that SIS was inferior to hysteroscopy in distinguishing submucous myomata from endometrial polyps (7).

Bernard et al. reported that SIS diagnosed only 40% of endometrial cancers in a study of 162 women with AUB. However, the accuracy in diagnosing intracavitary lesions was high (sensitivity of 98.9%; specificity of 76.4%) and SIS was able to identify lesions as small as 3 mm (30). Dijkhuizen et al. (31) reported a sensitivity of 100% and specificity of 85% in the diagnosis of intracavitary lesions, and Williams and Marshburn (32) found a sensitivity of 96% and a specificity of 100% for detection of intrauterine polyps and fibroids. In a study conducted by the latter team, there were no cases of missed pathologic condition (32).

Kamel et al. (25) found a sensitivity of 93.1% and specificity of 93.9% in the detection of polyps when compared to hysteroscopy. Combining SIS with TVS, the false positive rate improved from 25% to 2.9% and the false negative rate improved from 36.5% to 2.8% over TVS alone (25).

Bradley et al. (33) stated that SIS is superior to TVS, EMB, D&C, or hysteroscopy alone, and reported that excellent images and adequate distention were obtained with minimal fluid volumes (5–30 ml) at a rate of about 5–10 mL/min. However, if performed during the secretory phase, there was an increased risk of disrupting or shearing the endometrium, with the creation of wrinkles or polypoid appearing projections in the endometrial lining. Bradley et al. also noted that SIS was more precise than other techniques in predicting the size of fibroids. Despite the success of SIS in identifying lesions, the diagnosis could not be made by this modality alone due to the lack of tissue for pathologic evaluation. Therefore, the utility of SIS was limited (12,26).

Hysterosalpingogram (HSG)

HSG is of limited value in the evaluation of AUB. SIS provides essentially the same or more information than HSG with less risk, less discomfort, and less cost. With HSG, there is a high false positive rate (11–15%) and a high false negative rate (13–35%) compared with hysteroscopy, and the specificity has been reported to be as low as 15% (33). As with SIS and TVS, HSG does not provide a tissue diagnosis. Localization of lesions to the anterior or posterior uterine wall, identification of a stalk, and differentiation from uterine synechiae are difficult with this modality (25). Additionally, this procedure may cause a significant amount of pain and has the added risk of radiation exposure, making it less acceptable to patients (33).

Magnetic Resonance Imaging (MRI)

With MRI, the ability to help define uterine pathology is relatively good, but the expense and lack of tissue for diagnosis limit its use. It may be useful in distinguishing between adenomyosis and fibroids, and can detect and localize lesions as small as 0.3 cm. In cases where the need exists to distinguish between adenomyosis and fibroids, or when accurate localization of a lesion is required, MRI may be superior to TVS, SIS, or HSG (33).

Complications

Relatively few complications are associated with imaging of the uterine cavity. The most common problems are minor discomfort from the endovaginal probe, vasovagal reactions during infusion of fluid into the endometrial cavity with SIS or HSG, and anxiety, especially in claustrophobic patients undergoing MRI. These complications are rarely life threatening and are easily managed. Infection is a rare complication of both SIS and HSG (26).

Endometrial Sampling

As previously stated, definitive diagnosis of endometrial hyperplasia or neoplasia requires a tissue sample. Tissue sampling is indicated for confirmation or evaluation of chronic uterine infection, acute endometritis, tuberculosis, dating of the endometrium for infertility evaluation, and for the evaluation of abnormal uterine bleeding (34). However, because of technical limitations, blind sampling most often misses endometrial polyps or submucous fibroids. Methods of sampling must be tailored to the needs of the patient.

Contraindications are few, with the only absolute contraindication being pregnancy. Relative contraindications are profuse bleeding, cervicitis, endometritis, cervical cancer, and coagulopathy (34).

Endometrial Cytologic Sampling

Both cytologic and tissue sampling of the endometrium are possible. Cytologic sampling is generally well tolerated, but rarely yields sufficient tissue samples for evaluation. The technique uses a brush, introduced into the uterine cavity, to collect the cytologic sample. Inadequate samples are collected in as many as 16% of cases and for this reason, it is rarely used (34).

Endometrial Biopsy (EMB)

EMB uses abrasion or curettage with or without suction for sample collection. A small tube is passed into the uterine cavity and suction is applied while the tissue is aspirated. EMB has largely replaced operative D&C, mainly because of its ease of performance, relatively low complication rate, and the ability to perform the procedure in a less costly office setting with little or no anesthesia required. However, because it is undirected and provides only a small sample, EMB is only appropriate if one first demonstrates that the endometrial process is global and not focal.

Several different sampling techniques exist, including Pipelle® catheter, Vabra®, Tiss-u-trap®, Novak®, and Z-sampler (34). All of these sampling techniques are limited by their inability to sample the entire endometrium. The Pipelle catheter has been shown to sample as little as 4.5–15% of endometrial lining as compared to Vabra aspiration that samples 41%. With either of these techniques, 28–70% of biopsy samples may contain inadequate tissue to allow accurate histologic interpretation (33). Vabra aspirator was found to be

93% sensitive for cancer detection, and 95% sensitive for hyperplasia detection. Pipelle was 90% sensitive for cancer and 83–90% sensitive for hyperplasia detection (34). O'Connell et al. reported a sensitivity of 94% and a specificity of 96% with EMB alone, and a positive correlation with fractional curettage-hysteroscopy of 95% (6). However, there is a 4–10% likelihood of encountering cervical stenosis, making the procedure impossible to perform (33).

In Goldstein et al.'s study, 3 of 5 patients with endometrial polyps were missed, and Pipelle sampling missed the diagnosis in 7 of 18 patients (39%) with hyperplasia (35). Guido et al. studied Pipelle biopsy in patients with known carcinoma undergoing hysterectomy. Of 65 patients, Pipelle biopsy provided adequate tissue for diagnosis in 63 (97%), but malignancy was detected in only 54 (83%). Of the 11 false negatives, 5 (8%) had disease confined to endometrial polyps, and 3 (5%) had tumor localized to <5% of the surface area. Guido et al. concluded that undirected sampling, whether through curettage or other suction aspiration devices, is "fraught with error, especially in cases in which the abnormality is not global but focal" (35).

Others have shown that the Pipelle is not reliable in the preoperative evaluation of the patient with AUB. While it is a reasonably sensitive tool for diffuse multifocal endometrial cancer and endometrial hyperplasia, it has low sensitivity for detecting polyps and myomas (only 10%, compared with 33% for diagnosis of hyperplasia) (28).

Tahir et al. reported better results. Combining TVS with Pipelle sampling, the diagnosis of hyperplasia or malignancy was correctly made in 200 patients subsequently evaluated with hysteroscopy. However, some polyps and fibroids that were subsequently found on hysteroscopy were missed with TVS and Pipelle sampling. They concluded that TVS and Pipelle sampling should be a first line investigation in postmenopausal bleeding or in cases of irregular vaginal bleeding, knowing that this approach will occasionally miss polyps and fibroids. Hysteroscopy, they believed, should be a second line therapy in all cases (22).

Combining EMB and SIS has also been used to evaluate AUB. O'Connell et al. reported a sensitivity of 94% and a specificity of 96% when EMB was combined with SIS with a positive correlation with fractional curettage-hysteroscopy of 95% (6). Still, this technique does not allow for a directed biopsy and should be limited to patients with multifocal lesions.

Dilation and Curettage (D&C)

Recampier first introduced dilation and curettage in 1843, when he attempted to "scrape off uterine fungosities." For many years it was considered to be the gold standard diagnostic tool for evaluation of postmenopausal bleeding. However, by the early 1980s EMB had become readily available, and there were increasing published reports of deficiencies with D&C (6,34). Grimes found D&C to carry a higher risk of perforation, infection, and bleeding, and was significantly more expensive than EMB. In 1982, he suggested that D&C should no longer be the primary procedure for sampling the endometrium because less that one-half the uterine cavity was actually sampled in a majority of patients, and less than one-fourth of the endometrium was sampled in as many as 16% of the cases. The false negative rate with D&C ranges between 10% and 60% (36,37).

Other investigators have confirmed these findings. Towbin et al. reported that 60% of hysterectomy specimens, obtained immediately after curettage, showed that less than half of the endometrium was sampled and that the source of the bleeding was frequently missed (24). Stovall et al. found that 15% of endometrial carcinomas were missed by D&C.

Gebauer et al. found D&C to be no better in the diagnosis of polyps. When comparing curettage to hysteroscopy, they found that curettage alone was insufficient to detect endometrial polyps, especially when the endometrial stripe was thick, presumably because a thick stripe made locating the polyp more difficult (37). If the stripe was less than 10 mm, curettage was adequate; however, if the stripe was greater that 10 mm, hysteroscopic guidance was advocated for extraction of the tissue because D&C was found to be unsuccessful in a high percentage of cases (37). Bradley et al. stated that D&C should not be the criterion for evaluating any endometrial pathology (33). Emanuel et al. agreed, finding that D&C was a very limited tool in the diagnosis of endometrial polyps and submucous myomas, noting that the chance of finding such lesions was equal to the chance of missing them (38). Additional studies have found that the diagnosis was missed in 10% of cases, with 80% of these involving cases with polyps (35). Only Bettocchi et al. disagreed with these data, stating that the sensitivity of D&C was 46% with a specificity of 100%, a positive predictive value of 100% and a negative predictive value of 7.1% (39).

Complications Associated with Endometrial Sampling

Though uncommon, endometrial sampling techniques can be associated with more serious complications, including uterine perforation, bleeding, pain, and infection. Up to 5 per 1000 women will require a major surgical procedure as a result of complications related to performance of a D&C (22).

Perforation is a rare complication with an incidence of 1–2 per 1000. Word reported an incidence of perforation as high as 1 in 325 women. Injury to the uterus and surrounding pelvic viscera varied according to the instruments used, and was noted to be more serious with rigid or sharp devices (34). While most cases can be appropriately managed with observation as opposed to operative intervention, uterine perforation can lead to injury of the omentum and intra-abdominal organs. Patients in whom perforation is suspected should be watched for signs of infection or bleeding. Each case must be managed on an individual basis, with some women requiring abdominal exploration (laparoscopy or laparotomy) to determine the extent of damage.

Intraoperative or postoperative bleeding is sometimes associated with uterine perforation. Consequently, perforation should be considered any time excessive bleeding occurs or in cases of an unexplained drop in the patient's blood count (34). In such cases, the cervix should also be evaluated and cervical trauma should be considered. In cases of cervical stenosis, forceful mechanical dilation is often required, increasing the risk of cervical laceration or uterine perforation.

Vasovagal episodes may be a problem in the awake patient and are most commonly observed with excessive manipulation of the cervix. These reactions are generally self-limited and are treated symptomatically, but because of the risks of bradycardia, seizure activity, and cardiac arrest, resuscitation equipment should be available (33).

The potential for infection exists any time the uterine cavity is entered with a foreign body. Routine prophylaxis is not recommended except in women with a history of PID where there is the possibility of flushing bacteria, retrograde, into the tubes or abdominal cavity.

Hysteroscopy

Although hysteroscopy was first described more than 100 years ago, it was not until the 1980s and 1990s that its use in the office became practical because of improved, narrower profile, and flexible instrumentation (7). Advantages of hysteroscopy include immediate evaluation with the direct visualization of the endometrium and endocervix along with the ability to detect and biopsy small foci of pathology. Additionally, hysteroscopy has a low false negative rate of about 2–4%. The main contraindications to hysteroscopy are cervical cancer and active pelvic infection. Diagnostic hysteroscopy can be done in the office or as an outpatient surgical procedure. However, many physicians are not equipped to perform office hysteroscopy, and as few as 28% of gynecologists routinely perform this procedure (29), with the main reason being the cost in purchasing and maintaining the equipment (33). Despite the difficulties of cost and slight increases in patient's complaints of pain, Kremer et al. showed that women were just as accepting of office-based hysteroscopy as they were of day surgery for hysteroscopy (40). The outpatient surgical setting is preferred for women with cervical stenosis or with excessive anxiety about the procedure.

Anesthesia in the office-based setting can be achieved with paracervical block with 1-2% lidocaine (7). The choice of distention media depends on the goals of the procedure. For diagnostic hysteroscopy, CO_2 offers excellent visualization. CO_2 is colorless, nonvolatile, has few side effects, is readily available, inexpensive, and is highly soluble if absorbed intravascularly. Because it has a tendency to form bubbles, its use is limited in cases where blood fills the uterine cavity (7). For diagnostic cases complicated by heavy bleeding or in operative procedures, high viscosity or low viscosity fluids are preferred. A disadvantage of fluids for uterine distension is increased light refraction and fluid turbulence, which can complicate the interpretation of findings. Use of low viscosity fluids requires continuous flow sheathes and sophisticated monitoring systems to prevent and/or detect fluid overload. Because of space and cost considerations, these systems are not well suited to an office setting.

Hysteroscopes are available in rigid or flexible designs, and in diameters as narrow as 3.1 mm. The flexible scope is best suited to the office setting, where maximizing patient comfort and minimizing bleeding and trauma to the endocervical canal are top priorities. Biopsy forceps and lassos are available to accommodate the narrow operative channel, but are of limited therapeutic value (7).

The most common pathologies found at diagnostic hysteroscopy are myomata, polyps, hyperplasia, cancer, and adenomyosis (7). Towbin et al. studied 149 patients with office hysteroscopy for complaints of menorrhagia, metrorrhagia, or postmenopausal bleeding. In comparing hysteroscopy and TVS, they found that hysteroscopy was 79% sensitive and 93% specific in diagnosing intracavitary pathology. Therefore, hysteroscopy was deemed to be the desired modality for evaluation of AUB, since it allowed differentiation of polyps from myomas and polyps from polypoid endometrium (24).

Ben-Yehuda et al. compared the usefulness of hysteroscopy to D&C in the diagnosis of endometrial hyperplasia and endometrial cancer and found that hysteroscopy did not improve the sensitivity of D&C with this diagnosis. However, he did not address the potential for hysteroscopically directed biopsies, and therefore may have ignored a potential advantage of hysteroscopy. He did note that hysteroscopy was superior to D&C in the diagnosis of fibroids (41). Goldstein et al. felt that hysteroscopy with curettage should be reserved for those patients with a demonstrated focal abnormality on SIS who are in need of visually directed removal, or in those patients where TVS is either inadequate or uninterruptible (35).

Hysteroscopy/EMB

Hysteroscopy with directed biopsy remains the decisive diagnostic test for detecting polyps (25). As well as providing a real time look into the uterine cavity, Kamel et al. found that hysteroscopically directed biopsy had a sensitivity of 97–98% and a specificity of 93% (25). Gimpelson and Rappold, in 1988, studied 342 women symptomatic for AUB. First a D&C was done, followed by a hysteroscopy with directed biopsy. In those evaluated by D&C, the diagnosis was missed in 60 women. Hysteroscopy made the correct diagnosis in all cases. These studies provide evidence of the unquestioned superiority of hysteroscopy with appropriately directed biopsy in the evaluation of AUB, especially in cases where disease is focal in nature.

Complications Associated with Hysteroscopy

Inclusive of undesirable events and death, the complication rate of hysteroscopy ranges from 0.13% to 0.28% (42). Jansen noted 38 complications among 13,600 patients undergoing hysteroscopic procedures with diagnostic procedures having a significantly lower rate (0.13%) than operative procedures (0.95%); the most frequent complications were associated with uterine perforation (0.76%) of which over half were entry-related (42). The risk of perforation was increased in cases of Asherman's syndrome and cervical stenosis (43,44). When the hysteroscope was inserted under direct visualization, perforation of the uterus with a hysteroscopy was rare as compared to the incidence seen with blind insertion of uterine sounds and cervical dilators. Fully half of all injuries during hysteroscopy were thought to be related to the surgeon's inexperience (42).

Mechanical trauma is more commonly associated with the use of larger-gauge scopes in the presence of cervical stenosis. Use of narrow diameter scopes significantly decreased the risk of trauma (43). As with endometrial sampling, cervical lacerations from the tenaculum could occur, but these were generally easily treated (45). Laminaria placement, prior to the procedure, might help prevent trauma (45).

Because hysteroscopy is performed in the lithotomy position, there is an increased risk for peroneal or sciatic nerve injury, particularly during longer procedures. Nerve injury occurs in approximately 1 in 3600 women, and generally presents as persistent neuropathy secondary to undue stretching. The risk can be minimized with careful attention to proper positioning of the patient and padding of the legs (43).

Intraoperative hemorrhage, even with operative hysteroscopy, is a rare event, probably as a result of increased intrauterine pressure secondary to the liquid distention medium tamponading exposed vessels. However, postoperative bleeding may occur when this increased pressure is released (43,45). Treatments include vigorous massage of the uterine fundus, tamponade with uterine packing or intrauterine balloon, or dilute vasopressin injections into the cervical stroma. If unsuccessful, bilateral uterine artery embolization or emergency hysterectomy may be required. Vascular compartment expansion with fluids and blood products should be used as needed (43).

Pain, referred to the shoulder, is common with CO_2 distention of the uterine cavity as this gas passes freely to the abdominal cavity through patent Fallopian tubes (36). Cervical dilation may cause discomfort, but this can commonly be prevented with the use of a paracervical block or general anesthesia. Administration of a nonsteriodal anti-inflammatory 1 hour prior to the procedure may be of help in alleviating some of the cramping associated with uterine distention.

In addition to providing excellent visualization, CO_2 has a long history of safety for distention of the uterine cavity.

CO_2 offers a very low risk of gas embolism. Despite the fact that several case reports in the literature implicate its use with embolism as a cause of both nonfatal and fatal cardiac arrest, CO_2 offers little risk for gas embolization owing to its great solubility in blood. Use of inappropriate insufflation equipment (such as laparoscopic insufflators) increases the risk for embolism because of the high pressure used during insufflation. Insufflation equipment for hysteroscopy should limit maximum flow rates to 100 mL/min with a maximal distending pressure limited to 100 mmHg (36). Pretreatment with gonadotropin-releasing hormone agonists to reduce endometrial vascularity, avoidance of steep Trendelengburg position, and careful deaereation of equipment are suggested as methods to decrease the risk of gaseous embolism (43). Spontaneous ventilation is also thought to increase the risk of gas embolism because of the generation of negative pressure in the chest cavity (45).

Infection is a rare occurrence when fluid distention systems are used but might result when vaginal and cervical bacteria contaminate the uterus and tubes (36). The inability of the cilia of the Fallopian tubes to clear bacteria introduced during the procedure is felt to be a major factor in cases where infection follows hysteroscopy. Women with previous injury to one or both tubes, such as a previous history of PID, are at highest risk. Therefore, active pelvic infection is a contraindication to hysteroscopy. Risk factors for development of tubal infection post hysteroscopy include: secondary infertility, prior pelvic infection, prior pelvic surgery for infection, prior adnexal tenderness, prior adnexal mass, primary infertility, and undocumented history of salpingitis. These patients may present with endometritis, parametritis, or with a pyometra some time following a hysteroscopic procedure (45).

McCausland reported on a series of 700 patients, 200 of whom did not receive prophylactic antibiotics, and 4 of whom had previous history of PID. Of these four patients, three developed severe pelvic infections with tuboovarian abscesses following hysteroscopy. 500 patients received doxycycline prophylaxis starting at the time of laminaria tent insertion and continuing for 5 days post-op. Despite a past history of PID in

10 of these patients, none developed a pelvic infection (46). Excessive intravascular absorption of low viscosity fluids employed for uterine distension occurs in about 0.2% of cases. Significant morbidity and mortality may be associated with fluid overload, depending on the medium used (43). Limiting intrauterine pressure to the minimum required for adequate visualization is of utmost importance. Use of oxytocin or vasopressin as well as pretreatment with gonadotropin-releasing hormone agonist may be of value in preventing intravasation (45).

High viscosity fluids are associated with higher complication rates than that seen with low viscosity fluids. High viscosity fluids are rarely used during diagnostic hysteroscopy and are increasingly being replaced by low viscosity fluids for operative cases. Dextran 70 is one of the more commonly used high viscosity fluids employed for either diagnostic or operative hysteroscopy. Intravasation of Dextran 70 can cause pulmonary edema, coagulopathies, and allergic reactions, including anaphylaxis. For every 100 ml infused, the plasma volume expands 860 ml; therefore, intravasation of 350 ml of Dextran 70 in a 60–kg patient will essentially double her plasma volume (45).

Use of nonphysiologic, low viscosity fluids carries the risk of fluid overload along with hyponatremia. Young women are at greater risk for this complication than are postmenopausal women, perhaps because endogenous progesterone inhibits the enzyme sodium-potassium adenosine triphosphatase (45). Close monitoring of the patient's fluid status will help prevent hyponatremia. Termination of a hysteroscopic procedure should be immediately considered when significant discrepancies between infused and returned fluid are observed. Commonly employed low viscosity fluids include glycine, sorbitol, and mannitol. Glycine is of special concern because it is metabolized to ammonia. Consequently, with intravasation of glycine there exists the potential for hyperamonemia encephalopathy, transient blindness, muscle aches, and memory loss (45). Mannitol 5% may be the best choice of the available low viscosity, nonphysiologic solutions, owing to its properties as an osmotic diuretic.

Normal saline is isotonic, and when used for uterine distention offers less concern than do either high viscosity or low viscosity fluids. It is inexpensive and safe. Although excessive intravasation can lead to pulmonary edema and fluid overload, hyponatremic encephalopathy is avoided (7). Water should never be used for uterine distention as it causes hemolysis.

Dissemination of Tumor Cells

There have been several case reports of tumor cell dissemination after hysteroscopy. Endometrial cancer cells, found in the abdominal cavity, were suspected to be related to distention and irrigation of uterine cavity during fluid hysteroscopy. Obermair (47) reported on 113 women with endometrial carcinoma who had D&C prior to TAH/BSO. Seventy-four had hysteroscopy before D&C while 39 did not. Peritoneal cytology was suspicious or positive in 10 of 113 cases (8.8%), and 9 of these patients had undergone hysteroscopy prior to surgical staging. Positive washings were associated with a history of hysteroscopy ($p = 0.04$) but not myometrial invasion, histologic subtype, grade, or time between D&C and staging laparotomy. The investigator did not comment on whether or not prognosis was affected by the presence of positive or suspicious cytology (47). The viability of cancer cells when washed into the peritoneal cavity and whether or not their presence has any bearing on long-term survival continues to be debated (45).

The risk of flushing endometrial cancer cells through the Fallopian tubes also exists for SIS, HSG, and diagnostic hysteroscopy with CO_2 insufflation, but the risk is speculative. The low pressures and small volumes used during these procedures likely minimize the risk (33). The risk of flushing cells when CO_2 is used for distention appears to be of low magnitude (45).

Failed or Missed Diagnosis

The ultimate complication in the evaluation of AUB is the failure or inability to make the correct diagnosis. Because of its potential for direct viewing, hysteroscopy is the gold standard in making the diagnosis of intracavitary pathology, (i.e., polyps, myomata, multifocal hyperplasia, and carcinoma). However, without accurate tissue sampling, the diagnosis is difficult and it may not be possible to correctly direct treatment. In the case of a missed carcinoma, the consequences could be devastating.

REFERENCES

1. Cooper JM. Preface. Obstet Gynecol Clin North Am 2000; 27(2):xi–xiii.

2. Bravender T, Emans SJ. Menstrual disorders: dysfunctional uterine bleeding. *Pediatr Clin North Am* 1999; 46(3):545–553, viii.

3. Long CA. Evaluation of patients with abnormal uterine bleeding. *Am J Obstet Gynecol* 1996 Sep; 175(3 Pt 2):784–786.

4. Ewenstein BM. The pathophysiology of bleeding disorders presenting as abnormal uterine bleeding. *Am J Obstet Gynecol* 1996 Sep; 175(3 Pt 2):770–777.

5. Minjarez DA, Bradshaw KD. Abnormal uterine bleeding in adolescents. *Obstet Gynecol Clin North Am* 2000 Mar; 27(1):63–78.

6. O'Connell LP, Fries MH, Zerinjue E, Brehm W. Triage of abnormal postmenopausal bleeding: a comparison of endometrial biopsy and transvaginal sonohysterography versus fractional curettage with hysteroscopy. *Am J Obstet Gynecol* 1998 May; 178(5):956–961.

7. Cooper JM, Brady RM. Hysteroscopy in the management of abnormal uterine bleeding. *Obstet Gynecol Clin North Am* 1999 Mar; 26(1):217–236.

8. Anastasiadis PG, Koutlaki NG, Skaphida PG, Galazios GC, Tsikouras PN, Liberis VA. Endometrial polyps: prevalence, detection, and malignant potential in women with abnormal uterine bleeding. *Eur J Gynaecol Oncol* 2000; 21(2):180–183.

9. Torrejon R, Fernandez-Alba JJ, Camicer I, Martin A, Castro C, Garcia-Cabanillas J, Rodriguez-Cornejo J, Moreno LJ, Comino

R. The value of hysteroscopic exploration for abnormal uterine bleeding. *J Am Assoc Gynecol Laparosc* 1997; 4(4):453–456.

10. Chuong CJ, Brenner PF. Management of abnormal uterine bleeding. *Am J Obstet Gynecol* 1996 Sep; 175(3 Pt 2):787–792.

11. Munro MG. Medical management of abnormal uterine bleeding. *Obstet Gynecol Clin North Am* 2000; 27(2):287–304.

12. Brenner PF. Differential diagnosis of abnormal uterine bleeding. *Am J Obstet Gynecol* 1996 Sep; 175(3 Pt 2):766–769.

13. Paley PJ. Screening for the major malignancies affecting women: current guidelines. *Am J Obstet Gynecol* 2001 Apr; 184(5):1021–1030.

14. Sheehan DM. Herbal medicine, phytoestrogens and toxicity: risk:benefit considerations. *Proc Sc Exp Biol Med* 1998; 217(3):379–385.

15. Farquhar CM, Lethaby A, Sowter M, Verry J, Baranyai J. An evaluation of risk factors for endometrial hyperplasia in premenopausal women with abnormal menstrual bleeding. *Am J Obstet Gynecol* 1999; 181(3):525–529.

16. Byers LJ, Fowler JM, Twiggs LB. Uterus. In: Abeloff MD, Armitage JO, Lichter AS, Niederhuber JE, eds. *Clinical Oncology*, 2nd ed, New York: Churchill Livingstone, 2000, p.1987.

17. Shwayder JM. Pathophysiology of abnormal uterine bleeding. *Obstet Gynecol Clin North Am* 2000; 27(2):219–234.

18. Miller LG. Herbal medicinals: selected clinical considerations focusing on known or potential drug-herb interactions. *Arch Intern Med* 1998; 158(10):2200–2211.

19. Emanuel MH, Ankum WM, Verdel MJ, Hart AA. The reproducibility of the results of transvaginal sonography of the uterus in patients with abnormal uterine bleeding. *Ultrasound Obstet Gynecol* 1996; 8(5):346–349.

20. de Vries LD, Dijkhuizen FP, Mol BW, Brolmann HA, Moret E, Heintz AP. Comparison of transvaginal sonography, saline infusion sonography, and hysteroscopy in premenopausal women with abnormal uterine bleeding. *J Clin Ultrasound* 2000; 28(5):217–223.

21. Holbert TR. Transvaginal ultrasonographic measurement of endometrial thickness in postmenopausal women receiving estrogen replacement therapy. *Am J Obstet Gynecol* 1997; 176(6):1334–1339.

22. Tahir MM, Bigrigg MA, Browning JJ, Brookes ST, Smith PA. A randomised controlled trial comparing transvaginal ultrasound, outpatient hysteroscopy and endometrial biopsy with inpatient hysteroscopy and curettage [see comments.] *Br J Obstet Gynaecol* 1999 Dec; 106(12):1259–1264.

23. Saidi MH, Sadler RK, Theis VD, Akright BD, Farhart SA, Villanueva GR. Comparison of sonography, sonohysterography, and hysteroscopy for evaluation of abnormal uterine bleeding. *J Ultrasound Med* 1997 Sep; 16(9):587–591.

24. Towbin NA, Gviazda IM, March CM. Office hysteroscopy versus transvaginal ultrasonography in the evaluation of patients with excessive uterine bleeding [see comments.] *Am J Obstet Gynecol* 1996 June; 174(6):1678–1682.

25. Kamel HS, Darwish AM, Mohamed SA. Comparison of transvaginal ultrasonography and vaginal sonohysterography in the detection of endometrial polyps. *Acta Obstet Gynecol Scand* 2000; 79(1):60–64.

26. Laughead MK, Stones LM. Clinical utility of saline solution infusion sonohysterography in a primary care obstetric-gynecologic practice. *Am J Obstet Gynecol* 1997; 176(6):1313–1318.

27. Schwarzler P, Concin H, Bosch H, Berlinger A, Wohlgenannt K, Collins WP, Bourne TH. An evaluation of sonohysterography and diagnostic hysteroscopy for the assessment of intrauterine pathology. *Ultrasound Obstet Gynecol* 1998; 11(5):337–342.

28. Pasqualotto EB, Margossian H, Price LL, Bradley LD. Accuracy of preoperative diagnostic tools and outcome of hysteroscopic management of menstrual dysfunction. *J Am Assoc Gynecol Laparosc* 2000 May; 7(2):201–209.

29. Widrich T, Bradley LD, Mitchinson AR, Collins RL. Comparison of saline infusion sonography with office hysteroscopy for the evaluation of the endometrium. *Am J Obstet Gynecol* 1996; 174(4):1327–1334.

30. Bernard JP, Lecuru F, Daries C, Robin F, de Bievre P, Taurelle R. Saline contrast sonohysterography as first-line investiga-

tion for women with uterine bleeding. *Ultrasound Obstet Gynecol* 1997; 10(2):121–125.

31. Dijkhuizen FP, de Vries LD, Mol BW, Brolmann HA, Peters HM, Moret E, Heintz AP. Comparison of transvaginal ultrasonography and saline infusion sonography for the detection of intracavitary abnormalities in premenopausal women. *Ultrasound Obstet Gynecol* May 2000; 15(5):372–376.

32. Williams CD, Marshburn PB. A prospective study of transvaginal hydrosonography in the evaluation of abnormal uterine bleeding. *Am J Obstet Gynecol* 1998; 179(2):292–298.

33. Bradley LD, Falcone T, Magen AB. Radiographic imaging techniques for the diagnosis of abnormal uterine bleeding. *Obstet Gynecol Clin North Am* 2000; 27(2):245–276.

34. Cooper JM, Erickson M. Endometrial sampling techniques in the diagnosis of abnormal uterine bleeding. *Obstet Gynecol Clin North Am* 2000; 27(2):235–244.

35. Goldstein SR, Zeltser H, Horan CK, Snyder JR, Schwartz LB. Ultrasonography-based triage for perimenopausal patients with abnormal uterine bleeding. *Am J Obstet Gynecol* 1997 Jul; 177(1):102–108.

36. Serden SP. Diagnostic hysteroscopy to evaluate the cause of abnormal uterine bleeding. *Obstet Gynecol Clin North Am* 2000; 27(2):277–286.

37. Gebauer G, Hafner A, Siebzehnrubi E, Lang N. Role of hysteroscopy in detection and extraction of endometrial polyps: results of a prospective study. *Am J Obstet Gynecol* Jan 2001; 184(2):59–63.

38. Emanuel MH, Wamsteker K, Lammes FB. Is dilation and curettage obsolete for diagnosing intrauterine disorders in premenopausal patients with persistent abnormal uterine bleeding? *Acta Obstet Gynecol Scand* 1997; 76(1):65–83.

39. Bettocchi S, Ceci O, Vincino M, Marello F, Impedovo L, Selvaggi L. Diagnostic inadequacy of dilatation and curettage. *Fertil Steril* Apr 2001; 75(4):803–805.

40. Kremer C, Duffy S, Moroney AM. Patient satisfaction with outpatient hysteroscopy versus day case hysteroscopy: randomized controlled trial. *Br Med J* 2000; 320:279–282.

41. Ben-Yehuda OM, Kim YB, Leuchter RS. Does hysteroscopy improve upon the sensitivity of dilation and curettage in the diagnosis of endometrial hyperplasia or carcinoma? *Gynec Oncol* 1998; 68:4–7.

42. Jansen FW. Complications of hysteroscopy: a prospective, multicenter study. *Obstet Gynecol* 2000; 96(2):266–270.

43. Munro MG. Medical management of abnormal uterine bleeding. *Obstet Gynecol Clin North Am* 2000; 27(2):287–304.

44. Lindheim SR. Operative hysteroscopy in the office setting. *J Am Assoc Gynecol Laparosc* 2000 Feb; 7(1):65–69.

45. Loffer FD. Complications of hysteroscopy-their cause, prevention, and correction [see comments. *J Am Assoc Gynecol Laparosc* 1995 Nov; 3(1):11–26.

46. McCausland VM. Tuboovarian abscesses after operative hysteroscopy. *J Reprod Med* 1993 Mar; 38(3):198–200.

47. Obermair A. Does hysteroscopy facilitate tumor cell dissemination? Incidence of peritoneal cytology from patients with early stage endometrial carcinoma following dilatation and curettage (D and C) versus hysteroscopy and D and C. *Cancer* 2000 Jan 1; 88(1):139–143.

8

Conservative Treatment of Endometrial Hyperplasia and Early Endometrial Cancer

GENESIS BOWEN AND THOMAS RANDALL

Pennsylvania Hospital, Philadelphia, Pennsylvania, U.S.A.

INTRODUCTION

The standard primary treatment of women with endometrial adenocarcinoma is total abdominal hysterectomy with bilateral salpingo-oophorectomy. Radiation therapy has also been successfully used in patients with significant co-morbidities that preclude surgery. These options are acceptable in women who are postmenopausal or who do not wish to retain their childbearing potential. Neither radiation therapy nor surgery would be an attractive option for patients who wish to later become pregnant. Primary hormonal therapy has been studied as a means to preserve fertility or to treat patients with

229

major co-morbidities. This chapter offers a review of the literature of conservative management on endometrial carcinoma with particular emphasis on the premenopausal patient in whom preservation of fertility is desired.

CLINICAL CHARACTERISTICS

Endometrial hyperplasias are considered to be a spectrum of changes in the endometrium associated with the anovulatory state (1), most often occurring in the postmenopausal population. These changes usually begin as simple hyperplasia, in which there is glandular hyperplasia without evidence of cytologic atypia. As these lesions progress, more complex hyperplasia with crowding of glands and cytologic atypia is noted. If left unattended, these lesions will eventually develop into carcinoma in situ and frank adenocarcinoma. The ability to identify those at greatest risk will aid in the successful treatment of these pathologic changes.

Several studies have looked at the occurrence of endometrial cancer in premenopausal women (2–4). Although rare in this population (3–5% occurrence in women under 40) (3–6), there are certain characteristics associated with endometrial hyperplasia and cancer in these women (Table 1). The most common associations are related to hormonal abnormalities, the use of higher dose oral contraceptives (2) or other exogenous estrogens, infertility, nulliparity, and polycystic ovarian syndrome (PCOS). Certain medical conditions such as obesity, hypertension, and diabetes mellitus are also associated. In a

Table 1 Clinical Characteristics in Women Under Age 40 with Endometrial Carcinoma

	Peterson et al.	Silverberg et al.	Crissman et al.	Gitsch et al.	Total
Obese	81%	55%	37%	54%	57%
Nulliparous	53%	52%	37%	46%	47%
Menstrual irregularity/PCOS	81%	46%	0%	18%	36%

hospital record review at the University of Michigan, a clinical profile was established for women under 40 years of age with endometrial carcinoma (7). Of the 650 cases of endometrial cancer reviewed, 32 (5%) were under 40 years of age; 81% of these younger patients gave a history of amenorrhea or menstrual irregularity, 81% were overweight, 53% nulliparous, 22% had coexisting diabetes, and 19% had hypertension. Eighty-four percent of these patients were alive at follow-up. In the study by Silverberg et al. (2), which suggested a correlation between the use of sequential oral contraceptives and endometrial cancer in women under the age of 40, the clinical features traditionally associated with endometrial cancer were also present. Of the 20 patients studied and 123 patients gathered from literature review, 55% were obese, 52% nulliparous, 46% had evidence of PCOS on histology, 80% had grade 1 lesions, and 90% were alive at follow-up. Similarly, Crissman et al. (3) found 37% of their 32 premenopausal patients with endometrial cancer to be obese, 37% nulliparous, 25% hypertensive, and 81% presented with abnormal vaginal bleeding. All of the patients studied were found to have well-differentiated cancers. Six of 32 (19%) were found to have coexisting cancer of the ovary. Ninety-four percent were alive at follow-up. Gitsch et al. (4) found that in the 17 patients studied, 54% were obese, 46% were nulliparous, 18% had PCOS, and 30% had coexisting ovarian cancer. Fifty-eight percent of those studied had well-differentiated carcinomas, with 76% alive at follow-up 12–78 months after primary surgery. In another study (8), patients aged 45 and younger were found to have the same distribution of stage, histology, and survival as those women over 45 years of age, but these women were five times more likely to have synchronous ovarian cancer. The ovarian cancers in these women were all stage I and had good prognosis compared to older women; it was found that nulliparity, not age, was an independent risk factor for development of a synchronous ovarian malignancy.

Endometrial cancer often presents with abnormal vaginal bleeding. This directs the clinician toward early tissue sampling and diagnosis in postmenopausal patients, but diagnosis is often delayed in younger women for whom the distinction between anovulation and abnormal vaginal bleeding is more difficult. Fortunately, endometrial adenocarcinoma in young women is often associated with early stage disease, well-differentiated histology, minimal myometrial involvement, and thus a favorable prognosis (4,5). Using these clinical criteria to identify those young women predisposed to the development of endometrial carcinoma may encourage consideration of prophylaxis with weight reduction and progesterone therapy, along with earlier tissue diagnosis when abnormal bleeding is present. As for women of all ages, consideration of the diagnosis of endometrial carcinoma is important, as early diagnosis may be life saving and may even allow the preservation of fertility.

PROGESTIN THERAPY

The endometrium is very sensitive to the actions of estradiol and progesterone due to the presence of high-affinity steroid-specific receptors (9). Progesterone administration leads to a down-regulation of both estradiol and progesterone receptors. In addition, progesterone increases the synthesis and accumulation of glycogen and glycoproteins and inhibits the proliferation of endometrial epithelial cells. These actions aid in further differentiating endometrial epithelial cells into secretory cells. These effects of progestins and the presence of progesterone receptors are potential indicators of responsiveness of neoplastic endometrium to the effects of progesterone.

Ehrlich and colleagues (10) studied the effect of the presence of progesterone receptors in determining progestin responsiveness of recurrent or advanced endometrial cancers. Cytoplasmic progestin receptors were measured from biopsy specimens of women found to have endometrial hyperplasia or adenocarcinoma. Patients with advanced or recurrent endometrial carcinoma were treated with medroxyprogesterone acetate or megestrol for a minimum of 3 months or until progression of the endometrial adenocarcinoma was observed, and continued indefinitely in those who showed a response to treatment. They found that 80% of those tumors that were progestin receptor positive and 6% of the progestin receptor negative tumors responded favorably to progestin therapy. Alternatively, 94% of nonresponders were progestin receptor negative. Thus the presence of progesterone receptors appeared to predict the response to progestin treatment.

Progestins can induce regression of endometrial cancer. Histologically, specimens of endometrium in which hyperplasia was successfully treated with progesterone show early secretory changes including subnuclear vacuoles, arrest of mitotic activity, and a generally quiescent glandular epithelium (11). Medroxyprogesterone acetate has been shown to induce regression of well-differentiated adenocarcinoma with a histologic response closely related to the presence and levels of progesterone receptors (9,11). Several different treatment regimens have been studied (Table 2).

Progestational agents have been used in the past to treat patients with recurrent endometrial cancer, with an overall response rate of 25% (12). A number of different treatment regimens and doses using both oral and intramuscular preparations of progestins have been employed with similar response rates. Overall survival for all progestin-treated individuals is 1 year. In young patients and in those with well-dif-

Table 2 Treatment of Endometrial Carcinoma with Progestins

	No. of Patients	Agents Used	No. of Responses
Wentz et al.			
Group 1	20	Dimethisterone 100 mg qd x 6 weeks	20
Group 2	80	Megestrol acetate 20 mg qd x 6 weeks	80
Kim et al.	21	Megestrol acetate 160 mg qd x 3 months	13
Bokhman et al.	19	Oxyprogesterone acetate 50 mg qd x 3 months, then biw x 3 months	15
Randall and			
Kurman	12	Megesterol acetate or medroxy-progesterone acetate	9
Total	152		137

ferentiated cancers, however, therapy appears to be more effective.

Bokhman et al. (13) studied 19 patients with endometrial carcinoma who had clinical profiles similar to that previously described. These patients were treated with 500 mg of oxyprogesterone caproate (OPC) intramuscularly daily. At 3 month follow-up, endometrial biopsies were taken; those with evidence of adenocarcinoma were taken directly to hysterectomy (4 patients, 2 of which had microfoci of adenocarcinoma on histological examination), whereas those without evidence of adenocarcinoma on biopsy were treated for another 3 months with twice-weekly OPC injections. At the end of this 6 month period, successful atrophy and amenorrhea were noted in all remaining patients. These patients were then cycled on OCPs for 3–4 months and then ovulation was induced using clomiphene citrate. All of these patients experienced complete cure with no recurrences in the 3–9 year follow-up and 8 of the 15 patients had subsequent successful pregnancies.

In another study (11), high dose progestins were used for 3–6 cycles in women with cystic glandular or adenomatous endometrial hyperplasia, severe or atypical adenomatous hyperplasia, or endometrial adenocarcinoma. Results revealed that adenomatous hyperplasia in young women can revert back to normal and make subsequent pregnancies possible. This effect was observed in a 27-year-old woman who presented with infertility and severe adenomatous endometrial hyperplasia and successfully became pregnant after a 4 month treatment with cyclic progesterone. Alternatively, a 31-year-old woman who presented with infertility and severe atypical adenomatous hyperplasia and focal endometrial carcinoma was treated with high dose progesterone for 6 months with persistence of neoplastic glands on D&C specimen. Reluctant to undergo hysterectomy, the patient was treated with an additional 3 months of progesterone. The subsequent endometrial biopsy specimen showed extensive areas of secretory endometrium with persistent neoplastic endometrium, and hysterectomy specimen revealed one area of frankly invasive, moderately differentiated adenocarcinoma. It was concluded that the response to progesterone may not always involve the entirety of the endometrial neoplasm and findings of secretory changes in biopsy specimens did not always correlate with cure. Clones of hormone-resistant endometrial tumor were found to progress while extensive areas showed secretory changes. These clones can easily be missed on biopsy specimens and only a hysterectomy specimen can effectively rule out carcinoma.

Wentz (1) studied two groups of women using oral synthetic progestational agents. In the first group, 20 patients were exposed to 100 mg dimethisterone daily for 6 weeks and followed by frequent curettage or endometrial biopsy (17 of the 20 were followed for greater than 30 months). Histologic evaluations revealed a return to the normal state of endometrium in all patients, with no recurrence of hyperplasia in follow-up. The premenopausal patients returned to regular ovulatory state as indicated by the presence of secretory endometrium on the first day of menses. The postmenopausal patients continued to have atrophic endometrium with no further bleeding. In the second group, oral megesterol acetate was given to women with persistent adenomatous and atypical hyperplasia. The regimen used was 20 mg in four divided doses daily for 6 weeks. A total of 80 patients with adenomatous hyperplasia were used (27 premenopausal and 53 postmenopausal). Thirty of the patients presented with persistent atypical hyperplasia; no recurrences of hyperplasia were found in the follow-up period.

In a series performed by Randall and Kurman (14), treatment of atypical hyperplasia and well-differentiated carcinoma of the endometrium with progestins in young women (under age 40 years) again appeared to be a safe alternative to hysterectomy. These women were treated with either megestrol acetate or medroxyprogesterone acetate for 3 to 18 months followed by frequent endometrial sampling. Sixteen of the 17 women with atypical hyperplasia and 9 of the 12 women with well-differentiated carcinoma had regression of their lesions. Additionally, 5 of the 25 women in the series who attempted pregnancy were successful and carried their pregnancies to term. It was observed that the median duration of therapy needed to achieve a response was 9 months. Patients who were felt to have failed treatment had a median duration of treatment of 3 months. This was observed regardless of the dose of progestin administered. Thus, it might be concluded that it is the duration of treatment, not the dose intensity, which is most important in achieving a response to primary progestin therapy.

Kim et al. (6) also found progestin therapy to be a reasonable alternative to hysterectomy in treating women with grade 1 disease. Combining the data of their study with that obtained by literature review (7 patients treated plus 14 cases derived from literature review), 13 of 21 patients treated with progestins had an initial response. Eight patients showed no response to progestin therapy and underwent definitive treatment. Of the initial responders, three developed recurrent disease and one was found to have extrauterine disease at the time of surgery. No viable infants were delivered. The seven study patients were treated with a 3-month course of megestrol acetate at 160 mg/day.

The presence of hyperplasia with cytologic atypia places patients at an increased risk for progression to endometrial carcinoma. Cytologic atypia was found to be a highly accurate indicator of biologic response of hyperplastic endometrium to exogenous progestin therapy (15). Eighty percent of the 65 patients studied by Ferenczy and Gelfand (15) who had endometrial hyperplasia without atypia had good long-term response to progestin over the 7-year follow-up period with no progression to carcinoma. However, women with cytologically atypical lesions demonstrated a tendency toward persistence rather than regression after therapy and carried a significant potential for progression to carcinoma.

To evaluate the prevalence of conservative therapy among gynecologic cancer specialists, Trimble and Curtin (16) performed a survey of 524 members of the Society of Gynecologic Oncologists (SGO). Of the 312 members who responded, 59% reported using progestins as an alternative to radiation therapy or surgery in younger patients or those with significant co-morbidities. The usual regimen used in these patients involved 160 mg of megace daily for 3–6 months followed by endometrial biopsy or D&C to evaluate response. A total of 358 patients were treated, with 178 (49%) successful treatments. Twenty-five women subsequently became pregnant. While primary progestin treatment for endometrial cancer is not the most common approach, these investigators have shown that its utilization is fairly prevalent among gynecologic cancer experts.

ANTICIPATION OF TREATMENT FAILURE

Well-differentiated endometrial cancer in young patients has a favorable prognosis and tends to show high sensitivity to progestogens. In some cases, however, resistance to progestin therapy or recurrence of disease following a full course of therapy has been noted. Identification of risk factors for failure of primary progestin therapy would be desirable. Here we review several potential indicators of treatment failure. Though none of these indicators have been validated, they may help the practitioner and patient make a more informed decision about the initiation or continuation of primary progestin therapy.

It was found that the progesterone receptor concentration varies with the degree of tumor differentiation. Well-differentiated endometrial carcinomas tend to have high concentrations of progesterone receptors, with decreases in receptor concentration as the tumor becomes more anaplastic (10). Likewise, progesterone receptor immunohistochemistry constitutes a powerful independent prognosticator of lymph node metastasis (18). The status of progesterone receptors on preoperative endometrial biopsy specimens corresponds well to that of hysterectomy specimens, thus enabling physicians to estimate the risk of lymph node metastases preoperatively. Patients with negative preoperative progesterone receptor immunohistochemistry are at a higher risk of having lymph node metastases. Tumors in premenopausal women tend to be well-differentiated with high concentrations of progesterone receptors and thus are more likely to respond to treatment with progestins than those in older women and/or those with more advanced disease.

Several other molecular markers have been investigated as possible prognosticators of endometrial carcinoma, including DNA ploidy, estrogen receptor status, p53 expression, HER-2/neu, and bcl-2 (18,19). The presence of estrogen receptors on endometrial cancer specimens showed no significant correlation with lymph node metastases. Conversely, p53 expression tended to correlate significantly with lymph node metastasis. However, the p53 expression status of preoperative specimens was not in agreement with that of hysterectomy specimens, making it difficult to estimate risk for lymph node metastasis based on preoperative p53 expression status. The presence of vascular space invasion is the only other pathologic criterion found to be present significantly more frequently in those with nodal metastasis or recurrent carcinoma. Thus, careful histopathological evaluation of the degree of differentiation of a lesion, by an experienced gynecologic pathologist, appears to be the best prediction of response to progestin therapy.

Sood and colleagues studied the value of preoperative CA-125 as a predictor of extrauterine disease (19). There is a significant rise in CA-125 with increasing stage, grade, or depth of invasion. Increased CA-125 is associated with positive peritoneal cytology, lymph node metastasis, and poorer 5-year survival rates. In fact, CA-125 was found to be the most powerful predictor of poor survival followed by positive pelvic lymph nodes, depth of myometrial invasion, and histology, respectively. In this series, a preoperative CA-125 of less than 20 U/ml correlates to a 3% chance of finding extrauterine disease in the setting of favorable histology and low grade disease. (This risk increases to 6% with high grade disease with favorable histology and 17% with unfavorable histology.) CA-125 values between 20 and 65 U/ml correlates to a 14% risk of extrauterine disease with favorable histology and low grade, and greater than 65 U/ml alone correlates to a 49% risk of metastatic disease. The serum CA-125 measurement, therefore, appears to provide a non-invasive indication of extrauterine disease.

Management plans for endometrial carcinoma are often dictated by tumor size and by suspicion of myometrial invasion, tumor spread, and lymph node metastases. Clinical staging is often not compatible with surgical findings. A more effective preoperative staging technique would be valuable for planning appropriate therapy. Specifically, it would be useful to identify patients with metastatic disease for whom conservative treatment might be less appropriate. Both ultrasound and MRI have shown potential in the preoperative assessment of endometrial cancer. Cacciatore et al. (20) performed preoperative sonography on 93 patients with a histologic diagnosis of endometrial carcinoma. Sonography was used to evaluate both uterine size and endometrial echoes. Although uterine volume was often enlarged in those with endometrial carcinoma compared to controls, a poor correlation was found between uterine volume enlargement and myometrial invasion. However, a significant correlation was found to exist between endometrial echoes and myometrial invasion, with a correct prediction of myometrial invasion in 80% of cases. Accurate sonographic staging of endometrial cancer was found in 91% of cases. High intensity echoes were found to be present more often in well- or moderately differentiated carcinomas, while more heterogenic echo patterns were found in poorly differentiated carcinomas.

MRI is another radiographic technique that has been proved to have value in the preoperative evaluation of endometrial carcinoma (22). In a five-center NCI cooperative study, diagnostic accuracy of MRI was compared to FIGO surgical staging to evaluate the ability of MRI to determine depth of myometrial invasion and the presence of lymph node metastases. Eighty-eight patients with histologically documented endometrial carcinoma who were scheduled for surgical staging with lymph node sampling were subjected to an MRI imaging study preoperatively. MRI was found to have an 85% overall diagnostic accuracy at staging when compared to surgical specimens, but with only a 54% sensitivity for detecting deep myometrial invasion. MRI was also proven to be better at diagnosing lower stage lesions. The diagnosis of stage I and II lesions by MRI was correct with a probability of 0.87, while the assessment of stage III and IV disease was correct with a probability of 0.50. Both ultrasound and MRI are fairly accurate for the preoperative staging of endometrial cancer in the hands of experienced radiologists. Sonography is an economic and practical first-line imaging technique in the clinical evaluation of endometrial carcinoma. Patients suspected of having deep myometrial invasion, lymph node metastasis, or concomitant pelvic lesions should be referred for MRI evaluation.

TREATMENT REGIMENS

In our view, patients should receive primary progestin therapy only if they are not fit for surgery or if sufficiently committed to having a child that they are willing to share in the risk of foregoing definitive surgery. Both megestrol acetate and medroxyprogesterone acetate are effective over a variety of dosages and schedules. Endovaginal ultrasound or pelvic MRI may be helpful in detecting deep myometrial invasion and metastatic spread, both contraindications to conservative management. Additionally, tumor marker CA-125 can be used to predict the presence of extrauterine disease (Table 3).

If a patient has no evidence of metastatic disease and elects progesterone therapy, she may be prescribed 40 mg of megesterol acetate twice a day. Higher doses of megesterol acetate are frequently administered, but these doses are not associated with greater success and are more likely to cause side effects. After 3 to 6 months, patients should undergo

Table 3 Work-up of Young Women with Atypical Hyperplasia or Well-Differentiated Carcinoma

Review pathology of endometrial specimen (biopsy or curettage specimen):
    Differentiation of lesion
    Progesterone receptor status
Evaluate for extrauterine disease:
    Physical examination
    Pelvic MRI or transvaginal ultrasound
    CA-125 level

some type of endometrial sampling either by endometrial biopsy or D&C. Those patients with regression of disease after this initial treatment period should be maintained on a regimen to prevent de novo or recurrent carcinoma due to chronic anovulation. Patients can be cycled on either oral contraceptives or with medroxyprogesterone acetate 10 mg for 10 days per month. These patients should be followed with D&C or endometrial biopsy at 3- to 6-month intervals. Long-term surveillance is necessary to ensure that the proliferative process has been suppressed and that the endometrium is cycling either spontaneously or from exogenous hormone therapy (14). Patients who decline ongoing medical therapy should be offered hysterectomy once childbearing has been completed or abandoned.

For those patients in whom persistence is detected after the initial 3–6 month treatment period, megace may be given (80 mg twice a day) with repeat sampling in 3–6 months. Those with regression at this point can be cycled and allowed to attempt pregnancy as outlined above. Alternatively, these patients can be offered hysterectomy after the initial treatment failure. It is important to note that these high doses of progestogens are associated with side effects such as headache, bloating, decreased appetite, premenstrual tension and vaginal dryness that may lead to poor patient compliance. In fact, Ferenzcy and Gelfand (15) found a 40% occurrence of one or more of these side effects in their study. Patient discontinuation of hormonal therapy can lead to persistence and recurrence of disease, which carries a high risk of progression toward carcinoma. There have been many reports that endometrial cytologic atypia treated with oral progesterone is associated with a high rate of persistent disease and that the atypia tends to recur after the discontinuance of progestogen therapy. Thus, patient compliance should be closely monitored. Any patients with evidence of disease progression at any point in the treatment scheme should undergo hysterectomy with no further attempts at conservative management (Table 4).

In addition to close follow-up by frequent endometrial tissue sampling for detecting disease recurrences, it is impor-

Table 4 Treatment Regimen for Primary Hormonal Therapy of
Endometrial Cancer

Start progestin therapy (e.g., megesterol acetate, 40 mg bid)
Plan weight loss of 10% or more over 6 months
Test fasting glucose, insulin levels and consider use of insulin sensitive
agents
Sample endometrium at 3 months
  Regression → ovulation induction, oral contraceptives, or continue
    progestin therapy
  Persistence → continue progestin therapy
  Progression → surgery

---

tant to screen patients for co-existing disease. It has also been
found that women with endometrial cancer diagnosed before
the age of 50 are greater than three times as likely to develop
subsequent colorectal cancer than those without endometrial
cancer (23). It is extremely important to screen this population against colorectal cancer by encouraging more aggressive
colonoscopy-based screening in this group of patients. There
is some excess risk of colorectal cancer during the first 6
months of follow-up for all types of gynecologic malignancies,
so early screening is necessary.

Lastly, factors that promote the development of carcinoma may still be present after hormonal therapy (i.e., obesity,
hypertension, anovulation, etc.). It is important to identify and
treat these risk factors when possible by cycling patients with
OCPs, initiating weight-loss programs at the time of treatment, and treating hyperlipidemia and glucose intolerance.

REFERENCES

1. Wentz WB. Progestin therapy in endometrial hyperplasia.
    Gynecol Oncol 1974; 2:362–367.

2. Silverberg SG, Makowski EL, Rochie WD. Endometrial carci-
    noma in women under 40 years of age. *Cancer* 1977; 39:592–598.

3. Crissman JD, Azoury RS, Barnes AE, Schellhas HF.
    Endometrial carcinoma in women 40 years of age or younger.
    Obstet Gynecol 1981; 57:699–704.

4.   Gitsch G, Hanzal E, Jensen D, Hacker NF. Endometrial cancer in premenopausal women 45 years and younger. *Obstet Gynecol* 1995; 85:504–508.

5.   Vardi JR, Tadros GH, Zafaranloo S, Kapadia L, Alderete MN, Shebes M. Stage IV endometrial carcinoma in a 25–year-old woman: a case report and review of the literature. *Gynecol Oncol* 1989; 34:244–248.

6.   Kim YB, Holschneider CH, Ghosh K, Nieberg RK, Montz FJ. Progestin alone as primary treatment of endometrial carcinoma in premenopausal women. *Cancer* 1997; 79:320–327.

7.   Peterson EP. Endometrial carcinoma in young women: a clinical profile. *Obstet and Gynecol* 1968; 31:702–707.

8.   Evans-Metcalf ER, Brooks SE, Reale FR, Baker SP. Profile of women 45 years of age and younger with endometrial cancer. *Obstet Gynecol* 1998; 91:349–354.

9.   Podczaski E, Satyaswaroop PG, Mortel R. Hormonal interactions in gynecologic malignancies. In: Hoskins WJ, Perez CA, Young RC, eds. *Principles and Practice of Gynecologic Oncology*, Second Edition. Philadelphia: Lippincott-Raven, 1997,pp.211–229.

10. Ehrlich CE, Young PCM, Cleary RE. Cytoplasmic progesterone and estradiol receptors in normal, hyperplastic, and carcinomatous endometria: therapeutic implications. *Am J Obstet Gynecol* 1981; 141:539–546.

11. Deligdisch L. Hormone therapy on the endometrium. *Modern Pathol* 1993; 6:94–106.

12. Barakat RR, Park RC, Grigsby PW, Muss HD, Norris HJ. Corpus: epithelial tumors. In: Hoskins WJ, Perez CA, eds. *Principles and Practice of Gynecologic Oncology*, Second Edition. Philadelphia: Lippincott-Raven, 1997; pp. 859–883.

13. Bokhman JV, Chepick OF, Volkova AT, Vishnevsky AS. Can primary endometrial carcinoma stage I be cured without surgery and radiation therapy? *Gynecol Oncol* 1985; 20:139–155.

14. Randall TC, Kurman RJ. Progestin treatment of atypical hyperplasia and well-differentiated carcinoma of the endometrium in women underage 40. *Obstet Gynecol* 1997; 90:434–440.

15. Ferenczy A, Gelfand M. The biologic significance of cytologic atypia in progestogen-treated endometrial hyperplasia. *Am J Obstet Gynecol* 1989;160:126–131.

16. Trimble EL, Curtin JP. Conservative, hormonal management of endometrial adenocarcinoma: a survey of the Society of Gynecologic Oncologists, National Cancer Institute, Bethesda, MD, Sloan-Kettering Cancer Center, New York, NY.

17. Iwai K, Fukuda K, Hachisuga T, Mori M, Uchiyama M, Iwasaka T. Prognostic significance of progesterone receptor immunistochemistry for lymph node merasrases in endomerrial carcinoma. *Gynecol Oncol* 1999; 72:351–359.

18. Bell GJ, Minnick A, Reid GC, Judis J, Brownell M. Relationship of nonstaging pathological risk factors to lymph node metasiasis and recurrence in clinical stae 1 endometrial carcinoama. *Gynecol Oncol* 1997; 66:388–392.

19. Sood AK, Buller RE, Burger RA, Dawson JD, Sorosky JI, Berman M. Value of preoperative CA-125 level in the management of uterine cancer and prediction of clinical outcome. *Obset Gyncol* 1997; 90;441–447.

20. Cacciators B, Lehtovirta P, Wahlstom T, Ylostalo P. Preoperative sonographic evaluation of endometrial cancer. *Am J Obstet Gynecol* 1989; 160:133–137.

21. Hricak H, Rubinstein LV, Gherman GM, Karstaedt N. MR imaging evaluation of endometrial carcinoma: results of an NCI Cooperative Study. *Radiology* 1991; 179:829–832.

22. Weinberg DS, Newschaffer CJ, Topham A. Risk for colorectal cancer after gynecologic cancer. *Ann Intern Med* 1999; 131:189–193.

9

The Surgical Management of Early Endometrial Cancer

CHRISTINA S. CHU

University of Pennsylvania Medical Center,
Philadelphia, Pennsylvania, U.S.A.

INTRODUCTION

Endometrial cancer (EC) is the most common gynecologic malignancy in the United States (1,2). In the year 2001, approximately 36,000 new cases were diagnosed, and 6,500 women died as a result of the disease (3). Fortunately, most patients present with early stage disease and have an excellent prognosis. A combination of several large series reveals that 80% of patients are diagnosed in stages I and II (Table 1). For the medically operable candidate with early stage disease, surgery is the treatment of choice. While vaginal and laparoscopic routes have been used, the standard of therapy

Table 1   Distribution by Stage at Diagnosis[a]

Stage	No. of Patients	% of Patients
I	850	70.5
II	117	9.7
III	175	14.6
IV	59	4.9
Unstaged	4	0.3
Total	1205	100

Based on 1205 patients combined from 4 series (23, 47, 98, 99).

still remains total abdominal hysterectomy, bilateral salpingo-oophorectomy, and surgical staging (4–7). Some authors
have suggested that with surgical extirpation, a 90% survival
rate is obtainable (8,9), though others have reported a 5-year
survival rate closer to 75% for stage I disease (10). Despite the
good overall survival for patients with early stage disease,
local and distant recurrence continue to be problematic for
select patients with high-risk disease. This chapter provides
an overview of prognostic factors affecting outcome in
patients with early stage EC and discusses rationales for surgical staging and different surgical approaches.

STAGING

In 1988, the International Federation of Obstetrics and
Gynecology (FIGO) introduced a new surgical staging system
for EC (11). This staging classification is outlined in Table 2.
The prior clinical staging system established in 1971 was
abandoned based upon the emerging awareness of inaccura-
cies inherent in clinical assessment, and the identification of
risk factors associated with poor outcome. From 19–40% of
patients thought to have disease confined to the uterine corpus based on clinical staging parameters have been demonstrated to have extrauterine disease at laparotomy (1,12). The
current surgical staging system utilizes factors commonly
associated with prognosis including assessment of grade,
myometrial invasion, cervical involvement, peritoneal cytol-

Table 2 1988 FIGO Surgical Staging[a]

Stage	Definition
IA G123	Tumor limited to endometrium
IB G123	Invasion of less than half of the myometrium
IC G123	Invasion of more than half of the myometrium
IIA G123	Endocervical glandular involvement only
IIB G123	Cervical stromal invasion
IIIA G123	Invasion of serosa and/or adnexa and/or positive peritoneal cytology
IIIB G123	Vaginal metastases
IIIC G123	Metastases to pelvic and/or para-aortic lymph nodes
IVA G123	Tumor invasion of bladder and/or bowel mucosa
IVB G123	Distant metastases, including intraabdominal and/or inguinal lymph nodes

[a]Approved by FIGO, Rio de Janeiro, October, 1988.

ogy, and lymph node metastasis. Typically, surgical staging involves removal of the uterus, cervix, and adnexa, with peritoneal washings. Sampling of pelvic and paraaortic lymph nodes is also incorporated for selected patients.

Surgical staging is designed to provide valuable prognostic information. As reported by FIGO in 1994, overall 5-year survival is 86% for patients with stage I disease, 66% for stage II, 44% for stage III, and 16% for stage IV (13). Individual investigators have confirmed a difference in survival among patients with early stage disease. Descamps et al. (14) noted a 22% recurrence rate in patients with stage II disease compared to a 10% rate for stage I ($p = 0.02$). Tabernero et al. (15) reported a significant overall 5-year survival difference of 87% for 37 patients with stage II tumors compared to 100% for 148 patients with stage I.

In addition to prognostic benefit, some have suggested a therapeutic benefit to surgical staging (4,16–18), though others have disputed this finding based on increased complications (19) and lack of proven survival benefit (20,21). Despite criticism, the use of surgical staging procedures is the rule among gynecologic oncologists (22). In 1999, Kennedy et al. (23) reported that among 297 patients treated at 11 institutions participating in the Society of Gynecologists Outcomes

Task Force Study, 99% of patients were surgically staged, and 80% underwent lymph node sampling.

PROGNOSTIC FACTORS

Aside from stage, several clinicopathologic factors have been identified that provide significant predictive value for recurrence and survival in women with endometrial cancer (Table 3). Examination of these factors may help the clinician identify patients at higher risk for poor outcome and allow for appropriate individualization of therapy.

FIGO Grade

Histologic grade is one of the most important indicators of prognosis. In 1994, FIGO reported that overall 5-year survival for stage I patients was 94% for patients with grade 1 disease, 88% for grade 2, and 79% for grade 3 (13). Increasing grade is strongly associated with both poorer survival and increased rates of recurrence (Table 4). In addition, tumor differentiation is correlated with increased risk of lymph node metastases, adnexal metastases, malignant cytology, and deep myometrial invasion (24).

Myometrial Invasion

Depth of myometrial invasion is also consistently correlated with outcome. A summary of recurrence and survival rates based on depth of invasion is presented in Table 5. DiSaia et al. reported that the overall survival of patients with invasion

Table 3 Prognostic Factors in Endometrial Cancer

• FIGO stage	• Adnexal metastases
• FIGO grade	• Lymph-vascular space invasion
• Depth of myometrial invasion	• Tumor size
• Lymph node metastases	• Hormone receptor status
• Age	• DNA analysis (ploidy,
• Tumor histology	S-phase fraction,
• Peritoneal cytology	proliferative index)

Table 4 Histologic Grade and Prognosis

Author	n	Grade 1	Grade 2	Grade 3	Stages	Notes
			Survival			
DiSaia et al. (2)	222	95%	87%	71%	I, clinical	overall survival
Lindahl et al. (54)	136	100%	94%	89%	I, surgical	overall survival
Genest et al. (100)	241	96%	79%	70%	I, surgical	5-year survival
Taberno et al. (15)	157	92%*	92%*	71%	I-II, clinical	5-year survival
Kim et al. (96)	103	100%	83%	58%	I-III, surgical	5-year DFS
Touboul et al. (37)	437	92%	72%	71%	I-IV, surgical	10-year DFS
Mariani et al. (26)	142	95%*	95%*	80%	NS	5-year DFS**
			Recurrence			
DiSaia et al. (2)	222	4%	15%	41%	I, clinical	
Morrow et al. (25)	895	7%	16%	33%	I-II, clinical	
Descamps et al. (14)	201	13%	14%	41%	I-II, clinical	
Aalders et al. (42)	379	3%	55%	32%	I-IV, clinical	
Mundt et al. (101)	43	58%*	58%*	31%	I-IV, surgical	pelvic disease

DFS = disease-free survival, NS = not specified, * = rate combined for grades 1 and 2,
** = lymphatic failure

Table 5 Myometrial Invasion and Prognosis

Ref.	< 1/2	> 1/2	Stages	Notes
Mundt et al. (101)	26%	60%	I–IV, surgical	pelvic recurrence
Touboul et al. (37)	95%	75%	I–IV, surgical	10-year DFS
Kim and Neloff (96)	92–100%	68%	I–III, surgical	5-year DFS
Mariani et al. (26)	97%	78%	NS	5-year DFS**

Ref	< 1/3	mid 1/3	> 2/3	Stages	Notes
DiSaia et al. (2)	8–13%	12%	46%	I, clinical	recurrence
Descamps et al. (14)	13%	26.6%*	26.6%*	I–II, clinical	recurrence
Morrow et al. (25)	10%	17%	32%	I–II, clinical	recurrence
Taberno et al. (15)	98%	83%*	83%*	I–II, clinical	5-year DFS

DFS = disease-free survival; NS = not specified; * = rate combined for > 1/3 invasion; ** = lymphatic failure.

confined to the inner-third of the myometrium was 11%, compared to 12% and 36% for those with mid- and outer-third invasion, respectively (2). FIGO reported on 5342 patients with stage I disease, and noted survival to be 82.4% for patients with tumor invading less than one-third of the myometrium, 78% for one-third to one-half invasion, and 66.8% for greater than one-half invasion (13). Like FIGO grade, depth of invasion is related to other prognostic factors such as grade, lymph node metastases, and extrauterine metastases. The relationship between grade and myometrial invasion is shown in Table 6. Patients with well-differentiated tumors tend to have superficially invasive disease, while those with poorly-differentiated tumors are more likely to present with deeper invasion.

Lymph Node Metastases

Metastases to the pelvic and para-aortic lymph nodes occurs in approximately 10% and 6% of patients with disease clinically confined to the uterus, respectively (Table 7). Several authors have correlated the incidence of nodal disease with increased rates of recurrence and death. In patients with clinical stage I and II disease, Descamps et al. (14) reported

Table 6 Presentation of Patients with Stage I Disease Classified by FIGO Grade and Depth of Myometrial Invasion

Depth of Invasion	Grade 1	Grade 2	Grade 3
Clinical I (n = 621 patients)[a]			
Inner 1/3	15.5%	21.1%	8.7%
Middle 1/3	3.5%	11.1%	3.9%
Outer 1/3	2.9%	9.2%	10.3%
Surgical Stage I (n = 513 patients)[b]			
Endometrium	14.2%	5.8%	1.6%
Inner 1/2	33.3%	24.3%	5.7%
Outer 1/2	4.5%	7.8%	2.7%

[a]Adapted from Creasman et al., 1987 (1).
[b]Adapted from Straughn et al., 2002 (102).

recurrence in 52.6% of patients with lymph node metastases compared to only 9.9% of those without. In a similar population, Morrow et al. (25) found that recurrence occurred in 28 of 48 patients (58%) with para-aortic nodal disease, 18 of 63 (29%) with pelvic nodal involvement only, and only 104 of 784 patients (13%) with no nodal involvement. For patients with clinical stage I disease, DiSaia et al. (2) reported that deaths occurred in 52% versus only 5% of patients with positive versus to negative pelvic lymph nodes, and 53% versus 8% for para-aortic nodes, respectively. The incidence of lymph node metastases is related to other factors such as FIGO grade and depth of tumor invasion. Tables 8 and 9 summarize the frequency of lymph node metastases in relation to these factors.

Table 7 Incidence of Lymph Node Metastases in Patients with Clinical Stage I or II (Occult) Disease

Location	Patients
Pelvic	120/1212 (9.9%)
Para-aortic	98/1672 (5.9%)

[a]Total combined from 4 series (1,25,103,104).

Table 8   Incidence of Pelvic Node Metastases Based on FIGO
Grade and Myometrial Invasion (n = 621 patients)[a]

Depth of Invasion	Grade 1	Grade 2	Grade 3
Endometrium	0%	3%	0%
Superficial 1/3	3%	5%	9%
Middle 1/3	0%	9%	4%
Outer 1/3	11%	19%	34%

[a]Adapted from Creasman et al., 1987 (1).

Tumor Histology

Certain histologic subtypes of EC are recognized to have a
worse prognosis. Creasman et al. (1) reported a significantly
higher incidence of para-aortic lymph node metastases in
patients with non-endometrioid cell types. Similarly, Mariani
et al. (26) examined lymphatic failures in 142 patients and
reported 5-year recurrence-free survival to be 78% for
patients with non-endometrioid compared to 94% for
endometrioid histologies (p = 0.001). A large series from the
Mayo Clinic investigated 388 patients with endometrial cancer (27); 13% of patients were noted to have non-endometrioid
cell types (including 14 patients with papillary serous, 11
with clear cell, 20 with adenosquamous, and 7 with undifferentiated histologies). Of these patients, 62% were already
found to have extrauterine disease at the time of staging.
Overall survival for patients with endometrioid histology was
92% compared to only 33% for those with other cell types.

Table 9   Incidence of Para-aortic Node Metastases Based on
FIGO Grade and Myometrial Invasion (n = 621 patients)[a]

Depth of Invasion	Grade 1	Grade 2	Grade 3
Endometrium	0%	3%	0%
Superficial 1/3	1%	4%	4%
Middle 1/3	5%	0%	0%
Outer 1/3	6%	14%	23%

[a]Adapted from Creasman et al., 1987 (1).

Despite adjuvant therapy, only 10% of these high risk patients survived for 5 years.

Papillary serous carcinomas of the endometrium have been noted to have a distinct, aggressive behavior. Mannel et al. (28) described 17 patients with papillary serous tumors, none of whom survived 5 years. Hendrickson et al. (24) examined 256 patients with endometrial cancer and noted that 50% of all the treatment failures occurred in patients with papillary serous histologies, though this subtype comprised only 10% of the entire study population. These tumors may present with extrauterine spread despite the absence of deep myometrial invasion (29–31) and have a predilection for upper abdominal recurrence (24,32). One large series of 50 patients with papillary serous tumors was reported by Goff et al. (33) who found that 72% of patients presented with extrauterine disease at the time of staging. Of the 14 patients with no myometrial invasion, 36% had metastases to lymph nodes, 43% had intraperitoneal disease, and 50% had positive peritoneal cytology. Even among patients with no lymph-vascular space invasion, 58% had extrauterine disease.

Another cell type with particularly poor prognosis is clear cell carcinoma (34,35). In a study of 56 patients with clear cell histology, Christopherson et al. reported 5-year survival to be only 44% (36). Touboul et al. (37) noted that clear cell histology was an independent poor prognostic factor for disease-free survival on multivariate analysis.

Unlike papillary serous and clear cell histologies, adenocarcinomas with squamous differentiation (adenosquamous tumors or adencanthomas) do not appear to have a worse prognosis. Zaino et al. compared 465 patients with endometrioid histologies and 175 patients with squamous differentiation, and noted that biologic behavior was more a reflection of the grade and depth of invasion of the glandular component (38).

Age

Not all studies have been consistent in evaluating age as a prognostic factor. Several authors have not found age to be a useful predictor of survival (39,40) or recurrence (25,26).

However, Chambers et al. (41) examined 60 patients with clinical stage I grade 3 disease and confirmed that age at diagnosis of greater than 65 years was a significant poor prognostic factor. Similarly, Descamps et al. (14) examined 201 patients with clinical stage I and II disease and reported age to be a statistically significant predictor of recurrence on both univariate and multivariate analysis. Though these authors reported age to be an independent prognostic variable, in other studies, improved prognosis for younger women seems to be related to the presence of lower grade lesions and less invasive tumors. Malkasian et al. (9) noted grade 3 lesions in only 3.5% of premenopausal women as compared to 12.5% of postmenopausal women. In a study of stage I disease, Aalders et al. (42) compared 246 women aged 60 or older and 294 women under 60 years of age and noted that deep myometrial invasion occurred more frequently in the older women (46.3% versus 24.1%).

Peritoneal Cytology

Positive peritoneal cytology is generally accepted as a sign of poor prognosis, though the evidence is mixed. A summary of recurrence rates for patients with early stage endometrial cancer based on cytologic findings is presented in Table 10. Several authors have not found malignant cytology to significantly affect recurrence rates (43–46). However, in the largest series by Morrow et al. (25) which examined 1180 women with clinical stage I and II disease, of those with adequate follow up, 29.1% of patients with positive washings recurred compared to only 10.5% of those with negative findings. Notably, of those who recurred, 68% failed outside of the peritoneal cavity. Similarly, Tang et al. (47) found a statistical difference on multivariate analysis in 5-year survival for patients with benign and malignant cytology (90% versus 72%, respectively). Descamps et al. (14) studied 201 patients with clinical stage I and II disease, and found that positive cytology was an independent predictor of recurrence. For the 14 patients with positive cytology, 25% of patients recurred, as opposed to only 10% of those with negative cytology. Turner et al. (48)

Table 10 Peritoneal Cytology in Early Stage Endometrial Cancer

Ref.	Total Patients	Positive Cytology	% Positive Cytology	Clinical Stage	Recurrence Rate	
					Positive Cytology	Negative Cytology
Creasman and Rutledge (105)	167	26	16%	I	38%	10%
Creasman and Rutledge (1)	621	76	12%	I	—	—
Konski et al. (43)	134	19	14%	I	10%	5%
Szpak et al. (51)	54	12	22%	I	50%	0%
Yazigi et al. (45)	93	10	11%	I	10%	7%
Harouny et al. (49)	276	47	17%	I	29%	3%
Hirai et al. (46)	173	25	15%	I	12%	10%
Lurain et al. (44)	157	30	19%	I	17%	9%
Turner et al. (48)	567	28	5%	I	32%	7%
Kadar et al. (50)	269	34	13%	I, II	13%*	73%*
Zuna and Behrens (106)	98	6	6%	I	11 mo**	131 mo**
	24	5	21%	II	7 mo**	129 mo**
Morrow et al. (25)	1180	97	8%	I, II	29%	11%
Descamps et al. (14)	201	14	7%	I, II	35%	10%

* = 5-year survival for patients with extrauterine disease; ** = median survival in months.

reported a 5-year survival rates of 84% and 96% for 567 stage I patients with malignant and benign findings, respectively ($p = 0.001$). Recurrence rates were also significantly different at 32% versus 7%, respectively ($p = 0.002$). Cytology remained a significant independent predictor of survival and progression free interval on multivariate analysis.

Positive cytology has been generally associated with high FIGO grade, deep myometrial invasion, adnexal metastases, and lymph node metastases (1,44–46,49–51). Creasman et al. (1) studied 621 clinical stage I patients. Of the 76 (12%) with positive washings, 35% were noted to have extrauterine disease at staging. The rate of pelvic lymph node metastases was 25% versus 7% for patients with positive and negative washings, respectively ($p < 0.0001$). Para-aortic lymph node metastases were noted in 19% versus 4%, respectively ($p < 0.0001$). Milosevic et al. (52) reviewed 17 studies of peritoneal cytology. Of the 3280 patients included, 11% displayed malignant cytology. The association of poor prognosis with malignant cytology appeared to be related to other factors: Of the patients with positive washings, 8.3% had FIGO grade 1 disease, 12.1% grade 2, and 15.9% grade 3; superficial myometrial invasion was noted in 7.6%, and deep in 7.6%, and deep invasion in 17.2%.

Adnexal Metastases

About 5–6% of patients with disease clinically limited to the uterus will have adnexal metastases upon pathologic examination (1). Morrow et al. (25) reported that of 902 patients with clinical stage I and II disease, less than 1% had gross adnexal disease, and 6% had occult metastases. Adnexal metastases are associated with increased frequency of nodal involvement and disease recurrence. Morrow et al. reported the incidence of para-aortic lymph node metastases to be 42.8% for patients with gross adnexal involvement, 23.5% for occult involvement, and 9.3% for no involvement (25). Similarly, Creasman et al. (1) noted that among clinical stage I and stage II (occult) patients, the rate of positive para-aortic lymph nodes was 20% versus 5%

for those with and without adnexal metastases, respectively, and that the rate of positive pelvic lymph nodes was 32% and 8%, respectively. Mariani et al. (26) examined lymphatic recurrences in 142 patients and noted that the 5-year recurrence-free survival for patients with adnexal metastases was 67% as opposed to 94% for those without adnexal involvement ($p < 0.0001$).

Lymph-Vascular Space Invasion (LVSI)

Approximately 15% of patients with early stage disease show evidence of tumor invasion of the lymphatic and capillary spaces (1,53). Several authors have demonstrated LVSI to be an important predictor of prognosis. LVSI is commonly associated with deep invasion, poorly differentiated tumors, and lymph node metastases. Hanson et al. (53) examined 111 patients with stage I disease and noted that LVSI was found in 5% of patients with superficial-third myometrial invasion and 70% of those with outer-third involvement. Only 2% of patients with grade 1 tumors, compared to 42% with grade 3, displayed LVSI. In another study of 621 patients with clinical stage I and II disease (1), the rates of pelvic and para-aortic lymph node metastases was 27% and 19% for those with LVSI compared to 7% and 9% for those without, respectively ($p = 0.0001$ for both comparisons).

The presence of LVSI is also predictive of poorer rates of recurrence and survival. Lindahl et al. (54) noted that for 139 patients with stage I disease with myometrial invasion, the death rate was 27.8% versus 3.9% for those with and without LVSI ($p = 0.0001$). Similarly, Aalders et al. (55) found the recurrence and death rate among 540 stage I patients to be 26.7% compared to 9.1% for those with and without evidence of LVSI ($p < 0.01$). Several authors have also reported the presence of LVSI to be an independent prognostic factor on multivariate analysis. Hanson et al. (53) noted recurrence rates to be 44% for stage I patients without, and only 2% for those with LVSI ($p < 0.0001$) independent of histologic grade. Ambros and Kurman (56) found on multivariate analysis that depth of invasion, DNA ploidy, and vascular invasion associated changes (vascular invasion by tumor and/or myometrial perivascular lymphocytic infiltrate) were independently correlated to survival.

Tumor Size

Tumor size as a prognostic factor has been examined by a few authors. Touboul et al. (37) examined patients of various stages and compared 237 patients with tumors 3 cm or less in diameter to 198 patients with tumors of greater than 3 cm and noted the probability of 10-year disease-free survival to be 96% and 73%, respectively ($p < 0.0001$). This difference remained significant on multivariate analysis ($p = 0.015$). Schink et al. (57) examined 91 patients with disease clinically confined to the uterus and noted tumor size to be independently associated with lymph node metastases ($p = 0.022$). Tumors less than 2 cm had a 5.7% rate of lymph node metastases, and those greater than 2 cm had a rate of 21%. For tumors involving the entire cavity, the rate of lymph node positivity was 40%.

Hormone Receptor Status

In general, decreased levels of cytoplasmic estrogen receptor (ER) and progesterone receptor (PR) have been associated with poor prognosis, with PR exerting a stronger effect than ER. Receptor content has been noted to be inversely correlated to FIGO grade (58–60), as well as to extrauterine metastases (61,62). Several studies have demonstrated that levels of ER and PR are independent prognostic factors for disease-free survival as well as overall survival (62–64). For patients with stage I and II disease, Creasman et al. (62) found both ER and PR content to be significant predictors of disease-free survival on multivariate analysis. Another study of early stage patients was conducted by Ehrlich et al. (61) who reported that recurrence rates were 37.2% compared to 4% for patients with low and high PR content, respectively ($p < 0.001$), and 41% compared to 12.7% for patients with low and high ER content, respectively ($p = 0.02$). Overall survival was also noted to be significantly superior for patients with high levels of PR. Of particular interest, Liao et al. (60) noted that elevated receptor content afforded an improved survival, even to patients with lymph node metastases.

DNA Analysis

Several small studies have confirmed the importance of DNA ploidy, S-phase fraction, and proliferative index as independent predictors of survival and recurrence. About 25% of ECs are aneuploid (65–67), and approximately 30–49% display elevated S-phase fractions (66, 68). Ambros and Kurman (56) demonstrated that among 57 patients with stage I ECs, ploidy was a significant predictor of survival on both univariate and multivariate analysis. Similarly, Iversen (67) examined 52 patients with EC and concluded that aneuploidy was correlated with increased recurrence and death, and decreased disease-free interval and median survival. Stendahl et al. (65) conducted a larger series examining 185 EC specimens with flow cytometry for aneuploidy and S-phase fraction, which were found to be correlated significantly with increased death rate ($p < 0.002$ and $p < 0.0001$, respectively), and the incidence FIGO grade 3 tumors. Similarly, Von Minckwitz et al. (66) examined 161 patients with stage I disease, and confirmed that increased S-phase fractions predicted recurrence and death, and that aneuploidy was independently associated with both decreased overall survival and disease-free survival. Sorbe et al. (69) conducted the largest study using flow cytometry to analyze specimens from 227 patients and also noted elevated S-phase fraction to be an independent prognostic factor. Podratz et al. (68) found an elevated proliferative index to be the most significant predictor of death and recurrence on multivariate analysis. Despite the strong evidence for the usefulness of DNA analysis techniques, given the small size of studies, the lack of agreement over the definition of elevated S-phase, and controversy over whether testing should be performed on paraffin-embedded or fresh-frozen tissue, further investigation needs to be conducted before these indices may be of widespread clinical use.

SURGICAL APPROACHES

Unlike early cervical cancer, patients with EC undergoing surgical treatment with hysterectomy, either alone or combined with radiation, fare significantly better than those treated with radiation alone (70,71). Many different treatment plans have been advocated for the treatment of early stage EC. The Outcomes Task Force of the Society of Gynecologic Oncologists examined patients with endometrial cancer at 11 institutions and noted that 77% of patients underwent total abdominal hysterectomy, 8% radical abdominal hysterectomy, 9% laparoscopic hysterectomy, and 1% vaginal hysterectomy (23). Maggino et al. (22) conducted a survey of 62 gynecologic oncology centers in North America and noted that lymphadenectomy was used routinely in 54% of centers and selectively in another 43%. Radical surgery was performed in 65% of centers for indications such as cervical involvement, and vaginal hysterectomy was employed at 94% for specific clinical indications such as obesity and poor performance status. Currently, total abdominal hysterectomy with bilateral salpingo-oophorectomy remains the standard of treatment, though sometimes combined with radiotherapy, and occasionally, chemotherapy.

After the diagnosis of EC has been established by endometrial biopsy or dilation and curettage, thorough evaluation should be undertaken to assess a patient's suitability for major abdominal surgery. If surgery is deemed appropriate, a standard abdominal staging procedure should include exploratory surgery through an incision sufficient to allow adequate exploration of the abdomen and pelvis, as well as pelvic and para-aortic lymphadenectomy if necessary. After opening, peritoneal washings should be obtained for cytology. Next, a thorough exploration of the peritoneal cavity should be undertaken with biopsy of any suspicious lesions. Some authors have advocated routine biopsy of the omentum. Two series examined a total of 181 patients with clinical stage I disease and found 13 (7.2%) with omental metastases, 9 (69%) of which were occult (72,73). Metastases were associated with papillary serous histology, grade 3 tumors, and deep myometrial invasion. Extra-fascial hysterectomy and bilateral salp-ingo-oophorectomy should be performed after clamping or occluding the fallopian tubes with surgical clips to prevent trans-tubal spillage of cancer cells. It is not necessary to remove the vaginal cuff. The uterus should be opened intra-operatively, away from the surgical site, to determine depth of tumor invasion. Frozen section analysis may be performed by pathology to confirm depth of maximal invasion as well as tumor grade.

Alternatives to traditional abdominal hysterectomy exist. For selected patients at high risk for perioperative complications, vaginal hysterectomy has been employed (74,75). While vaginal hysterec-tomy may afford a low-morbidity approach, the performance of thor-ough peritoneal exploration, peritoneal cytology, bilateral salpingo-oophorectomy, and lymphadenectomy may be precluded. Laparoscopic-assisted vaginal hysterectomy combined with laparo-scopic lymphadenectomy has been suggested in order to overcome these limitations (76). Several investigators have reported shorter hospital stays, and equivalent rates of postoperative complications, lymph node counts, estimated blood loss, recurrence, and survival when compared to abdominal hysterectomy (77–80). For patients with known or suspected cervical involvement, the use of radical hys-terectomy is generally accepted to be safe and effective and may pro-vide an alternative to simple hysterectomy with adjuvant radiation (28,81–83), Boothby et al. (81) reported 5-year survivals to be 68.5%, 36.5%, and 46.1% for stage II patients undergoing surgery only, radi-ation only, or combined radiation and surgery, respectively, though these differences were not statistically significant. Mariani et al. (82) noted that radical hysterectomy alone appeared to be therapeutic in patients with stage II disease and negative nodes, given the absence of recurrence in this group regardless of adjuvant radiation. Five-year recurrence-free survival was 50% for patients treated with sim-ple hysterectomy compared to 71% for radical hysterectomy (p = 0.04) though survival was not significantly different.

After removal of the uterus, the surgeon must determine whether to proceed with lymphadenectomy. Clinical determina-tion of lymph node status is inaccurate. Metastases may be small; Girardi et al. (84) examined lymph node specimens in 76 patients and found that 37% of lymph node metastases were 2 mm or less in diameter. Additionally, lymph node metastases less than 1 cm in size may not be adequately detected with pre-operative magnetic resonance imaging (MRI), computer-assisted tomography (CT), or lymphangiography (85–87). Palpation at the time of surgery is associated with a sensitivity of only 72% (88). Adequate surgical staging is clearly the only way of providing accurate assessment of nodal status. However, concerns for safety exist, particularly in elderly patients or those with co-morbidities affecting functional status. Lymph node sampling has been reported to present significant risk for increased operative time, blood loss, and length of hospital stay. (89) However, the vast majority of studies have shown that the experienced surgeon may safely perform hysterectomy and lymph node dissection safely (90–92), with increases in mean operative time limited to approximately 30 minutes (89, 93). Giannice et al. (94) compared morbidity and mortality in 36 patients over the age of 70 with endometrial and ovarian carcinoma undergoing surgery with lymphadenectomy compared to 72 matched controls undergoing surgery without lymphadenectomy. While mean operative time was increased by about 60 minutes for patients undergoing lymphadenectomy, no significant differences were noted in mean blood loss, transfusion rate, intraoperative complications, ileus, hospital stay, or post-operative complications such as fever, sepsis, infection, thromboembolic events, or cardio-pulmonary problems. The authors concluded that lymphadenectomy was safe in elderly patients without increase in morbidity or mortality.

Though lymphadenectomy is safe and feasible, the benefit of routine use in all patients has been questioned (20,21,84,95,96). However, Kilgore et al. (16) documented a significant survival advantage for patients undergoing multiple-site node sampling. Overall, the 212 patients with multiple sites sampled had a significantly better survival than the 208 patients without sampling and the 205 patients with only limited pelvic sampling ($p = 0.0002$) Both patients designated as low risk (disease confined to the corpus) and high risk (disease spread to the cervix, adnexa, serosa, or washings) appeared to derive a significant survival advantage from multiple-site node sampling (high risk, $p = 0.0006$; low risk, $p = 0.026$).

While some surgeons may advocate routine retroperitoneal dissection for all patients based on the potential therapeutic benefit, most surgeons would advocate lymphadenectomy only in selected patients with risk factors for extrauterine disease. Pelvic and para-aortic lymph node sampling should be performed in all patients with gross extrauterine disease, enlarged lymph nodes, and cervical involvement. Other indications include FIGO grade 3 disease, greater than 50% myometrial invasion, and high risk tumor types such as clear cell and papillary serous histologies. Regardless of grade, tumors confined to the endometrium do not require lymph node sampling because fewer than 1% demonstrate nodal spread (1). Similarly, grade 1 tumors only require sampling when the tumor has invaded to the outer half of the myometrium, since only 3% of patients demonstrate nodal disease (1). A more disputed area remains those patients with grade 2 and 3 tumors with less than 50% myoinvasion. These patients have a 5% or less chance of lymph node metastases (1,25). Retroperitoneal sampling is favored in these patients if any question as to the depth of invasion exists (97). A summary of indications is provided in Table 11.

CONCLUSIONS

About 70–80% of patients with EC present with early stage disease, and for the vast majority of these women, the mainstay of therapy remains hysterectomy and bilateral salpingo-oophorectomy. While vaginal and laparoscopic-assisted routes are also

Table 11 Indications for Lymphadenectomy

- FIGO grade 3 lesions
- FIGO grade 2 lesions demonstrating myometrial invasion
- Greater than 50% myometrial invasion, regardless of FIGO grade
- Clear cell or papillary serous histology
- Cervical involvement
- Enlarged lymph nodes
- Gross extrauterine spread

employed, the abdominal approach remains the current standard. Surgical staging should be performed in all patients, with pelvic and para-aortic lymphadenectomy used for selected patients after a thorough evaluation of each individual's risk factors for poor prognosis. Those with risk factors such as deep myometrial invasion, high grade disease, cervical involvement, and aggressive tumor types such as papillary serous and clear cell histologies should undergo lymph node sampling. Excellent survival rates of 90% may be achieved with surgery; however, those at increased risk for recurrence should be considered for adjuvant radiation or chemotherapy.

REFERENCES

1. Creasman WT, Morrow CP, Bundy BN, Homesley HD, Graham JE, Heller PB. Surgical pathologic spread patterns of endometrial cancer. A Gynecologic Oncology Group Study. *Cancer* 1987; 60:2035–2041.

2. DiSaia PJ, Creasman WT, Boronow RC, Blessing JA. Risk factors and recurrent patterns in stage I endometrial cancer. *Am J Obstet Gynecol* 1985; 151:1009–1015.

3. Greenlee RT, Murray T, Bolden S, Wingo PA. Cancer statistics, 2000. *CA Cancer J Clin* 2000; 50:7–33.

4. Chen SS. Operative treatment in stage I endometrial carcinoma with deep myometrial invasion and/or grade 3 tumor surgically limited to the corpus uteri. No recurrence with only primary surgery. *Cancer* 1989; 63:1843–1845.

5. Frick HC 2nd, Munnell EW, Richart RM, Berger AP, Lawry MF. Carcinoma of the endometrium. *Am J Obstet Gynecol* 1973; 115:663–676.

6. Graham J. The value of preoperative or postoperative treatment by radium for carcinoma of the uterine body. *Surg Gynecol Obstet* 1971; 132:855–860.

7. Kadar N, Malfetano JH, Homesley HD. Determinants of survival of surgically staged patients with endometrial carcinoma histologically confined to the uterus: implications for therapy. *Obstet Gynecol* 1992; 80:655–659.

8. Keller D, Kempson RL, Levine G, McLennan C. Management of the patient with early endometrial carcinoma. *Cancer* 1974; 33:1108–1116.

9. Malkasian GD Jr, Annegers JF, Fountain KS. Carcinoma of the endometrium: stage I. *Am J Obstet Gynecol* 1980; 136:872–888.

10. Annual Report on the Results of Treatment in Gynecologic Cancer: International Federation of Gynecology and Obstetrics. Stockholm: FIGO, 1985.

11. FIGO Stages—1988 Revision. *Gynecol Oncol* 1989; 35:125–127.

12. Chen SS. Extrauterine spread in endometrial carcinoma clinically confined to the uterus. *Gynecol Oncol* 1985; 21:23–31.

13. Pettersson F. Annual report on the results of treatment in gynecological cancer. Vol. 22. Stockholm: International Federation of Gynecology and Obstetrics, 1994.

14. Descamps P, Calais G, Moire C, Bertrand P, Castiel M, Le Floch O, Lansac J, Body G. Predictors of distant recurrence in clinical stage I or II endometrial carcinoma treated by combination surgical and radiation therapy. *Gynecol Oncol* 1997; 64:54–58.

15. Tabernero JM, Alonso MC, Ojeda B, Fuentes J, Balart J, Badia J, Climent MA, Delgado E. Endometrial cancer stages I and II. Analysis of survival and prognostic factors. *Eur J Gynaecol Oncol* 1995; 16:18–25.

16. Kilgore LC, Partridge EE, Alvarez RD, Austin JM, Shingleton HM, Noojin F 3rd, Conner W. Adenocarcinoma of the endometrium: survival comparisons of patients with and without pelvic node sampling. *Gynecol Oncol* 1995; 56:29–33.

17. Mariani A, Webb MJ, Galli L, Podratz KC. Potential therapeutic role of para-aortic lymphadenectomy in node-positive endometrial cancer. *Gynecol Oncol* 2000; 76:348–356.

18. Mohan DS, Samuels MA, Selim MA, Shalodi AD, Ellis RJ, Samuels JR, Yun HJ. Long-term outcomes of therapeutic pelvic lymphadenectomy for stage I endometrial adenocarcinoma. *Gynecol Oncol* 1998; 70:165–171.

19. Petereit DG. Complete surgical staging in endometrial cancer provides prognostic information only. *Semin Radiat Oncol* 2000; 10:8–14.

20. Blythe JG, Hodel KA, Wahl TP, Baglan RJ, Lee FA, Zivnuska FR. Para-aortic node biopsy in cervical and endometrial cancers: does it affect survival? *Am J Obstet Gynecol* 1986; 155:306–314.

21. Corn BW, Lanciano RM, Greven KM, Schultz DJ, Reisinger SA, Stafford PM, Hanks GE. Endometrial cancer with para-aortic adenopathy: patterns of failure and opportunities for cure. *Int J Radiat Oncol Biol Phys* 1992; 24:223–227.

22. Maggino T, Romagnolo C, Landoni F, Sartori E, Zola P, Gadducci A. An analysis of approaches to the management of endometrial cancer in North America: a CTF study. *Gynecol Oncol* 1998; 68:274–279.

23. Kennedy AW, Austin JM Jr, Look KY, Munger CB. The Society of Gynecologic Oncologists Outcomes Task Force. Study of endometrical cancer: initial experiences. *Gynecol Oncol* 2000; 79:379–398.

24. Hendrickson M, Ross J, Eifel PJ, Cox RS, Martinez A, Kempson R. Adenocarcinoma of the endometrium: analysis of 256 cases with carcinoma limited to the uterine corpus. Pathology review and analysis of prognostic variables. *Gynecol Oncol* 1982; 13:373–392.

25. Morrow CP, Bundy BN, Kurman RJ, Creasman WT, Heller P, Homesley HD, Graham JE. Relationship between surgical-pathological risk factors and outcome in clinical stage I and II carcinoma of the endometrium: a Gynecologic Oncology Group study. *Gynecol Oncol* 1991; 40:55–65.

26. Mariani A, Webb MJ, Keeney GL, Aletti G, Podratz KC. Predictors of lymphatic failure in endometrial cancer. *Gynecol Oncol* 2002; 84:437–442.

27. Wilson TO, Podratz KC, Gaffey TA, Malkasian GD, Jr., O'Brien PC, Naessens JM. Evaluation of unfavorable histologic subtypes in endometrial adenocarcinoma. *Am J Obstet Gynecol* 1990; 162:418–423; discussion 423–416.

28. Mannel RS, Berman ML, Walker JL, Manetta A, DiSaia PJ. Management of endometrial cancer with suspected cervical involvement. *Obstet Gynecol* 1990; 75:1016–1022.

29. Lauchlan SC. Tubal (serous) carcinoma of the endometrium. *Arch Pathol Lab Med* 1981; 105:615–618.

30. Sherman ME, Bitterman P, Rosenshein NB, Delgado G, Kurman RJ. Uterine serous carcinoma. A morphologically diverse neoplasm with unifying clinicopathologic features. *Am J Surg Pathol* 1992; 16:600–610.

31. Chambers JT, Merino M, Kohorn EI, Peschel RE, Schwartz PE. Uterine papillary serous carcinoma. *Obstet Gynecol* 1987; 69:109–113.

32. Jeffrey JF, Krepart GV, Lotocki RJ. Papillary serous adenocarcinoma of the endometrium. *Obstet Gynecol* 1986; 67:670–674.

33. Goff BA, Kato D, Schmidt RA, Ek M, Ferry JA, Muntz HG, Cain JM, Tamimi HK, Figge DC, Greer BE. Uterine papillary serous carcinoma: patterns of metastatic spread. *Gynecol Oncol* 1994; 54:264–268.

34. Kurman RJ, Scully RE. Clear cell carcinoma of the endometrium: an analysis of 21 cases. *Cancer* 1976; 37:872–882.

35. Silverberg SG, De Giorgi LS. Clear cell carcinoma of the endometrium. Clinical, pathologic, and ultrastructural findings. *Cancer* 1973; 31:1127–1140.

36. Christopherson WM, Alberhasky RC, Connelly PJ. Carcinoma of the endometrium: I. A clinicopathologic study of clear-cell carcinoma and secretory carcinoma. *Cancer* 1982; 49:1511–1523.

37. Touboul E, Belkacemi Y, Buffat L, Deniaud-Alexandre E, Lefranc JP, Lhuillier P, Uzan S, Jannet D, Uzan M, Antoine M, Huart J, Ganansia V, Milliez J, Blondon J, Housset M, Schlienger M. Adenocarcinoma of the endometrium treated with combined irradiation and surgery: study of 437 patients. *Int J Radiat Oncol Biol Phys* 2001; 50:81–97.

38. Zaino RJ, Kurman R, Herbold D, Gliedman J, Bundy BN, Voet R, Advani H. The significance of squamous differentiation in

endometrial carcinoma. Data from a Gynecologic Oncology Group study. *Cancer* 1991; 68:2293–2302.

39. Phelan C, Montag AG, Rotmensch J, Waggoner SE, Yamada SD, Mundt AJ. Outcome and management of pathological stage I endometrial carcinoma patients with involvement of the lower uterine segment. *Gynecol Oncol* 2001; 83:513–517.

40. Podczaski E, Kaminski P, Gurski K, MacNeill C, Stryker JA, Singapuri K, Hackett TE, Sorosky J, Zaino R. Detection and patterns of treatment failure in 300 consecutive cases of "early" endometrial cancer after primary surgery. *Gynecol Oncol* 1992; 47:323–327.

41. Chambers SK, Kapp DS, Peschel RE, Lawrence R, Merino M, Kohorn EI, Schwartz PE. Prognostic factors and sites of failure in FIGO Stage I, Grade 3 endometrial carcinoma. *Gynecol Oncol* 1987; 27:180–188.

42. Aalders JG, Abeler V, Kolstad P. Recurrent adenocarcinoma of the endometrium: a clinical and histopathological study of 379 patients. *Gynecol Oncol* 1984; 17:85–103.

43. Konski A, Poulter C, Keys H, Rubin P, Beecham J, Doane K. Absence of prognostic significance, peritoneal dissemination and treatment advantage in endometrial cancer patients with positive peritoneal cytology. *Int J Radiat Oncol Biol Phys* 1988; 14:49–55.

44. Lurain JR, Rumsey NK, Schink JC, Wallemark CB, Chmiel JS. Prognostic significance of positive peritoneal cytology in clinical stage I adenocarcinoma of the endometrium. *Obstet Gynecol* 1989; 74:175–179.

45. Yazigi R, Piver MS, Blumenson L. Malignant peritoneal cytology as prognostic indicator in stage I endometrial cancer. *Obstet Gynecol* 1983; 62:359–362.

46. Hirai Y, Fujimoto I, Yamauchi K, Hasumi K, Masubuchi K, Sano Y. Peritoneal fluid cytology and prognosis in patients with endometrial carcinoma. *Obstet Gynecol* 1989; 73:335–338.

47. Tang X, Tanemura K, Ye W, Ohmi K, Tsunematsu R, Yamada T, Katsumata N, Sonoda T. Clinicopathological factors predicting retroperitoneal lymph node metastasis and survival in endometrial cancer. *Jpn J Clin Oncol* 1998; 28:673–678.

48. Turner DA, Gershenson DM, Atkinson N, Sneige N, Wharton AT. The prognostic significance of peritoneal cytology for stage I endometrial cancer. *Obstet Gynecol* 1989; 74:775–780.

49. Harouny VR, Sutton GP, Clark SA, Geisler HE, Stehman FB, Ehrlich CE. The importance of peritoneal cytology in endometrial carcinoma. *Obstet Gynecol* 1988; 72:394–398.

50. Kadar N, Homesley HD, Malfetano JH. Positive peritoneal cytology is an adverse factor in endometrial carcinoma only if there is other evidence of extrauterine disease. *Gynecol Oncol* 1992; 46:145–149.

51. Szpak CA, Creasman WT, Vollmer RT, Johnston WW. Prognostic value of cytologic examination of peritoneal washings in patients with endometrial carcinoma. *Acta Cytol* 1981; 25:640–646.

52. Milosevic MF, Dembo AJ, Thomas GM. The clinical significance of malignant peritoneal cytology in stage I endometrial carcinoma. *Int J Gynecol Cancer* 1992; 2:225–235.

53. Hanson MB, van Nagell JR Jr, Powell DE, Donaldson ES, Gallion H, Merhige M, Pavlik EJ. The prognostic significance of lymph-vascular space invasion in stage I endometrial cancer. *Cancer* 1985; 55:1753–1757.

54. Lindahl B, Einarsdottir M, Iosif C, Ranstam J, Willen R. Endometrial carcinoma: results of primary surgery on FIGO stages Ia-Ic and predictive value of histopathological parameters. *Anticancer Res* 1997; 17:2297–2302.

55. Aalders J, Abeler V, Kolstad P, Onsrud M. Postoperative external irradiation and prognostic parameters in stage I endometrial carcinoma: clinical and histopathologic study of 540 patients. *Obstet Gynecol* 1980; 56:419–427.

56. Ambros RA, Kurman RJ. Identification of patients with stage I uterine endometrioid adenocarcinoma at high risk of recurrence by DNA ploidy, myometrial invasion, and vascular invasion. *Gynecol Oncol* 1992; 45:235–239.

57. Schink JC, Lurain JR, Wallemark CB, Chmiel JS. Tumor size in endometrial cancer: a prognostic factor for lymph node metastasis. *Obstet Gynecol* 1987; 70:216–219.

58. Creasman WT, McCarty KS, Sr., Barton TK, McCarty KS, Jr. Clinical correlates of estrogen- and progesterone-binding proteins in human endometrial adenocarcinoma. *Obstet Gynecol* 1980; 55:363–370.

59. Creasman WT, Soper JT. Assessment of the contemporary management of germ cell malignancies of the ovary. *Am J Obstet Gynecol* 1985; 153:828–834.

60. Liao BS, Twiggs LB, Leung BS, Yu WC, Potish RA, Prem KA. Cytoplasmic estrogen and progesterone receptors as prognostic parameters in primary endometrial carcinoma. *Obstet Gynecol* 1986; 67:463–467.

61. Ehrlich CE, Young PC, Stehman FB, Sutton GP, Alford WM. Steroid receptors and clinical outcome in patients with adenocarcinoma of the endometrium. *Am J Obstet Gynecol* 1988; 158:796–807.

62. Creasman WT, Soper JT, McCarty KS Jr, McCarty KS Sr, Hinshaw W, Clarke-Pearson DL. Influence of cytoplasmic steroid receptor content on prognosis of early stage endometrial carcinoma. *Am J Obstet Gynecol* 1985; 151:922–932.

63. Martin JD, Hahnel R, McCartney AJ, Woodings TL. The effect of estrogen receptor status on survival in patients with endometrial cancer. *Am J Obstet Gynecol* 1983; 147:322–324.

64. Palmer DC, Muir IM, Alexander AI, Cauchi M, Bennett RC, Quinn MA. The prognostic importance of steroid receptors in endometrial carcinoma. *Obstet Gynecol* 1988; 72:388–393.

65. Stendahl U, Wagenius G, Strang P, Tribukait B. Flow cytometry in invasive endometrial carcinoma. Correlations between DNA content S-phase rate and clinical parameters. *In Vivo* 1988; 2:123–127.

66. Von Minckwitz G, Kuhn W, Kaufmann M, Feichter GE, Heep J, Schmid H, Bastert G. Prognostic importance of DNA-ploidy and S-phase fraction in endometrial cancer. *Int J Gynecol Cancer* 1994; 4:250–256.

67. Iversen OE. Flow cytometric deoxyribonucleic acid index: a prognostic factor in endometrial carcinoma. *Am J Obstet Gynecol* 1986; 155:770–776.

68. Podratz KC, Wilson TO, Gaffey TA, Cha SS, Katzmann JA. Deoxyribonucleic acid analysis facilitates the pretreatment identification of high-risk endometrial cancer patients. *Am J Obstet Gynecol* 1993; 168:1206–1213; discussion 1213–1205.

69. Sorbe B, Risberg B, Thornthwaite J. Nuclear morphometry and DNA flow cytometry as prognostic methods for endometrial carcinoma. *Int J Gynecol Cancer* 1994; 4:94–100.

70. Surwit EA, Joelsson I, Einhorn N. Adjunctive radiation therapy in the management of stage I cancer of the endometrium. *Obstet Gynecol* 1981; 58:590–595.

71. Grigsby PW, Perez CA, Camel HM, Kao MS, Galakatos AE. Stage II carcinoma of the endometrium: results of therapy and prognostic factors. *Int J Radiat Oncol Biol Phys* 1985; 11:1915–1923.

72. Chen SS, Spiegel G. Stage I endometrial carcinoma. Role of omental biopsy and omentectomy. *J Reprod Med* 1991; 36:627–629.

73. Saygili U, Kavaz S, Altunyurt S, Uslu T, Koyuncuoglu M, Erten O. Omentectomy, peritoneal biopsy and appendectomy in patients with clinical stage I endometrial carcinoma. *Int J Gynecol Cancer* 2001; 11:471–474.

74. Bloss JD, Berman ML, Bloss LP, Buller RE. Use of vaginal hysterectomy for the management of stage I endometrial cancer in the medically compromised patient. *Gynecol Oncol* 1991; 40:74–77.

75. Scarselli G, Savino L, Ceccherini R, Barciulli F, Massi GB. Role of vaginal surgery in the 1st stage endometrial cancer. Experience of the Florence School. *Eur J Gynaecol Oncol* 1992; 13:15–19.

76. Childers JM, Surwit EA. Combined laparoscopic and vaginal surgery for the management of two cases of stage I endometrial cancer. *Gynecol Oncol* 1992; 45:46–51.

77. Gemignani ML, Curtin JP, Zelmanovich J, Patel DA, Venkatraman E, Barakat RR. Laparoscopic-assisted vaginal hysterectomy for endometrial cancer: clinical outcomes and hospital charges. *Gynecol Oncol* 1999; 73:5–11.

78. Malur S, Possover M, Michels W, Schneider A. Laparoscopic-assisted vaginal versus abdominal surgery in patients with endometrial cancer—a prospective randomized trial. *Gynecol Oncol* 2001; 80:239–244.

79. Scribner DR, Jr., Walker JL, Johnson GA, McMeekin SD, Gold MA, Mannel RS. Surgical management of early-stage endometrial cancer in the elderly: is laparoscopy feasible? *Gynecol Oncol* 2001; 83:563–568.

80. Eltabbakh GH, Shamonki MI, Moody JM, Garafano LL. Laparoscopy as the primary modality for the treatment of women with endometrial carcinoma. *Cancer* 2001; 91:378–387.

81. Boothby RA, Carlson JA, Neiman W, Rubin MM, Morgan MA, Schultz D, Mikuta JJ. Treatment of stage II endometrial carcinoma. *Gynecol Oncol* 1989; 33:204–208.

82. Mariani A, Webb MJ, Keeney GL, Calori G, Podratz KC. Role of wide/radical hysterectomy and pelvic lymph node dissection in endometrial cancer with cervical involvement. *Gynecol Oncol* 2001; 83:72–80.

83. Massi G, Savino L, Susini T. Three classes of radical vaginal hysterectomy for treatment of endometrial and cervical cancer. *Am J Obstet Gynecol* 1996; 175:1576–1585.

84. Girardi F, Petru E, Heydarfadai M, Haas J, Winter R. Pelvic lymphadenectomy in the surgical treatment of endometrial cancer. *Gynecol Oncol* 1993; 49:177–180.

85. Hann LE, Crivello MS. Imaging techniques in the staging of gynecologic malignancy. *Clin Obstet Gynecol* 1986; 29:715–727.

86. King LA, Talledo OE, Gallup DG, el Gammal TA. Computed tomography in evaluation of gynecologic malignancies: a retrospective analysis. *Am J Obstet Gynecol* 1986; 155:960–964.

87. Piver MS, Barlow JJ. Para-aortic lymphadenectomy, aortic node biopsy, and aortic lymphangiography in staging patients with advanced cervical cancer. *Cancer* 1973; 32:367–370.

88. Arango HA, Hoffman MS, Roberts WS, DeCesare SL, Fiorica JV, Drake J. Accuracy of lymph node palpation to determine need for lymphadenectomy in gynecologic malignancies. *Obstet Gynecol* 2000; 95:553–556.

89. Larson DM, Johnson K, Olson KA. Pelvic and para-aortic lymphadenectomy for surgical staging of endometrial cancer: morbidity and mortality. *Obstet Gynecol* 1992; 79:998–1001.

90. Orr JW Jr, Orr PF, Taylor PT. Surgical staging endometrial cancer. *Clin Obstet Gynecol* 1996; 39:656–668.

91. Orr JW. Surgical staging of endometrial cancer: does the patient benefit? *Gynecol Oncol* 1998; 71:335–339.

92. Podratz KC, Mariani A, Webb MJ. Staging and therapeutic value of lymphadenectomy in endometrial cancer. *Gynecol Oncol* 1998; 70:163–164.

93. Fanning J, Firestein S. Prospective trial evaluating morbidity of lymphadenectomy in endometrial cancer (abstract). *Gynecol Oncol* 1996; 60:126.

94. Giannice R, Susini T, Ferrandina G, Poerio A, Margariti PA, Carminati R, Marana E, Mancuso S, Scambia G. Systematic pelvic and aortic lymphadenectomy in elderly gynecologic oncologic patients. *Cancer* 2001; 92:2562–2568.

95. Larson DM, Broste SK, Krawisz BR. Surgery without radiotherapy for primary treatment of endometrial cancer. *Obstet Gynecol* 1998; 91:355–359.

96. Kim YB, Niloff JM. Endometrial carcinoma: analysis of recurrence in patients treated with a strategy minimizing lymph node sampling and radiation therapy. *Obstet Gynecol* 1993; 82:175–180.

97. Barakat RR, Grigsby PW, Sabbatini P, Zaino RJ. Corpus: Epithelial Tumors. In: Hoskins WJ, Perez CA, Young RC, eds. *Principles and Practice of Gynecologic Oncology*. Philadelphia: Lippincott Williams and Wilkins, 2000:919–959.

98. Vardi JR, Tadros GH, Anselmo MT, Rafla SD. The value of exploratory laparotomy in patients with endometrial carcinoma according to the new International Federation of Gynecology and Obstetrics staging. *Obstet Gynecol* 1992; 80:204–208.

99. Petersen RW, Quinlivan JA, Casper GR, Nicklin JL. Endometrial adenocarcinoma—presenting pathology is a poor guide to surgical management. *Aust N Z J Obstet Gynaecol* 2000; 40:191–194.

100. Genest P, Drouin P, Gerig L, Girard A, Stewart D, Prefontaine M. Prognostic factors in early carcinoma of the endometrium. *Am J Clin Oncol* 1987; 10:71–77.

101. Mundt AJ, McBride R, Rotmensch J, Waggoner SE, Yamada SD, Connell PP. Significant pelvic recurrence in high-risk pathologic stage I—IV endometrial carcinoma patients after adjuvant chemotherapy alone: implications for adjuvant radiation therapy. *Int J Radiat Oncol Biol Phys* 2001; 50:1145–1153.

102. Straughn JM Jr., Huh WK, Kelly FJ, Leath CA 3rd, Kleinberg MJ, Hyde J Jr., Numnum TM, Zhang Y, Soong SJ, Austin JM Jr., Partridge EE, Kilgore LC, Alvarez RD. Conservative management of stage I endometrial carcinoma after surgical staging. *Gynecol Oncol* 2002; 84:194–200.

103. Boronow RC, Morrow CP, Creasman WT, Disaia PJ, Silverberg SG, Miller A, Blessing JA. Surgical staging in endometrial cancer: clinical-pathologic findings of a prospective study. *Obstet Gynecol* 1984; 63:825–832.

104. Morrow CP, Di Saia PJ, Townsend DE. Current management of endometrial carcinoma. *Obstet Gynecol* 1973; 42:399–406.

105. Creasman WT, Rutledge F. The prognostic value of peritoneal cytology in gynecologic malignant disease. *Am J Obstet Gynecol* 1971; 110:773–781.

106. Zuna RE, Behrens A. Peritoneal washing cytology in gynecologic cancers: long-term follow-up of 355 patients. *J Natl Cancer Inst* 1996; 88:980–987.

10

The Role of Laparoscopy in the Management of Endometrial Cancer

JOAN L. WALKER AND ROBERT S. MANNEL

University of Oklahoma, Oklahoma City,
Oklahoma, U.S.A.

This chapter is dedicated to a pioneer of laparoscopic surgery in gynecologic oncology who tragically died in a motorcycle accident on Valentine's Day, Joel Childers (1955–2002).

DEMAND FOR LAPAROSCOPIC SURGERY

The public demand for minimally invasive surgical approaches exists in the community, as evidenced by the acceptance of the laparoscopic approach for cholecystectomy, adnexal surgery, and hysterectomy. Many surgeons are finding themselves in a competitive environment where they are perceived as inferior if they are not "keeping up" with these advances (36). Hopkins (37) wrote a thorough critique of laparoscopic surgery that he documents some of the controversies and myths, which he believes are communicated by advocates of the procedures. His major objections are the potential dissemination of cancer cells and the inability to utilize all of the surgeon's senses during the operation, especially the sense of touch. Academic caution has been exemplified by authors like David Grimes, in his review "Frontiers of operative laparoscopy: A review and critique of the evidence" (30). He concludes with the statement "Mechanisms are urgently needed to evaluate surgical innovations in gynecology with the same degree of rigor currently afforded medical innovations." The Gynecologic Oncology Group met this challenge and opened the randomized trial comparing laparotomy to laparoscopy for the surgical treatment and staging of endometrial cancer (EC). The goal is to validate the efficacy and safety of this innovative technique to surgically treat this disease. The study has enrolled over 1000 women, with two-thirds initially approached laparoscopically. The authors endorse the plea of Drs. Grimes and Hopkins—that gynecologic oncologists should enroll all women interested in the laparoscopic approach for the treatment of EC in this prospective trial until data are available to generalize this approach to standard community practice. Clinical Outcomes of Surgical Therapy (COST) Study Group (78) has published the short-term, quality-of-life outcomes for their randomized trial comparing laparoscopic approach to open colectomy for colon cancer. They reveal disappointing results; laparoscopy was only able to affect the hospitalized pain medication requirements and the 2-week post-surgery global rating scale. There was no difference at the 2-month time point. The length of stay was 6.4 days for the open technique, 5.6 days for those assigned to laparoscopy, and 5.1 days for those who successfully completed the laparoscopic approach. They document that 74% of the attempted laparoscopic procedures were completed without conversion to laparotomy. The associated editorials (51) ask why are we considering this an advance in surgical technique if there is no quantifiable quality of life or cost benefit? This may be the wrong operation to utilize the laparoscopic technique since the prolonged ileus of colon resection cannot be easily overcome by laparoscopic techniques. The survival and sites for recurrence of colon cancer treated in this clinical trial will be reported at a later date.

The length of stay and quality of life advantage should be more dramatic for laparoscopic treatment of EC due to the fact that the bowel is not directly manipulated by the surgeon, and discharge should not be delayed by ileus as seen in colectomy. The expectation is that the length of stay could be as short as 1–2 days for laparoscopy compared to 4 days for the open techniques. The largest abdominal incision to accomplish the laparoscopic approach should be 1 inch for EC rather than the 6 cm needed for colectomy for the treatment of colon cancer.

Historical Perspective: The Development of the Laparoscopic Approach

The Gynecologic Oncology Group (GOG) performed a surgical–pathologic study documenting the frequency and sites of metastatic disease in women with EC who were clinical stage I or II. This landmark surgical staging protocol was published by Creasman et al. in 1987 (17), and the survival outcomes and sites of recurrence were published by Morrow et al. in 1991 (45). The surgical staging procedure was standardized to include washings of the pelvis for cytology, and dissection of the para-aortic lymph nodes and bilateral pelvic lymph nodes including the obturator, external iliac, internal iliac and common iliac, lymph nodes. The para-aortic lymph nodes were described as "nodes, which are along the common iliac artery proximal to the midpoint and overlying the vena cava and aorta" (17). In retrospect it is believed that patients were less likely to have left para-aortic lymph nodes evaluated on this protocol than patients surgically staged today. The dissection was also not likely to extend to the insertion of the ovarian vein into the vena cava on the right or renal vein on the left. They found that 9% of women had positive pelvic nodes and 6% had nodes from the para-aortic sampling demonstrating metastasis, and that nodal metastasis strongly predicated outcome. The characteristics of the primary tumor, which pre-dicted outcome, included histologic cell type, grade, and depth of invasion and these were correlated with the risk of nodal spread and survival. There was not any standardized adju-vant treatment prescribed during this study. The treating physician individualized treatment protocol for the patient. The lowest risk group was defined as women with grade 1 endometrioid cell type and less than 66% invasion, grade 2 with less than 33% invasion, and grade 3 with no invasion. It was suggested that performing lymph node evaluation on these women would not be of much value, even though they documented the risk of the procedure to be low. Based on these data, many gynecologic oncologists have adapted an algorithm to perform lymphadenectomy only on women with a frozen section diagnosis of intermediate- or high-risk factors for metastatic disease. The FIGO (International Federation of Obstetrics and Gynecology) staging for EC was also changed to a surgical staging system as a result of the above data. FIGO simplified the results to stage IA (endometrium only), IB (inner-half myometrial invasion), and IC (outer-half myometrial invasion).

Since these publications three controversies have arisen:

1. Should lymphadenectomy be performed in all women with EC to yield accurate staging and possibly improve survival, or should we select women who may be at increased risk of metastasis based on the histology of the endometrial biopsy and a frozen sec-tion at the time of surgery?
2. Should bilateral para-aortic lymphadenectomy be performed on all patients where the decision to per-form pelvic lymphadenectomy has been made?
3. Is there therapeutic value to the lymphadenectomy itself, or is it only prognostic, therefore beneficial only due to the improved ability to tailor adjuvant therapy?

Current surgical management of EC must take into con-sideration the issues outlined in these controversies. These three controversies are independent of the operative approach to this disease chosen by the surgeon although the development of the laparoscopic technique brought these controversies to the forefront.

Improvement of laparoscopic equipment in the early 1990s led to the ability to perform surgical staging utilizing the minimally invasive laparoscopic approach. Childers and Surwit (11) reported in 1992 on the use of laparoscopy for surgical treatment of EC, setting into motion an increased level of interest in the development of the techniques to accomplish an equivalent or superior result compared to laparotomy. Laparoscopic lymphadenectomy originally included only the right para-aortic lymph nodes when reported by Childers et al. in 1993 (12). Criticism arose from other investigators that the technique needed to be expanded to include the left para-aortic in order to make this procedure an acceptable and equivalent technique. Flanagan et al. documented that there was an equal distribution of metastasis to the left para-aortic lymph nodes in EC and concluded that accurate surgical staging for gynecologic malignancies must include bilateral pelvic and para-aortic lymphadenectomy (23). Subsequent to this debate, Childers et al. published a successful technique for left-sided para-aortic lymphadenectomy (13).

Childers and the Gynecologic Oncology Committee of the GOG worked together to establish a prospective trial to document surgical competence for laparoscopic surgical staging for EC (GOG LAP 1). The subsequent GOG protocol (GOG LAP 2) was a randomized prospective clinical trial designed to document the safety and adequacy of the laparoscopic surgical approach compared to traditional laparotomy. Training for gynecologic oncologists employing laparoscopic surgical staging of EC was organized by the Society of Gynecologic Oncology (SGO) and industry sponsors to promote the minimally invasive approach to gynecologic cancers. Subsequent to the opening of the LAP 2 study, its objectives were changed to include the long-term follow-up of these women to identify sites of recurrent disease, progression-free survival, and overall survival rates. The target enrollment is 2200 women, where 2 out of 3 will undergo the laparoscopic approach. This study should be completed in 2005.

SURGICAL TECHNIQUES FOR LAPAROSCOPIC TREATMENT OF ENDOMETRIAL CANCER

LAVH/BSO

The traditional surgical approach to EC has been total abdominal hysterectomy bilateral salpingo-oophorectomy with peritoneal cytology, which is the current community standard of care as documented by Partridge in his review for the American College of Surgeons, Commission on Cancer. This was the surgical procedure performed on 80% of American women with EC (50). Few women currently undergo thorough surgical staging. Transvaginal hysterectomy, bilateral salpingo-oophorectomy is an accepted technique in the United States in women with medical co-morbidities or morbid obesity (5). The limitations of the transvaginal approach when compared to the abdominal approach include: 1) inability to complete the bilateral salpingo-oophorectomy in some patients; 2) failure to inspect the peritoneal cavity or the retroperitoneum for metastatic disease; and 3) failure to perform peritoneal cytology. The addition of laparoscopy to the vaginal hysterectomy overcame many of the aforementioned limitations; however, laparoscopically assisted vaginal hysterectomy bilateral salpingo-oophorectomy (LAVH/BSO) has it own learning curve and complications unrelated to a cancer diagnosis (1,2,32). Current studies now show that LAVH/BSO allows for a shorter hospital stay (1 to 2 days) and a more rapid return to normal activities than the traditional laparotomy approach. Concerns still exist that metastatic disease can be missed using the laparoscopic approach due to the inability to palpate and inspect the entire abdominal cavity.

Pelvic Lymphadenectomy

The surgical technique for laparoscopic pelvic lymphadenectomy was developed by both urology and gynecologic oncology simultaneously. The fact that it could be done was established in the early 1990s, but the answer whether it *should* be done has remained controversial. Cervix cancer was the first obvious use for the technique because of the use of radiation for primary treatment of this disease and the uncertain extent of the field, which should be irradiated in the absence of surgical staging. The combination of laparoscopic surgical staging and radiation therapy was potentially safer with fewer bowel adhesions and radiation induced bowel injuries (24). Querleu et al. were the first to report pelvic lymphadenectomy for cervix cancer in 1991 (54); Nezhat reported in 1992 the use of laparoscopic pelvic and para-aortic lymphadenectomy with radical hysterectomy in cervix cancer (48).

The use of pelvic lymphadenectomy for EC was begun by many surgeons simultaneously, but most actively promoted for use by Childers in 1992 (11). Subsequently many investigators documented the safety and adequacy of laparoscopic pelvic lymphadenectomy for EC. The adoption of this technique was limited due to an increasing body of literature documenting the frequency of metastasis to para-aortic lymph nodes in women with EC. Multiple reports demonstrated similar node counts for open and laparoscopic technique in the surgical staging of endometrial cancer (6,29). Possover et al. reporting on 150 patients undergoing pelvic and para-aortic lymphadenectomy, demonstrated the adequacy of lymph node counts utilizing the laparoscopic procedure. The average pelvic lymph node count was 26 per patient and ranged between 10 and 56 (53). Spirtos et al. (70) documented 40 women who his group attempted to stage surgically, limiting the size to a quintalet (BMI = height in meters^2 divided by weight in kg) of 30. Thirty-five completed the procedure and 2 of those failed to have left para-aortic nodes sampled resulting in an 82.5% success rate in a relatively thin group of women. The node count was 12–42 with 27.7 being the average nodes per patient, and 20.8 pelvic nodes (11 right, 9.8 left). There were an average of 7.9 aortic nodes (3.8 right, 4.1 left). Two patients had microscopically positive lymph nodes—one only pelvic, the other both pelvic and para-aortic

Para-aortic Lymphadenectomy

The laparoscopic right para-aortic lymphadenectomy was introduced for the management of EC by Childers and

Surwit (11) utilizing a transperitoneal approach. This procedure initiated the dissection by incising the peritoneum over the right common iliac artery to gain access to the retroperitoneum. The limits of the dissection were from the halfway point between the bifurcation of the aorta and the origin of the internal iliac artery, and the proximal extent was the renal vein, the duodenum, or the inferior mesenteric artery. The precaval nodes and right para-aortic nodes could be easily resected with the boundaries being the right ureter, genitofemoral nerve, and psoas muscle laterally, and the aorta medially. Presentation of this technique at the Western Association of Gynecologic Oncologists created controversy since the left sided para-aortic lymph nodes were not being removed. Data on lymph node metastasis rates by site were subsequently presented making it clear that the left para-aortic was equally important (25). McMeekin subsequently reported on 607 endometrial cancer patients where 47 were identified as having FIGO stage IIIC disease (44). Stage IIIC disease was defined by positive pelvic lymph nodes alone in 43%, positive pelvic and para-aortic metastasis in 40%, and positive para-aortic disease alone in 17%. This report concluded that the status of para-aortic lymph nodes cannot be reliably predicted based on negative pelvic lymph nodes, and the left side nodes were equally important to those on the right side.

In response to the debate over location of EC nodal metastasis, Childers et al. (13) developed a technique for left-sided para-aortic lymphadenectomy with successful results in 12 women. Querleu et al. (54) reported on four women, two of whom had ovarian cancer. Subsequently numerous surgeons reported on their experience with this procedure.

The left-sided technique was initially described as elevating the inferior mesenteric artery and dissecting left of the aorta and left common iliac only in the caudad direction. Elevation of the inferior mesenteric artery, with careful identification of the ovarian artery and vein as well as the ureter, did allow for left-sided dissection. The boundaries of the procedure were the inferior mesenteric artery cephalad, left ureter and psoas laterally, and the same distal margin.

There are others who continue cephalad up to the renal vessels from the midline, transperitoneal approach. This technique involves the mobilization of the duodenum off of the aorta and retracting it cephalad, then dissecting laterally over to the psoas and above and around the inferior mesenteric vessel as well as cephalad to the renal vessels. The ovarian vessels are encountered and can be sacrificed to aid in this dissection. Hemoclips can be used on the ovarian artery at its origin on the aorta. Most surgeons do not sacrifice the inferior mesenteric artery intentionally. The ureter and renal vessels must be protected from injury during this dissection.

The lateral approach is also described reflecting the descending colon and sigmoid medially, but this is difficult in an obese EC patient. The left common iliac nodes are approached by this technique and carried as far cephalad as technically feasible. Care must be taken to prevent bleeding from the vessels to the psoas and the vertebral veins.

Another technique advocated by Querleu et al. (54) is the retroperitoneal left-sided approach. This technique insufflates the retroperitoneum from just above and medial to the anterior superior iliac spine through a small 1–2 cm incision through the skin and fascia, with development of the retroperitoneal space initially with the surgeon's finger. Observation of the dissection with an umbilical laparoscope aids the successful dissection of the correct planes. The left common, para-aortic dissection can be more easily accomplished using this technique and is especially advantageous in the obese patient. They recommend conversion to the transperitoneal approach to complete the right para-aortic and pelvic lymphadenectomy.

The adequacy of the pelvic and para-aortic lympadenectomy has been documented by Scribner et al (62) in 103 patients, showing the average para-aortic lymph node count by laparoscopic technique to be 6.8, matching the open technique, which is 6.8 also. The pelvic lymph node counts were 18 and 17.3, respectively.

CURRENT TREATMENT ALGORITHMS UTILIZING LAPAROSCOPY IN EC

The majority of women in the United States currently undergoing total abdominal hysterectomy bilateral salpingo-oophorectomy with peritoneal cytology could be managed with a minimally invasive alternative. The multiple treatment algorithms currently utilized for open surgical staging can be adopted utilizing laparoscopic techniques. Four examples are listed below.

1. Laparoscopic surgical staging for all women with EC who are appropriate surgical candidates.
2. Laparoscopic hysterectomy, bilateral salpingooophorectomy with peritoneal cytology can be completed, and then the pathologist evaluates the surgical specimen for depth of invasion, grade of tumor, and cervical involvement. Intraperitoneal disease would be cause for conversion to laparotomy, debulking of disease and thorough surgical staging. Patients with grade 1 endometriod adenocarcinoma and less than 50% myometrial invasion may not require lymphadenectomy. All others would proceed to thorough laparoscopic surgical staging (49).
3. Laparoscopic hysterectomy with bilateral salpingo-oophorectomy and peritoneal cytology by the general obstetrician-gynecologist. Referral of women with high risk factors to gynecologic oncologists for restaging (35).
4. Vaginal hysterectomy alone for women with major health problems.

Surgeons can modify these algorithms to meet their community standards.

SURGICAL CANDIDATE SELECTION

Laparoscopic surgery can be limited by surgical experience, obesity, age, and co-morbidities. Contraindications include pelvic kidney, previous retroperitoneal surgery, pelvic radiation therapy, and a uterus that is too large to be removed intact transvaginally. The same medical contraindications to laparotomy and abdominal hysterectomy apply to laparoscopic surgical staging, since laparotomy may be required.

Obesity

Obesity is the most common co-morbidity in EC patients since the secondary effect of obesity is estrogen excess. The etiologic pathway of Type I endometrioid adenocarcinoma may involve the unopposed estrogen additive effects of anovulation and obesity. Obesity is therefore the most common patient related limitation on the successful completion of a laparoscopic surgical procedure. Unfortunately, obesity is increasing in the U.S. population, and will undoubtedly cause an increase in EC.

Childers et al. (13) reported that obesity prevented the completion of 5 out of 61 attempted laparoscopic para-aortic lymphadenectomy procedures. He reported that 180 pounds was the point at which poor exposure hindered the surgeon. Steep Trendelenberg, placement of the bowel into the upper abdomen, and peritoneal tenting were the major techniques to gain access to the para-aortic region. The use of laparoscopic retractors and more than four ports may allow surgery on heavier patients. Most authors limited their surgical candidates to 180 pounds or BMI index of ≤ 30 after this report.

Spirtos et al. (70) excluded women with BMI index (weight in kg/height in meters^2) of greater than 30 in his series of 40 patients published in 1995 where he demonstrated thorough left para-aortic lymphadenectomy. Five of the procedures could not be completed laparoscopically; two were opened for bleeding, two for intraperitoneal tumor spread, and one for equipment failure. He used shoulder braces to improve visualization using steep Trendelenburg without patients sliding down the table.

Ettabbakh et al. (22) reported on 42 obese women (BMI ≥ 28; mean, 35.8) managed laparoscopically for their EC. Though 93% underwent a successful pelvic lymphadenectomy, only 17% had completed the para-aortic procedure. Recently

Scribner et al. (62) reported on 55 patients with BMI of ≥ 28 (mean of 40) who underwent a planned laparoscopic pelvic and para-aortic lymphadenectomy. Complete staging was successful laparoscopically in 64% of the cases, with obesity the cause of the conversion to laparotomy in 24%. Morbid obesity (BMI ≥ 35) was associated with a 44% success compared to 82% success when BMI was between 28 and 35. Compared to a similar laparotomy group, the laparoscopy patients had a shorter length of stay, fewer postoperative fevers, and a shorter postoperative ileus. There was an increase in operating room time. The authors conclude that obesity should not be a *contraindication* to a planned laparoscopy.

Elderly

The elderly require careful attention to the risks and benefits of any cancer treatment. The elderly population is growing both in numbers and in proportion to the general population. In the 1980s approximately 11% of the population were 65 years of age and older. It is predicted that by 2005 this group will approach 25% of the female population. The elderly are more likely to have medical co-morbidities, and are at higher risk of cardiac and pulmonary complications. Patients in this age group have tremendous fear of the diagnosis of cancer and the potential consequences major surgery may have on their quality of life and independence. These women may not be able to return home after major surgery since they are often widowed and living alone. Part of the surgeon's responsibility during the preoperative evaluation is to understand the physical and social consequences that surgical treatment may have on the living situation of the often-fragile elderly woman. Social support must be arranged to deal with the disability caused by the treatment choices. Compromises in surgical treatment are often made in the elderly cancer population in order to cope with the medical co-morbidities, physical limitations, and social support available (5). Laparoscopy may be the optimal choice in the elderly for this reason.

EC is one of the most common malignancies in the elderly with a median age of 63.1 years at the time of diagnosis.

It has been demonstrated that with traditional surgery, elderly patients are at a higher risk of postoperative complications, longer hospital stays, and increased risk of loss of independence after surgery. In a study of 125 patients ≥ 65 years of age, Scribner et al. (60) retrospectively compared surgical managements and identified a significantly decreased length of stay, fewer fevers, less postoperative ileus, and fewer wound infections with laparoscopy. Laparoscopically assisted vaginal hysterectomy, bilateral salpingo-oophorectomy and pelvic and para-aortic lymphadenectomy was successfully completed in 78% of the elderly women where it was attempted. Obesity was the major reason for failure to complete the procedure laparoscopically. Age was not a factor for laparoscopic success or failure, but there were women with significant co-morbid conditions where vaginal hysterectomy alone was preferentially performed.

Bloss et al. (5) reported on the use of transvaginal hysterectomy alone in this population to help avoid major complications and loss of independence. Reasons for avoiding laparotomy are listed as obesity (87%), hypertension (58%), diabetes mellitus (35%), and cardiovascular diseases (26%). Those authors prescribed postoperative radiation therapy to 35% of the patients due to a lack of surgical staging information, and only 35% of the adnexa were successfully removed.

The potential benefit of laparoscopic surgical staging in the elderly has been reported by Scribner et al. (60). He compared three surgical approaches for the treatment of endometrial cancer in the elderly. The transvaginal hysterectomy group (n = 13) had an average age of 77 years and the median length of hospital stay was 2.1 days. The average weight of this group was 96 kg. The laparoscopically surgical staged group (n = 67) had a mean weight of 75.4 kg and the postoperative stay increased to a median of 3 days. This is compared to the traditional open laparotomy (n = 45) for surgical staging having a mean weight of 74 kg and a median length of stay of 5 days. The major issue in the elderly is that they have poor mental and physiologic reserve, and the consequences of complications can be tragic. Two deaths occurred in the laparoscopy group both of which were unrelated to the surgical staging of EC. The insertion of the trocar at the beginning of the procedure lacerated the hypogastric vein causing hemorrhage, which was difficult to control even after laparotomy. The second was a lateral 12 mm trocar site in a morbidly obese woman that herniated a loop of small bowel. She was admitted and operated on again for a small bowel obstruction, but later died of a pulmonary embolus. The use of laparoscopy in gynecology, unfortunately, has demonstrated how important training and experience are to reduce trocar complications. Some authors advocate the "open" trocar insertion technique to avoid bowel and vessel injuries, and the use of only 5 mm trocars in the lateral location to avoid hernias. Larger trocars should be kept in the midline, where the fascia is easier to successfully close.

TRAINING

Surgical training of gynecologic oncologists in this country does not always include laparoscopic surgery for EC. Several studies have shown that surgical training including animal laboratory practice, laparoscopic simulators, and workshops can improve surgeon performance and outcomes.

Eltabbakh et al. (22) reported on 75 consecutive women with clinical stage 1 EC that underwent laparoscopic surgical staging and documented a significant decrease in operative time from a mean of 3 hours and 51 minutes for the first 25 patients, and 1 hour and 48 minutes for the last 25. There was a significant increase in node count from 7.8 to 11.9 with experience. There was no difference in estimated blood loss, rate of conversion to laparotomy, complications, and length of stay. Operative time is dependent on the experience of the surgeon and tends to go down as numbers of cases increases. The average operative time reported by Spirtos et al. (70) in the first 15 cases was 3 hours and 13 minutes and fell to 2 hours and 26 minutes in the last 25 cases. Dottino et al. (19) also documented increasing node counts with experience.

POTENTIAL BENEFITS OF LAPAROSCOPIC SURGERY

Decrease in Wound Disruption and Infection

Scribner et al. (62) found a decreased wound complication rate with laparoscopic surgical techniques. Soper et al. documented an 11.3% incidence of wound infections in women undergoing abdominal hysterectomy (68). Depth of subcutaneous tissue was the strongest independent predictor of infection. This complication contributed to fevers and longer hospital stay. Women with subcutaneous tissue depth of > 6 cm had a 40% probability of wound infections. They were unable to suggest an appropriate intervention. The use of laparoscopic techniques may assist in preventing this outcome. Gallup et al. performed a randomized trial of standard wound closure versus closed suction drain technique in the obese population (27). The women with drains had a 20% wound complication rate compared to 31% without a drain ($p = 0.09$). Prophylactic antibiotics were given to 46% of the drain group and 51% of those without a drain.

Decrease in Adhesion Formation

Chen et al. demonstrated decrease in adhesion formation in a porcine model in 1998. They performed 40 extraperitoneal lymphadenectomies and 40 laparoscopic lymphadenectomies with peritoneal incisions overlying the vessels and 10 with the traditional laparotomy technique used in EC surgery. The adhesion rate was 100% in the laparotomy cases, 30% in the laparoscopy cases, and 21% in the extraperitoneal cases. This benefit could decrease long-term complications, especially in women requiring postoperative radiation therapy.

Decreased Hospital Stay

A randomized trial of 70 patients performed in Germany by Malur demonstrated similar complication rates and faster return of bowel function. Yet their hospital stays were excessive by U.S. standards (8.6–11.7 days). The only recurrence in the laparoscopy group was in the brain (43).

Gemignani et al. (29) reported on laparoscopically assisted vaginal hysterectomy for EC with an average length of stay of 2.0 days compared to 6.0 days for TAH/BSO. Room charges were significantly lower for the procedure ($3130 versus $6960) as well were the total charges ($11,826 versus $15,189).

Patient Satisfaction

The known patient demand for minimally invasive surgical techniques needs to be evaluated in a prospective fashion to determine the true quality-of-life benefit. The data available from the laparoscopic treatment of colon cancer are not encouraging, with only a minimal pain reduction at the 2-week time point only. Quality of life is a major endpoint of the GOG randomized clinical trial, which will prove very informative when data are made available. Length of stay is the only surrogate we have at this time and that indicates recovery will be improved for the laparoscopic group. The average hospital stay reported by Spirtos was 2.7 days with a range of 1 to 6 (71). The first 15 patients stayed 2.8 days and the last 20 stayed 2.4 days, with a range of 0.5 to 4.5.

Cost Containment

Cost effectiveness could be a benefit of laparoscopic surgical staging. Length of stay, operating room time, and instrument costs remain the three major sources of cost in the comparison of laparotomy and laparoscopy in the surgical treatment and staging of EC. Laparoscopic surgery can be very expensive if surgeons choose to use disposable instruments and the most recent technology. The choices are many, including robotics, argon beam, harmonic scalpel, surgical stapling devices, and other disposable instruments. Some surgeons utilize all reusable equipment and unipolar cautery and thus achieve similar success with minimal cost over laparotomy. The cost of the laparoscopic procedure will go down as the institution and the surgeon gain experience and the number of completed cases rises.

Evidence suggests that there would be a cost savings, along with a survival benefit, if a gynecologic oncologist surgically staged all EC cases. This savings may double if laparoscopic surgery proves safe and cost effective. The savings would come from the elimination of re-operation to surgically stage women who want to avoid radiation therapy, yet were found to have unexpected risk factors for metastatic disease on the final pathology review after simple hysterectomy. Savings would also come from an estimated 25% reduction in the need for adjuvant radiation therapy in women who choose not to be restaged for uterine high risk factors, and are of unknown stage.

COMPLICATIONS OF LAPAROSCOPY

Complications of laparoscopic surgery for EC can be divided into two broad categories: those that occur with laparoscopy in general, and those that are related to the specific staging surgery performed for cancer. The complications of laparoscopy are well defined in the literature when used for other conditions and these are mainly trocar insertion injuries, hernias, bowel complications, and urinary tract complications. The overall rates reported range from 0.22% for reproductive endocrinologists to 10% for organ removal by gynecologists. The Finnish gynecologists report 0.4% major complications (12.6/1000 cases) with operative laparoscopy, and 42% of the complications occurred with LAVH. The injuries were 48% ureteral, 19% bladder, 13% intestinal, 7% incisional hernias, and 2% large vessel injury (32). Electrosurgical injury usually occurs in the small bowel at the rate of 2.5/1000. In a series of 100 consecutive patients undergoing planned laparoscopic pelvic and para-aortic lymphadenectomy, Scribner (62) reported reasons for conversion to laparotomy including obesity (12%), intraperitoneal disease (5%), intraabdominal adhesions (5%), bleeding (4%), and urinary tract injury (1%). Complications relating only to the laparoscopic lymphadenectomy itself are very rare. Vascular injury requiring laparotomy has been reported to range from 0.5–5%.

Vascular lacerations also occur in the open procedures. This can be managed with the surgeon's digit holding pressure over the injury in the majority of cases of vena cava bleeding from small perforating vessels. Laparoscopically, bleeding can readily hamper the visualization of the operative field. Many surgeons place a sponge in the abdomen during the dissection to allow for rapid compression of a vessel laceration. Childers et al. (12) reported having to open 1 patient out of 57 for hemorrhage. Spirtos et al. (70) reported 2 patients out of 40 requiring laparotomy to control bleeding. One case involved a venous perforator arising from the vena cava, that could not be controlled laparoscopically, and the other, a perforator from a right iliac vessel (accessory obturator), that required laparotomy. Two patients also had inadequate left para-aortic lymph node sampling but did not undergo laparotomy for completion of the procedure.

The sites of venous injury appear to be the anterior perforators from the vena cava, the vessels that are located at the bifurcation of the common iliac and run laterally to the psoas muscle, as well as the accessory obturator vein which runs off the inferior aspect of the external iliac vein distally. Care must be taken when dissecting the lymph nodes in these areas to avoid tearing the major veins, leading to difficulty controlling the hemorrhage. Catastrophic hemorrhage is not usually encountered under direct visualization during surgical dissection; it is with blind trocar insertion that this problem is more likely to occur.

The ureter must be visualized during the lymphadenectomy throughout its course to avoid injury. The right ureter is generally easy to identify and retract laterally during the para-aortic lymphadenectomy. The left is more challenging and care must be taken to locate the ureter and psoas muscle in order to identify the margins for resection of lymphatic tissue. The ureter and the inferior mesenteric artery should be elevated to separate it from the nodal bundle. The most frequently reported laparoscopic urinary tract injury is cystostomy when dissecting the bladder from the cervix. This is evident when the Foley bag fills up with gas. Some authors recommend avoiding this dissection from above, and prefer the vaginal approach.

The unusual complication of laparoscopic surgical treatment of EC is the retention of carbon dioxide identified by the anesthesiologists during the procedures. This can be occurring due to subcutaneous emphysema when the CO_2 migrates out of the abdomen into the abdominal wall or through retroperitoneal spaces. The direct puncture technique helps decrease this problem as well as limiting intraabdominal pressures. There can also be small holes in the veins, which allow CO_2 to embolize into the venous system. The procedure must be converted to laparotomy when this complication is observed.

Extreme Trendelenburg for a long period of time does cause edema of the face, which is worrisome to the patient and family, so they should be alerted to this outcome ahead of time. It usually resolves within 24 hours. Sometimes ventilation pressures also rise, causing conversion to laparotomy.

Bowel herniation into trocar sites after operative laparoscopy is a known complication. Boike et al. (7) reported on 19 patients with 21 bowel herniation, which were identified at 11 institutions. The average age was 50.5 (41–75) years. The operative procedures included LAVH (6), LAVH plus lymphadenectomy (5), oophorectomy (2), adhesiolysis (2), myomectomy (2), lymphadenectomy alone (1), and ovarian cystectomy (1). Two patients had incisional herniation simultaneously at two port sites. Average time until reoperation was 8.5 (2–45) days from the preceding procedure. The port size was 12 mm in 57%, 10 mm in 38%, and one with an 11 mm port size. Fascial screws were used in 57%. An attempt to close the fascia was made in 43% of the cases. The location of the port was extraumbilical in 76% of the cases. There were 5 cases at the umbilicus. The bowel involved was small bowel in 18, cecum in 2, and ascending colon in 1. CT scan made the diagnosis in 8, clinical exam in 6, upper gastrointestinal series in 3 of the cases. The incidence was estimated at one of the institutions to be 1% These authors give guidance for prevention of this complication: wherever possible use 5 mm trocars; avoid fascial screws; use a 12 mm port midline suprapubically if a large second trocar is required; closure of the fascial defect is required for large port sites. Devices available to perform fascial closure when the fascia cannot be visualized include: Grice suture needle (Ideas for Medicine, Clearwater, Flordia), Carter-Thomason needlepoint suture passer (Advanced Surgical Education, San Clemente, California), and the EndoClose instrument (United States Surgical Corp, Norwalk, Connecticut).

Early identification of bowel injury requires a high degree of suspicion when there is a slow return of bowel function or intermittent nausea and vomiting. These injuries can be from hernias, bowel obstructions, or electrical injuries, which may take 5 days to become symptomatic. The patients will be home when they become symptomatic so some authors recommend a routine postoperative telephone call to identify those women who are not progressing appropriately. Describing to those patients those symptoms requiring early office attention is also recommended.

Theoretical Cancer Recurrence and Survival Risk

Many theoretical concerns occur in the cancer patient that are not an issue in benign laparoscopic surgery. The procedure itself can cause the spread of cancer into the peritoneal cavity, into an episiotomy site, or to the trocar sites. Will the technique of the surgical procedure cause new and unusual sites of recurrence? Will new sites of recurrence be harder to salvage than the expected vaginal cuff site recurrences seen with traditional abdominal hysterectomy? These are the questions that will surely be answered by forthcoming research.

Sonoda et al. (67) reported that 10.3% of their patients undergoing LAVH for EC were found to have positive peritoneal cytology. This is compared to 2.8% of the women who had the traditional open technique. They believed this was due to the uterine manipulation performed during the surgery. The authors used an inflatable intrauterine manipulator device rather than an acorn cannula in the cervix. They do not discuss whether the washings were always obtained at the beginning of the procedure before any uterine manipulation has occurred. They identified 2 of the 14 cases that had laparoscopy and positive cytology also had undergone hysteroscopy preoperatively. They theorize that hysteroscopy, or even dilation and curettage, could also disseminate cancer cells from the endometrial cavity retrograde out the fallopian tubes into the peritoneal cavity. None of the 7 cases of positive cytology that underwent an abdominal hysterectomy had a preoperative hysteroscopy. The meaning of positive peritoneal cytology is not known. The avoidance of dilation and curettage procedures and hysteroscopy has not been advocated, even though retrograde dissemination of endometrial cells has been demonstrated (64).

The regress of EC cells into the peritoneal cavity during uterine manipulation can be theoretically avoided by the use of the bipolar cautery on the fallopian tubes before uterine manipulation is initiated. Another option is to avoid inserting a manipulator into the uterine cavity. The uterus can be moved with a Babcock above the cornua including the round ligament and the uterine ovarian ligament and the adnexa.

Avoiding the contamination of the peritoneal cavity and the port sites with tumor from the uterus is advocated. Separate instrument stands for the laparoscopy and the vaginal procedures should be mandated to avoid cross contamination. The occlusion of the fallopian tubes at the beginning of the procedure can be performed. The avoidance of using the same gloved hand on the uterine manipulator and the laparoscopic equipment is expected. Changing of the surgical team's gloves should occur between the vaginal hysterectomy portion of the case and the reinsufflation step to look for hemostasis in the peritoneal cavity, as well as at the time of port site closure (77).

The technique utilized to remove the lymph nodes from the peritoneal cavity during the laparoscopy has not been standardized. The majority of surgeons assume the lymph nodes that look benign do not contain tumor. Therefore, they grasp them with spoon forceps and withdraw them through a 12 mm port site cannula. The grossly positive nodes should be placed in a laparoscopy bag and withdrawn without disruption of the nodal structure so that tumor is not extruded into the peritoneal cavity. This author advocates laparotomy whenever gross metastatic disease is encountered.

Colon cancer literature has documented a 2% port site recurrence rate. An isolated port site recurrence in an EC patient has been reported by Muntz et al. (47). The patient had a laparoscopic staging and the surgical stage was IA, grade 2 endometroid adenocarcinoma; when recurrence was noted, there was no other site of disease except the lateral port site. The abdominal wall was resected and thorough restaging performed. She remains free of disease after adjuvant radiation therapy. These authors have only been able to identify three other reported cases of port site recurrences in EC. Wang (77) reported a port site and episiotomy site recurrence in a woman with stage IIIC grade 3 adenocarcinoma of the endometrium, with three pelvic and one para-aortic node metastases and a negative peritoneal cytology. This patient refused any further treatment and the disease recurred in the umbilicus and episiotomy site at 6 months. Poor reporting of adverse outcomes is a problem of our literature, and there are undoubtedly many such cases.

These authors have completed 300 cases laparoscopically and recently experienced the first port site recurrence. This patient had endometrioid adenocarcinoma stage IB grade 2. We also have a known case of umbilicus recurrence after laparotomy for stage IB grade 1 EC; she is alive and well after surgical resection. Barter et al. (4) also reported an isolated abdominal wound recurrence. This information, in the form of case reports, cannot provide adequate assessment of the risk involved for these potential complications. The GOG will overcome this reporting bias in the literature with the prospective trial of 2200 cases randomized between traditional and laparoscopic treatment and then followed for recurrence sites and survival.

The mechanism of port site recurrences could be a combination of increased intraabdominal pressure, CO_2 gas used for insufflation, and dissemination of intraperitoneal tumor cells into irrigation fluids into the peritoneal cavity. Hopkins et al. (36) developed a rat model system to evaluate these possibilities and determined that the combination of increased abdominal pressure and the use of CO_2 gas was worse than either alone. The laparotomy incision sites had fewer cancer cells grow in them than the simulated trocar sites. The COST study (78) has not published long-term follow-up, but a smaller study ($n = 219$) in Barcelona, Spain showed improved survival of colon cancer patients randomized to laparoscopy.

This was a surprise finding reported by Lacy in 2002, which is reassuring in that laparoscopy may not decrease survival or increase recurrence. The statistical analysis of the comparability of the two groups is not yet available.

GOG Experience

The Gynecologic Oncology Group will enroll 2200 patients on to a phase III randomized trial of laparoscopy versus laparotomy for the surgical treatment and staging of EC. The randomization is 2:1 where laparoscopy is being performed twice as often. The quality of life component to this protocol has completed accrual and the analysis is underway. The success rate for completion of laparoscopy is being judged by the rate of conversion to laparotomy and the causes for the conversion. The adequacy of lymph node dissection is being assessed by whether the pathologists found nodes in all required specimens, and the operative note describes an adequate dissection, which conforms to the surgical manual.

The main study endpoints include quality of life assessments preoperatively; 1, 3, and 6 weeks postoperatively; and at the 6-month postsurgery visit. The surgical outcomes include length of stay, estimated blood loss, operative time, node counts, conversion to laparotomy, and other complications. The sites of recurrence, progression-free survival, and overall survival will be the long-term endpoints. Seventy-eight percent of the women completed all five of the quality-of-life assessments. To avoid bias, the quality of life results will be published when the last participant has been randomized in 2005.

REFERENCES

1. ACOG Committee Opinion Number 146–November 1994; Laparoscopically Assisted Vaginal Hysterectomy; Compendium 2001; American College of Obstetrics and Gynecology.

2. ACOG Educational Bulletin No. 239, August 1997; Operative Laparoscopy.

3. Bajaj PK, Barnes MN, Robertson MW, Shah P, Austin Jmiii, Partridge EE, Austin JM Jr. Surgical management of endome-

trial adenocarcinoma using laparoscopically assisted staging and treatment. *Southern Med J* 1999; 92(12):1174–1177.

4. Barter JF, Hatch KD, Orr JW, Shingleton HM. Isolated abdominal wound recurrence of an endometrial adenocarcinoma confined to a polyp. *Gynecol Oncol*; 1986; 25(3):372–375.

5. Bloss JD, Berman ML, Bloss LP, Buller RE. Use of vaginal hysterectomy for the management of stage I endometrial cancer in the medically compromised patient. *Gynecol Oncol* 1991; 40:74–77.

6. Boike G, Lurain J, Burke J. A Comparison of laparoscopic management of endometrial cancer with traditional laparotomy (abstr). *Gynecol Oncol* 1994; 52:105.

7. Boike GM, Miller CE, Spirtos NM, Mercer LJ, Fowler JM, Summitt R, Orr JW. Incisional bowel herniations after operative laparoscopy: a series of nineteen cases and review of the literature. *Am J of Obstet and Gynecol* 1995; 172(6):1726–1733.

8. Bonjer HJ, Hazebroek EJ, Kazemier G, Giuffride MC, Meijer WS, Lange JF. Open versus closed establishment of pneumoperitoneum in laparoscopic surgery. *Br J Surg* 1997; 84:599–602.

9. Childers JM, Aqua KA, Surwit EA, Hallum AV, Hatch KD. Abdominal-wall tumor implantation after laparoscopy for malignant conditions. *Obstet Gynecol* 1994; 84:765–790.

10. Childers JM, Hatch K, Surwit EA. The role of laparoscopic lymphadenectomy in the management of cervicalcarcinoma. *Gyneol Oncol* 1992; 47:38–43.

11. Childers JM, Surwit EA. Combined laparoscopic and vaginal surgery for the management of two cases of stage I endometrial cancer. *Gynecol Oncol* 1992; 45:46–51.

12. Childers JM, Brzechffa PR, Hatch KD, Surwit EA. Laparoscopically assisted surgical staging (LASS) of endometrial cancer. *Gynecol Oncol* 1993; 51:33–38.

13. Childers JM, Hatch KD, Tran A, Surwit EA. Laparoscopic para-aortic lymphadenectomy in gynecologic malignancies. *Obstet and Gynecol* 1993; 82(5):741–747.

14. Childers JM, Brzechffa PR, Surwit EA. Laparoscopy using the left upper quadrant as the primary trocar site. *Gynecol Oncol* 1993; 50:221–225.

15. Chu KK, Chang SD, Chen FP, Soong YK. Laparoscopic surgical staging in cervical cancer preliminary experience among Chinese. *Gynecol Oncol* 1997; 64:49–53.

16. Compendium 2001, American College of Obstetrics and Gynecology.

17. Creasman WT, Morrow CP, Bundy BN, Homesley HD, Graham JE, Heller PB. Surgical pathologic spread patterns of endometrial cancer. *Cancer* 1987; 60:2035–2041.

18. Djokovic JL, Hedley-Whyte J. Prediction of outcome of surgery and anesthesia in patients over 80. *J Amer Med Assoc* 979; 242(21):2301–2306.

19. Dottino PR, Tobias DH, Beddoe AM, Golden AL, Cohen CJ. Laparoscopic lymphadencectomy for gynecologic malignancies. *Gynecol Oncol* 1999; 73:383–388.

20. Eltabbakh GH: Effect of surgeon's experience on the surgical outcome of laparoscopic surgery for women with endometrial cancer. *Gynecol Oncol* 2000; 78:58–61.

21. Eltabbakh GH. Shamonki MI, Moody JM, Garafano LL. Laparoscopy as the primary modality for the treatment of women with endometrial carcinoma. *Cancer* 2001; 91(2):378–387.

22. Eltabbakh GH, Shamonki MI, Moody JM, Garafano LL. Hysterectomy for obese women with endometrial cancer: laparoscopy or laparotomy? *Gynecol Oncol* 2000; 78:329–335.

23. Flanagan CW, Mannel RS, Walker JL, Johnson GL. Incidence and location of para-aortic lymph node metastasis in gynecologic malignancies. *J Amer College Surg* 1995; 181:72–74.

24. Fowler JM, Carter JR, Carlson JW, Maslonkowski R, Byers LJ, Carson LF, Twiggs LB. Lymph node yield from laparoscopic lymphadenectomy in cervical cancer:a comparative study. *Gynecol Oncol* 1993; 51:187–192.

25. Fowler JM. The role of laparoscopic staging in management of patients with early endometrial cancer (editorial). *Gynecol Oncol* 1999; 73:1–3.

26. Fuchtner C, Manetta A, Walker JL, Emma D, Berman M, DiSaia PJ. Radical hysterectomy in the elderly patient: analysis of morbidity. *Amer J of Obstet Gynecol* 1992; 166:593–597.

27. Gallup DC, Gallup DG, Nolan TE, Smith RP, Messing MF, Kline KL. Use of subcutaneous closed drainage system and antibiotics in obese Gynecologic patients. *Amer J of Obstet Gynecol* 1996; 175:358–362.

28. Geisler JP, Geisler HE. Radical hysterectomy in the elderly female:a comparison to patients age 50 or younger. *Gynecol Oncol* 2001; 80:258–261.

29. Gemignani ML, Curtin JP, Zelmanovich J, Patel DA, Venkatraman E, Barakat RR. Laparoscopic-assisted vaginal hysterectomy for endometrial cancer: clinical outcomes and hospital charges. *Gynecol Oncol* 1999; 73:5–11.

30. Grimes DA. Frontiers of operative laparoscopy: a review and critique of the evidence. *Amer J Obstet Gynecol* 1992; 166:1062–1071.

31. Grimes DA. Shifting indications for hysterectomy: nature, nurture or neither? *Lancet* 1994; 344 (Dec 17):1652–1653.

32. Harkki-Siren P, Sjoberg J, Kurki T. Major complications of laparoscopay: a follow-up Finnish study. *Obstet and Gynecol* 1999; 94:94–98.

33. Hicks ML, Philips JL, Parham G, Andrews N, Jones WB, Shingleton HM, Menck HR. The National Cancer Data Base Report on endometrial carcinoma in African-American women. *Cancer* 1998; 83(12):2629–2637.

34. Holub Z, Bartos P, Jabor A, Eim J, Fischlová D, Kliment L. Laparoscopic surgery in obese women with endometrial cancer. *J Amer Assoc of Gynecol Laparoscopists* 2000; 7(1):83–88.

35. Homesley HD. Management of endometrial cancer. *Amer J Obstet Gynecol* 1996; 174:529–534.

36. Hopkins, MP, Dulai RM, Occhino A, Holda S. The effects of carbon dioxide pneumoperitoneum on seeding of tumor in port sites in a rat model. *Amer J Obstet Gynecol* 1999; 181:1329–1334.

37. Hopkins MP. The myths of laparoscopic surgery. *Amer J Obstet Gynecol* 2000; 183:1–5.

38. Johnstone PAS, Rhode DC, Swattz SE, Fetter JE, Wexner SD. Port site recurrences after laparoscopic and thorascopic procedures in malignancy. *J Clin Oncol* 1996; 14:1950–1956.

39. Kadar N. Laparoscopic pelvic lymphadenectomy in obese women with gynecologic malignancies. *J Amer Assoc Gynecol Laparoscopists* 1995; 2(2):163–167.

40. Kilgore LC, Partridge EE, Alvarez RD, Autstin M, Shingleton HM, Noojin Fiii, Conner W. Adenocarcinoma of the endometrium: survival comparisons of patients with and without pelvic node sampling. *Gynecol Oncol* 1995; 56:29–33.

41. Kirschner CV, DeSerto TM, Isaacs JH. Surgical treatment of the elderly patient with gynecologic cancer. *Surgery Gynecol Obstet* 1990; 170(5):379–384.

42. Magrina JF, Mutone NF, Weaver AL, Magtibay PM, Fowler S, Cornella JL. Laparoscopic lymphadenectomy and vaginal or laparoscopic hysterectomy with bilateral salpingo-oophorectomy for endometrial cancer: morbidity and survival. *Amer J Obstet Gynecol* 1999; 181:376–381.

43. Malur S, Possover M, Michels W, Schneider A. Laparoscopic-assisted vaginal versus abdominal surgery inpatients with endometrial cancer prospective randomized trial. *Gynecol Oncol* 2001; 80:239–244.

44. McMeekin DS, Lashbrook DR, Gold MA, Scribner DR Jr, Kamelle SA, Tilmanns TD, Mannel RS. Nodal distribution and its significance in FIGO stage IIIC endometrial cancer. *Gynecol Oncol* 2001; 82:375–379.

45. Morrow CP, Bundy BN, Kurman FJ, Creasman WT, Heller P, Homesley HD, Graham JE. Relationship between surgical-pathological risk factors and outcome in clinical stage I and II carcinoma of the endometrium: a Gynecologic Oncology Group Study. *Gynecol Oncol* 1991; 40:55–65.

46. Munkarah A. Is there a role for surgical cytoreduction in stage IV endometrial cancer? *Gynecol Oncol* 2000; 78:83–84.

47. Muntz HG, Goff BA, Madsen BL, Yon JL. Port-site recurrence after laparoscopic surgery for endometrial carcinoma. *Obstet Gynecol* 1999; 93(5):807–809.

48. Nezhat CR, Burrell MO, Nezhat FR, Benigno BB, Welander CE. Laparoscopic radical hysterectomy with para-aortic and pelvic node dissection. *Amer J Obstet Gynecol* 1992; 166(3):864–865.

49. Orr JW Jr, Roland PY, Leichter D, Orr PF. Endometrial cancer: is surgical staging necessary? *Current Opinions in Oncology* 2001; 13:408–412.

50. Partridge EE, Shingleton HM, Menck HR. The National Cancer Data Base Report on endometrial cancer. *J Surgeons Oncol* 1996; 61:111–123.

51. Petrelli NJ. Clinical trials are mandatory for improving surgical cancer care (editorial). *J Amer Med Assoc* 2002; Jan 13:377

52. Pierson RL, Figge PK, Buchsbaum HJ. Surgery of gynecologic malignancy in the aged. *Obstet Gynecol* 1975; 46(5):523–527.

53. Possover M, Krause N, Plaul K, Kühne-Heid R, Schneider A. Laparoscopic para-aortic and pelvic lymphadenectomy: experience with 150 patients and review of the literature. *Gynecol Oncol* 1998; 71:19–28.

54. Querleu D, Leblanc E, Castelain B. Laparoscopic pelvic lymphadenectomy in the staging of early carcinoma of the cervix. *Amer J Obstet Gynecol* 1991; 164(2):579–581.

55. Ramshaw BJ. Laproscopic surgery for cancer patients. *CA: A Cancer Journal for Clinicians* 1997; 47:327–350.

56. Romano S, Shimoni Y, Muralee D, Shaley E. Retrograde seeding of endometrial carcinoma during hysteroscopy. *Gynecol Oncol* 1992; 44:116–118.

57. Rose PG. Endometrial carcinoma. *N Eng J Med* 1996; 335(9):640–649.

58. Schlaerth JB, Spirtos NM, Boike GM, Fowler JM. Laparoscopic retroperitoneal lymphadenectomy followed by laparotomy in women with cervical cancer. (abstract). *Gynecol Oncol* 1999; 72:443–527.

59. Schneider A, Possover M, Kamprath S, Endisch U, Krause N, Nöschel. Laparoscopy-assisted radical vaginal hysterectomy modified according to Schauta-Stoeckel. *Obstet Gynecol* 1996; 88(6):1057–1060.

60. Scribner DR Jr, Walker JL, Johnson GA, McMeekin DS, Gold MA, Mannel RS. Surgical management of early-stage endometrial cancer in the elderly: is laparoscopy feasible? *Gynecol Oncol* 2001; 83:563–568.

61. Scribner DR Jr, Mannel RS, Walker JL, Johnson GA. Cost analysis of lapaorscopy versus laparotomy for early endometrial cancer. *Gynecol Oncol* 1999; 75:460–463.

62. Scribner DR Jr, Walker JL, Johnson GA, McMeekin DS, Gold MA, Mannel RS. Laparoscopic pelvic and para-aortic lymph node dissection: analysis of the first 100 cases. *Gynecol Oncol* 2001; 82:498–503.

63. Scribner DR Jr, Walker JL, McMeekin DS, Gold MA, Mannel RS. Laparoscopic pelvic and para-aortic lymph node dissection in the obese. *Gynecol Oncol* March 2002:84(3):426–430.

64. Shim JU, Rose PG, Reale FR, Soto H, Tak WK, Hunter RE. Accuracy of frozen-section diagnosis at surgery in clinical stage I and II endometrial carcinoma. *Amer J Obstet Gynecol* 1982; 166:1335–1338.

65. Shuster PA, Barter JF, Potkul RK, Barnes WA, Delago G. Radical hysterectomy morbidity in relation to age. *Obstet Gynecol* 1991; 78(1):77–79.

66. Schmitz MJ, Nahhas WA. Hysteroscopy may transport malignant cells into the peritoneal cavity. *European J Gynaecol Oncol* 1994:152:121–124

67. Sonoda Y, Zerbe M, Smith A, Lin O, Barakat RR, Hoskins WJ. High incidence of positive peritoneal cytology in low-risk endometrial cancer treated by laparoscopically assisted vaginal hysterectomy. *Gynecol Oncol* 2001; 80:378–382.

68. Soper DE, Bump RC, Hurt WG. Wound infection after abdominal hysterectomy: effect of the depth of subcutaneous tissue. *Amer J Obstet Gynecol* 1995; 173:465–471.

69. Spirtos NM, Schlaerth JB, Kimball RE, Leiphart VM, Ballon SC. Laparoscopic radical hysterectomy (type III) with aortic and pelvic lymphadenectomy. *Am J Obstet Gynecol* 1996; 174(6):1763–1768.

70. Spirtos NM, Schlaerth JB, Spirtos TW, Schlaerth AC, Indman PD, Kimball RE. Laparoscopic bilateral pelvic and paraaortic lymph node sampling: an evolving technique. *Am J Obstet Gynecol* 1995; 173(1):105–111.

71. Spirtos NM, Schlaerth JB, Gross GM, Spirtos TW, Schlaerth AC, Ballon SC. Cost and quality-of-life analyses of surgery for

early endometrial cancer: laparotomy versus laparoscopy. *Am J Obstet Gynecol* 1996; 174(6):1795–1800.

72. Stocchi L, Nelson H, Young-Fadok TM, Larson DR, Ilstrup DM. Safety and advantages of laparoscopic vs. open colectomy in the elderly: matched-control study. *Diseases Colon & Rectum* 2000; 43:326–332.

73. Susini T, Scambia G, Margariti PA, Giannice R, Signorile P, Panici PB, Mancuso S. Gynecologic oncologic surgery in the elderly: a retrospective analysis of 213 patients. *Gynecol Oncol* 1999; 75:437–443.

74. Van Itallie TB. Health implications of overweight and obesity in the United States. *Ann Internal Med* 1985; 103(6 pt2): 983–988.

75. Vidaurreta J, Bermúdez A, di Paola G, Sardi J. Laparoscopic staging in locally advanced cervical carcinomaa new possible philosophy? *Gynecol Oncol* 1999; 75:366–371.

76. Walsh TH. Audit of outcome of major surgery in the elderly. *Br J Surg* 1996; 83:92–97.

77. Wang PH, Yen MS, Yuan CC, Chao KC, Ng HAT, Lee WT, Chao HAT. Port site metastasis after laparoscopic-assisted vaginal hysterectomy for endometrial cancer: possible mechanisms and prevention. *Gynecol Oncol* 66(1):151–155.

78. Weeks JC, Nelson H, Gelber S, Sargent D, Schroeder G. Clinical Outcomes of Surgical Therapy (COST) Study Group. Short-term quality-of-life outcomes following laparoscopic-assisted colectomy vs. open colectomy for colon cancer: a randomized trial. *J Amer Med Assoc* Jan 16, 2002; 287(3):321–328.

79. Wise WE Jr, Padmanabhan A, Meesig DM, Arnold MW, Aguilar PS, Stewart WRC. Abdominal colon and rectal operations in the elderly. *Diseases Colon & Rectum* 1991; 34(11):959–963.

80. Chen MD, Teigen GA, Reynolds HT, Johnson PR, Fowler JM. Laparoscopy versus laparotomy: an evaluation of adhesion formation after pelvic and paraaortic lymphadenectomy in a porcine model. *Am J Obstet and Gyn* 1998; 178(3):499–503.

11

The Role of Primary Surgery in Advanced Endometrial Cancer

ROBERT E. BRISTOW AND F.J. MONTZ
The Johns Hopkins Medical Insititutions,
Baltimore, Maryland, U.S.A.

INTRODUCTION

Endometrial corpus cancer (EC) is the fourth most common malignancy among United States women and the eighth most common cause of cancer-related death (1). The American Cancer Society estimated that 38,300 new cases of uterine corpus cancer were diagnosed during 2001 (1). Of these, 21% (or 8,043 women) had regional or distant spread of disease. Surgical staging and adjuvant therapy protocols for early-stage EC have been studied extensively and are associated with excellent long term survival outcomes. Patients with advanced disease, on the other hand, account for the majority of tumor-related deaths and present a significant clinical challenge. Effective management strategies for this group have yet to be precisely defined. The therapeutic armamentarium for metastatic EC includes surgery, chemotherapy, irradiation, hormonal therapy, or some combination of these modalities. The focus of this chapter, however, is the surgical management of advanced-stage EC, with the specific objectives being to: 1) review the existing data on primary cytoreductive surgery for patients with stage III and IV disease, and 2) summarize the recent literature addressing the surgical management of uterine papillary serous carcinoma (UPSC).

THEORECTICAL BASIS FOR CYTOREDUCTIVE SURGERY

The concept of surgical cytoreduction, selectively applied, dictates that "debulking" of a metastatic malignant neoplasm can potentially augment the response to subsequent adjuvant therapy (2). While not curative, cytoreductive surgery is thought to reduce cellular kinetic and pharmacologic barriers to maximal tumor cytotoxicity (2–5). Larger tumor masses are necessarily associated with an increasing number of cell divisions and may be more likely to harbor chemotherapy resistant tumor cell clones (4). Cytoreductive surgery may enhance the response to subsequent chemotherapy by removing tumor masses that potentially harbor drug resistant cells. Surgical cytoreduction may also enhance the effects of adjuvant therapy by reducing tumor volume and recruiting previously dormant tumor cells into the active phase of the cell cycle (increased growth fraction), theoretically making them more susceptible to cytotoxic therapy (5). Finally, larger tumor masses generally contain poorly perfused anoxic areas that are inaccessible to cytotoxic agents and resistant to radiation effects. By removing large hypoxic tumor masses, cytoreductive surgery is believed to enhance response rates to adjuvant therapy by leaving a population of cells with improved vascularization (6,7).

Cytoreductive surgery has been advocated for tumors of the testis, kidney, adrenal gland, gastrointestinal tract, central nervous system, and Burkitt's lymphoma; however, the largest body of literature addressing this approach to widespread malignancy comes from the experience with advanced ovarian cancer. These data demonstrate that ovarian cancer survival is inversely related to the maximal diameter of residual disease (8–10). In addition, surgery fails to have any appreciable effect on survival if the largest residual tumor dimension exceeds 2 cm, irrespective of the degree of surgical effort. These studies also illustrate that factors other than the cytoreductive surgical outcome are important determinants of survival (9). There is now a growing body of literature addressing the principles of surgical cytoreduction as applied to advanced metastatic EC.

STAGE III ENDOMETRIAL CANCER

The International Federation of Gynecology and Obstetrics (FIGO) stage III EC requires surgico-pathologic confirmation of tumor spread to the uterine serosa, adnexae, vagina, parametria, pelvic/para-aortic lymph nodes, or positive cytology in peritoneal fluid (11). For patients unable to undergo surgical staging, the FIGO 1971 clinical staging system is invoked in which stage III reflects extra-uterine spread of disease that is clinically confined to the true pelvis (11).

Despite heterogeneous patient populations and somewhat imprecise estimations of postoperative tumor burden, several studies provide evidence suggesting that survival outcome is related to the amount of residual disease in the setting of locally advanced metastatic EC. In 1984, Aalders et al. retrospectively evaluated 108 patients with clinical stage III EC and 67 patients with surgical stage III disease (12). The majority (87%) of clinically evident stage III was vaginal or parametrial, while the most frequent (81%) site of subclinical extrauterine intrapelvic extension was to the adnexae. For patients with clinical stage III disease, surgical eradication of all macroscopic tumor was of major prognostic significance. Although complete cytoreduction was only possible in 13% of these patients, the associated 5-year survival rate was 41%.

This was significantly better than the 5-year survival rate of 11% when all visible disease could not be resected. In 1985, Mackillop and Pringle reported on 36 patients with surgical stage III endometrial cancer, 30 of whom received postoperative radiation therapy (13). Twenty patients underwent a "complete" operation, leaving no evidence of residual disease, and had a 5-year survival rate of 79.5%. This was significantly better than the 5-year survival rate of 23.0% for patients who had "incomplete" surgery and were left with gross residual disease. Taken together, these early studies suggest that complete surgical removal of locally advanced disease is associated with prolonged survival and should be attempted whenever possible.

Adnexal Metastasis

Additional data indicate that, as an isolated finding, adnexal metastasis from endometrial cancer is associated with a favorable prognosis. In the series of Mckillop and Pringle, the 5-year survival rate for patients with isolated adnexal involvement was 82.3%, which was statistically significantly longer than the 27.7% 5-year survival for patients with other sites of intrapelvic spread (13). Connell et al. recently reported their retrospective experience with 40 cases of EC metastatic to the adnexae, which accounted for 10.5% of patients in their population (14). As an isolated finding, adnexal involvement occurred in just 3.2% of all patients but was associated with a 5-year disease-free survival rate of 71%. When the retroperitoneal lymph nodes had been sampled (and presumably negative), the 5-year disease-free survival rate improved to 82%. Perhaps more importantly, 50% of all patients with adnexal involvement were found to have a more advanced surgical stage of disease. FIGO stage IV disease was present in 35% of all patients with adnexal metastasis, while 15% had retroperitoneal nodal spread. For comparison, the classic study of clinical stage I EC reported by Creasman et al. for the Gynecologic Oncology Group (GOP) found that adnexal metastasis were associated with positive pelvic and para-aortic nodes in 32% and 20% of cases, respectively (15). It appears, therefore, that while adnexal involvement does not have a significant independent adverse effect on survival, it may be a harbinger of more advanced-stage disease in a large proportion of patients and should prompt a comprehensive exploration of the peritoneal cavity and retroperitoneal nodal areas.

In the setting of known EC, clinical or radiographic detection of an adnexal mass warrants surgical exploration for diagnostic as well as therapeutic purposes. An adnexal mass in this setting may represent a metastatic lesion from the endometrial primary, a second (synchronous) primary cancer of the ovary, or a benign condition such as an inflammatory mass. At the time of surgical exploration, attention should be initially directed to the adnexal tumor, which is excised and sent for frozen section analysis. An intra-operative diagnosis will assist the surgeon in determining the nature of the staging procedure, which should be dictated by both the operative findings and the surgeon's clinical judgment. Some would argue that if the frozen section is consistent with metastatic EC, then only retroperitoneal lymph node sampling, as per EC staging protocol, should be performed (16). If the adnexal mass is malignant and demonstrates endometrioid histology, we favor performing the extended surgical staging operation utilized for ovarian carcinoma (omentectomy, peritoneal biopsies, in addition to lymph node sampling), as the distinction between an endometrial lesion metastatic to the ovary and a synchronous primary ovarian cancer (also endometrioid histology) may only be possible on permanent section pathologic analysis. In the UCLA series of synchronous endometrial and ovarian primary cancers, 45% of ovarian cancers were of endometrioid histology (17). Obviously, if the ovarian histology is dissimilar to the primary endometrial tumor, then an extended staging procedure is warranted.

Lymph Node Metastasis

Several studies have addressed the therapeutic value of pelvic and/or para-aortic lymphadenectomy for patients with node-positive EC (FIGO stage IIIC). Larson et al. observed only one recurrence among 18 patients with node-positive disease after undergoing complete pelvic and para-aortic lymphadenectomy followed by either systemic chemotherapy or progestational agents (18). Mariani and co-workers from the Mayo Clinic recently described their experience with 51 patients with stage IIIC EC (19). Thirteen of these patients underwent a therapeutic para-aortic lymphadenectomy, defined as removal of at least 5 para-aortic lymph nodes. Patients undergoing para-aortic lymphadenectomy had a significant advantage in 5-year overall survival (77%) compared to patients with biopsy only or unsampled para-aortic nodes (42%) (Fig.1). Similarly, 5-year recurrence-free survival rates were 76% and 36% for patients with and without para-aortic lymphadenectomy, respectively. On multivariate analysis, the performance of para-aortic lymphadenectomy was a significant and independent predictor of both overall and progression-free survival in node positive patients. Notably, no patient undergoing therapeutic para-aortic dissection experienced recurrent disease in node-bearing areas. In contrast,

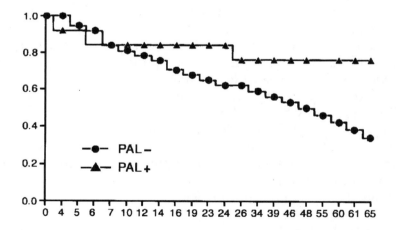

Figure 1 Overall survival in 51 patients with EC harboring node metastasis (excluding stage IV) disease, according to the extent of para-aortic lymphadenectoy: without (PAL−, n = 38) and with (PAL+, n = 13) (p = 0.05). (From Ref.19.)

nodal recurrence occurred in 37% of patients without para-aortic lymphadenectomy. Limitations of this study include the retrospective design, the non-random selection of patients for para-aortic lymphadenectomy, and the fact that only 33% of all patients received extended-field radiation therapy. Since two-thirds of the non-lymphadenectomy group had no para-aortic nodal biopsies, it seems likely that undetected and non-irradiated microscopic para-aortic nodal disease may have contributed to the poor survival outcome of this group.

Therapeutic lymphadenectomy has also been incorporated into aggressive adjuvant treatment programs for patients with node-positive disease. So-called "tri-modality therapy" utilizes not only surgery and radiation therapy, but chemotherapy as well. Onda et al. reported a series of 30 patients with stage IIIC endometrial cancer treated with pelvic and para-aortic lymphadenectomy followed by chemotherapy (cyclophosphamide, doxorubicin, cisplatin) and directed irradiation (20). The 5-year survival rate for all 30 patients was 84%. Using this regimen, 5-year survival was 100% when only pelvic nodes were involved and 75% when para-aortic nodes harbored metastatic disease. Katz et al. also reported favorable results using an aggressive multi-modality approach for 22 patients with stage IIIC disease. In this series, the mean overall survival time was 48 months after therapeutic pelvic and para-aortic lymphadenectomy followed by directed radiation therapy and the selective use of carboplatin and paclitaxel chemotherapy (21). Neither of these studies addressed the management of grossly enlarged nodes, however.

Indirect evidence supporting surgical debulking of grossly evident retroperitoneal adenopathy comes from two studies evaluating the efficacy of radiation therapy in node-positive EC. These reports demonstrate superior local control and survival rates for patients beginning treatment with small-volume residual nodal disease (22,23). Rose and colleagues studied 26 patients with histologically proven metastasis to the para-aortic lymph nodes (22). Seventeen patients received postoperative radiation therapy to the para-aortic fields and, not surprisingly, enjoyed a statistically significant advantage in median survival

(27 months) compared to the 9 patients not receiving radiation therapy (13 months). Notably, these authors found no statistically significant difference in overall survival between patients with microscopic para-aortic nodal metastasis and those with grossly positive para-aortic nodes that were completely resected. Similarly, Corn et al. described their experience with 50 patients treated with extended-field para-aortic radiation therapy, 26 of whom had undergone debulking of grossly enlarged nodes while the remaining 24 patients had only radiographic confirmation of nodal involvement and presumably initiated radiation therapy with bulky residual disease (23). The para-aortic failure rate was 19% for patients receiving combined surgery and radiation therapy, and 39% for those receiving only irradiation. Similarly, the overall survival rate for combined modality patients was 61% compared to 46% for radiation-only patients. While the numbers of patients studied are limited, these important studies suggest that, when combined with extended-field radiation, debulking of grossly enlarged para-aortic nodes may provide some benefit in terms of reduced nodal failure and improved overall survival.

STAGE IV ENDOMETRIAL CANCER

According to FIGO criteria, stage IVA EC represents locally advanced disease with invasion of the bladder or rectal mucosa. Patients with extra-pelvic peritoneal implants or distant metastasis meet criteria for stage IVB disease (11). Stage IV EC accounts for just 3–13% of all cases, yet is responsible for 23% of cancer-related deaths in the first year following diagnosis (11,24–26). In contrast to early-stage endometrial cancer, the 5-year survival rate for patients with stage IV disease ranges from 10% to 25% (24–26). The poor prognosis associated with stage IV disease is due, at least in part, to the limited efficacy of radiation therapy, chemotherapy, and hormonal therapy against large-volume tumors. With this in mind, cytoreductive surgery leaving patients with only minimal residual disease takes on potentially greater therapeutic importance.

In 1983, Greer and Hamberger reported 31 patients with intraperitoneal metastases of stage III and IV EC treated with post-operative whole abdominal radiation therapy (27). Ten patients with stage IV disease were left with residual disease ≤2 cm and had a 5-year survival rate of 70%. There were no 5-year survivors among patients with residual disease measuring >2 cm. Although this study included patients with both stage III and IV disease, was of limited size, and did not state the precise extent of initial or residual disease, it was one of the earliest to suggest that adjuvant therapy for advanced EC is more successful in the setting of small-volume residual disease.

More recent studies have demonstrated that without an attempt at surgical intervention, the prognosis for patients with stage IV EC is extremely poor. In 1994, Goff et al. reported their experience with 47 patients with stage IV EC (28). Twenty-nine patients underwent cytoreductive surgery leaving no "bulky" residual disease, although the specific diameter of tumor residuum was not directly stated. In this study, the group of patients submitted to cytoreductive surgery had a significantly longer median survival time (19 months) compared to the 18 patients who did not undergo primary surgical exploration (8 month median survival time) secondary to presumed unresectable disease. These data clearly demonstrate the prognostic value of cytoreductive surgery leaving "nonbulky" residual disease. Investigators from the University of Oklahoma recently reported similar results among 51 patients with stage IV EC, 44 of whom underwent surgery with 72% achieving optimal (<2 cm) disease status (29). The median survival time for patients undergoing surgery was 17 months, compared to 6 months when primary surgery was not undertaken. Collectively, these reports indicate that initial surgery has therapeutic as well as diagnostic value; however, the use of surgical selection criteria in these studies precludes an accurate assessment of true survival benefit.

Two large series have specifically evaluated the survival impact of cytoreductive surgery for stage IV EC. In 1997, Chi and colleagues from the Memorial Sloan-Kettering Cancer Center reported 55 patients with stage IV EC treated with primary surgery (30). These investigators found that overall survival was highly correlated with the amount of cytoreductive surgery performed. Forty-four percent of patients were left with optimal (≤2 cm) residual disease and had a median survival time of 31 months. This was a significant advantage compared to those patients who underwent cytoreduction but were left with suboptimal (>2 cm) residual disease (median survival, 12 months), and patients with unresectable carcinomatosis (median survival, 3 months). Furthermore, the authors found no statistically significant difference in survival between patients with small-volume metastatic disease (≤2 cm) prior to cytoreduction and those patients with initially large-volume disease (>2 cm) who were cytoreduced to an optimal residual volume (Fig. 2). These data suggest that surgery may at least partly counterbalance the prognostic influence of tumor biology, if initial tumor size is taken as a marker of biologic aggressiveness. Interestingly, no survival

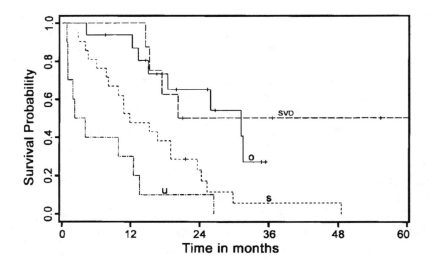

Figure 2 Survival of patients with stage IV EC based on the extent of tumor cytoreduction. SVD, optimally cytoreduced with initial small-volume metastatic disease; O, optimally cytoreduced with initial large-volume metastatic disease; S, suboptimally cytoreduced; U, unresectable. (From Ref. 30.)

advantage was detected for microscopic residual disease over and above that for residual disease ≤2 cm. The lack of significance may, however, reflect the fact that only 10 patients were left with no gross residual disease.

Investigators from the Johns Hopkins Hospital recently reported a retrospective series of 65 patients undergoing primary surgery for stage IVB EC (31). Optimal surgery, defined as residual tumor nodule ≤1 cm, was achieved in 55.4% of patients and was the strongest predictor of overall survival. Patients undergoing optimal cytoreduction had a median survival time of 34.3 months, compared to 11.0 months for those patients left with residual disease >1 cm (Fig. 3). In this study, patients left with only microscopic residual disease survived significantly longer (median survival, 40.6 months) than those patients with optimal but visible residual disease and those undergoing suboptimal surgery. In addition to sur-

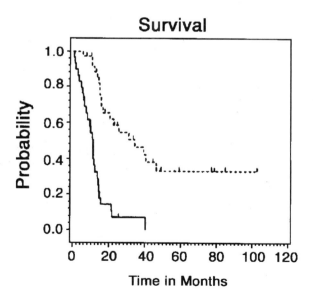

Figure 3 Overall survival of patients with stage IVB EC by residual disease status: ------, residual disease ≤ 1 cm (*n* = 36); ——— residual disease >1 cm (*n* = 29).

gical outcome, age ≤ 58 years and a more functional pre-operative GOG performance status were also independently associated with improved overall survival. From these data, the authors compiled a clinical profile of those patients most likely to experience prolonged survival: younger age, more functional performance status, and microscopic residual disease following primary surgery. Eleven patients fitting this clinical profile survived 40 months or longer. Finally, this study also suggested that combined modality adjuvant therapy consisting of both chemotherapy and radiation therapy may be of some therapeutic benefit for selected patients.

In summary, the available data suggest that optimal cytoreductive surgery can be accomplished in a significant proportion of patients (44%–72%) with stage IV EC and is consistently associated with a survival advantage (Table 1). Patients left with only microscopic residual disease appear to have the most favorable survival outcome. While the long-term prognosis for patients with stage IV EC remains guarded, identification of more active chemotherapeutic agents and the use of multi-modality adjuvant therapy may ultimately improve survival rates. Additional studies exploring the morbidity of aggressive surgery in this population as well as predictors of surgical outcome are warranted.

Table 1 Compiled Studies of Surgery for Stage IV Endometrial Cancer

Author (Ref.)	No. of Patients	Surgical Status	Median Survival	Significance
Goff et al. (28)	29	"No bulky residual"	18	$p < 0.01$
	18	No surgery	8	
McMeekin et al. (29)	44	Surgery (72% < 2 cm)	17	$p = 0.06$
	7	No surgery	6	
Chi et al. (30)	24	≤ 2 cm	31	$p < 0.01$
	21	> 2 cm	12	
	10	Unresectable	3	
Bristow et al. (31)	36	≤ 1 cm	34	$p < 0.01$
	29	> 1 cm	11	

UTERINE PAPILLARY SEROUS CARCINOMA/CANCER (UPSC)

The first collected series describing uterine papillary serous carcinoma (UPSC) as a distinct histopathologic variant of EC were reported independently by Lauchlan (32) and Hendrickson et al. (33) two decades ago. Histologically, these tumors more closely resemble serous carcinoma of the ovary and have a distinctly different clinical behavior compared to the more common endometrioid adenocarcinomas of the endometrium. UPSC has been characterized by a high risk of extra-uterine metastasis and recurrence (32,34–38). Numerous reports have described survival rates of 35% to 50% for surgical stage I/II, and 0 to 15% for stage III/IV disease (39). An important feature of most early studies of UPSC, however, is that survival statistics were generated from either outdated clinical staging parameters or only limited surgical staging information.

Two particularly troublesome features of UPSC have been the inability to predict extra-uterine extension of disease based on the primary tumor pathology and the unusual propensity of UPSC tumors for retroperitoneal, intraperitoneal, and upper abdominal spread (40–42). These observations have lead many authors to advocate routine extended surgical staging, as for ovarian carcinoma, when UPSC pathology is suspected. Those studies that describe patients undergoing omentectomy and peritoneal biopsy in addition to TAH/BSO, peritoneal cytology, and lymph node sampling consistently demonstrate extra-corporeal extension of UPSC in 69% to 87% of cases (40,41,43–45). According to these reports, lymph node metastasis will be documented in approximately 40% of patients (40,42). In the series reported by Goff et al., 72% of patients had extra-uterine disease and 42% had lymph node involvement (40). Notably, 36% of patients without myometrial invasion had retroperitoneal lymph node metastasis. Tumor spread to the omentum is discovered in approximately 20% of cases submitted to a rigorous surgico-pathologic evaluation (40,41,46). A comprehensive study by Geisler et al. detailed the surgico-pathologic findings of 65 patients with UPSC (41). These authors reported that 25% (12 of 48) patients without grossly evident upper abdominal disease had microscopic upper abdominal metastases that would not have been detected by the standard EC staging operation. Furthermore, 23.8% of patients with negative lymph nodes had microscopic disease detected in the omentum or abdominal peritoneum (41). In the setting of UPSC pathology, the additional information provided by extended surgical staging facilitates treatment planning utilizing directed radiation therapy and the selective use of chemotherapy. Contemporary series employing such an approach have reported 5-year survival rates of 64% to 95% for stage I/II disease and 31% to 69% for patients with stage III UPSC (44,47–49). It seems likely that the aggressive clinical course and high recurrence risk typical of UPSC may be at least partially due to metastatic disease going undetected, and therefore untreated, by the traditional EC staging procedure. Consequently, extended surgical staging is recommended for all cases in which UPSC pathology is suspected.

Depending upon the extent of initial exploration and surgico-pathologic sampling, stage IV disease will be discovered in 18% to 48% of patients with UPSC (34,35, 41,42,46, 47,49–51). The management of stage IV UPSC remains problematic, as evidenced by the reported 5-year survival rates of 0 to 5% (35,39,52). Nevertheless, recent data indicate that an intensive surgical approach can have a meaningful impact on the clinical course of disease. Investigators from the Johns Hopkins Hospital and the Massachusetts General Hospital reported a combined series of 31 patients with stage IV UPSC submitted to an aggressive attempt at primary cytoreductive surgery (45). Reflecting the overall poor prognosis of this disease, the median overall survival for all patients was just 14.4 months and 5-year survival was just 3.9%. Optimal cytoreduction, defined as residual disease ≤1 cm in maximal diameter, was achieved in 51.6% of patients and was the most significant predictor of survival outcome. Patients undergoing optimal surgery had a median survival time of 26.2 months compared to just 9.6 months for patients left with suboptimal residual disease. At 24 months, 57.1% of optimally cytoreduced patients were still alive, compared to just 6.7% of patients with large-volume residual disease. Further stratification according to residual tumor burden revealed that patients with only microscopic residual tumor had a significantly longer median survival time (30.4 months) compared to both patients with 0.1–1.0 residual disease (20.5 months) and those with suboptimal residual (Fig. 4). The administration of postoperative chemotherapy consisting of platinum plus paclitaxel was associated with a median survival time of 29.1 months, compared to 14.4 months for patients receiving other platinum-based combinations. While this difference did not reach statistical significance, likely due to small numbers of patients in each group, the survival advantage associated with platinum plus paclitaxel therapy is noteworthy and has been reported by others (51,53,54).

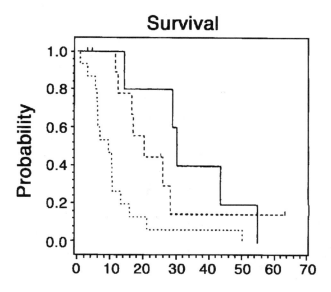

Figure 4 Stratification of survival curves by maximal diameter of residual disease: -------, microscopic residual (n = 6); ———, residual disease 0.1–1.0 cm (n = 10); ......, > 1 cm residual disease (n = 15), p = 0.004. (From Ref. 45.)

CONCLUSION

In summary, patients with apparent early-stage UPSC have a high risk of harboring extra-uterine disease and should undergo an extended surgical staging procedure similar to that for ovarian cancer. Directed multi-modality therapy based on the anatomic extent of disease may result in improved survival rates for patients with local or regional metastases. As for advanced EC in general, an aggressive attempt at primary cytoreductive surgery is warranted for patients with stage IV UPSC, as minimal residual disease is associated with prolonged survival. Additional studies are needed to define the most effective adjuvant treatment protocol following a maximal surgical effort; however, preliminary data indicate that platinum/paclitaxel-based chemotherapy may be an appropriate regimen.

REFERENCES

1. Greenlee RT, Hill-Harmon MB, Murray T, Thun M. Cancer statistics 2001. *CA Cancer J Clin* 2001; 51:15–36.

2. Silberman AW. Surgical debulking of tumors. *Surg Gynecol Obstet* 1982; 155:577–585.

3. Skipper HE. Adjuvant chemotherapy. *Cancer* 1978; 41:936–940.

4. Goldie JH, Coldman JA. A mathematical model for relating the drug sensitivity of tumors to their spontaneous mutation rate. *Cancer Treat Rep* 1979; 63:1727–1733.

5. Norton L, Simon R. Tumor size, sensitivity to therapy, and design of treatment schedules. *Cancer Treat Rep* 1977; 61:1307–1317.

6. Delcos L, Quinlan EJ. Malignant tumors of the ovary managed with postoperative megavoltage irradiation. *Radiology* 1969; 93:659–663.

7. Greco FA, Julian CG, Richardson RL, Burnett L, Hande KR, Oldham RK. Advanced ovarian cancer: brief intensive combination chemotherapy and second-look operation. *Obstet Gynecol* 1981; 58:199–205.

8. Hoskins WJ, Bundy BN, Thigpen JT, Omura GA. The influence of cytoreductive surgery on recurrence-free interval and survival in small-volume stage III epithelial ovarian cancer: A Gynecologic Oncology Group study. *Gynecol Oncol* 1992; 47:159–166.

9. Hoskins WJ, McGuire WP, Brady MF, Homesley HD, Creasman WT, Berman M, et al. The effect of diameter of largest residual disease on survival after primary cytoreductive surgery in patients with suboptimal residual epithelial ovarian carcinoma. *Am J Obstet Gynecol* 1994; 170:974–980.

10. Hoskins WJ. Epithelial ovarian carcinoma: Principles of primary surgery. *Gynecol Oncol* 1994; 55:S91–S96.

11. Creasman W, Odicino F, Maisonneuve P, Benedet J, Sheperd J, Sideri M, Pecorelli S. Carcinoma of the corpus uteri In International Federation of Gynecology and Obstetrics Annual Report on the Results of Treatment in Gynecologic Cancer: Pecorrelli S, Creasman WT, Pettersson F, Benedet JL, Sheperd JH. eds. *J Epidemiol Biostat* 1998; 3:35–62.

12. Aalders JG, Abeler V, Kolstad P. Clinical (Stage III) as compared to subclinical intrapelvic extrauterine tumor spread in endometrial carcinoma: A clinical and histopathologic study of 175 patients. *Gynecol Oncol* 1984; 17:64–74.

13. Mackillop WJ, Pringle JF. Stage III endometrial carcinoma: A review of 90 cases. *Cancer* 1985; 56:2519–2523.

14. Connell PP, Rotmensch J, Waggoner S, Mundt AJ. The significance of adnexal involvement in endometrial carcinoma. *Gynecol Oncol* 1999; 74:74–79.

15. Creasman WT, Morrow CP, Bundy BN, Homesley HD, Graham JE, Heller PB. Surgicopathologic spread patterns of endometrial cancer: a Gynecologic Oncology Group study. *Cancer* 1987; 60:2035–2041.

16. Chi DS. Barakat RR. Surgical management of advanced or recurrent endometrial cancer. *Surg Clin N Amer* 2001; 81:885–898.

17. Eisner RF, Nieberg RK, Berek JS. Synchronous primary neoplasms of the female reproductive tract. *Gynecol Oncol* 1989; 33:335–339.

18. Larson DM, Broste SK, Krawisz BR. Surgery without radiotherapy for primary treatment of endometrial cancer. *Obstet Gynecol* 1998; 91:355–359.

19. Mariani A, Webb MJ, Galli L, Podratz KC. Potential therapeutic role of para-aortic lymphadenectomy in node-positive endometrial cancer. *Gynecol Oncol* 2000; 76:348–356.

20. Onda T, Yoshikawa H, Mizutani K, Mishima M, Yokota H, Nagano H, et al. Treatment of node-positive endometrial cancer with complete node dissection, chemotherapy, and radiation therapy. *Br J Cancer* 1997; 75:1836–1841.

21. Katz LA, Andrews SJ, Fanning J. Survival after multimodality treatment for Stage IIIC endometrial cancer. *Am J Obstet Gynecol* 2001; 184:1071–1073.

22. Rose PG, Cha SD, Tak WK, Fitzgerald T, Reale F, Hunter RE. Radiation therapy for surgically proven para-aortic node metastasis in endometrial carcinoma. *Int J Radiat Oncol Biol Phys* 1992; 24:229–233.

23. Corn BW, Lanciano RM, Greven KM, Schultz DJ, Reisinger SA, Stafford PM, et al. Endometrial cancer with para-aortic adenopathy: Patterns of failure and opportunities for cure. *Int J Radiat Oncol Biol Phys* 1992; 24:223–227.

24. Wolfson AH, Sightler SE, Markoe AM, Schwade JG, Averette HE, Ganjei P, Hilsenbeck SG. The prognostic significance of surgical staging for carcinoma of the endometrium. *Gynecol Oncol* 1992; 45:142–146.

25. Vardi JR, Tadros GH, Anselmo MT, Rafla SD. The value of exploratory laparotomy in patients with endometrial carcinoma according to the new International Federation of Gynecology and Obstetrics staging. *Obstet Gynecol* 1992; 80:204–208.

26. Pliskow S, Penalver M, Averette HE. Stage III and stage IV endometrial carcinoma: A review of 41 cases. *Gynecol Oncol* 1990; 38:210–215.

27. Greer BE, Hamberger AD. Treatment of intraperitoneal metastatic adenocarcinoma of the endometrium by the whole-abdomen moving strip technique and pelvic boost irradiation. *Gynecol Oncol* 1983; 16:365–373.

28. Goff BA, Goodman A, Muntz HG, Fuller AF, Nikrui N, Rice LW. Surgical stage IV endometrial carcinoma: A study of 47 cases. *Gynecol Oncol* 1994; 52:237–240.

29. McMeekin DS, Garcia M, Gold M, Johnson G, Walker J, Mannel R. Stage IV endometrial cancer: Survival, recurrence, and role of surgery. American Society of Clinical Oncology 2001 Annual Meeting, abstract 821.

30. Chi DS, Welshinger M, Venkatraman ES, Barakat RR. The role of surgical cytoreduction in Stage IV endometrial carcinoma. *Gynecol Oncol* 1997; 67:56–60.

31. Bristow RE, Zerbe MJ, Rosenshein NB, Grumbine FC, Montz FJ. Stage IVB endometrial carcinoma: The role of cytoreductive surgery and determinants of survival. *Gynecol Oncol* 2000; 78:85–91.

32. Lauchlan SC. Tubal (serous) carcinoma of the endometrium. *Arch Pathol Lab Med* 1981; 105:615–618.

33. Hendrickson M, Ross J, Eifel P, Martinez A, Kempson R. Uterine papillary serous carcinoma. A highly malignant form of endometrial carcinoma. *Am J Surg Pathol* 1982; 6:93–108.

34. Chambers JT, Merino M, Kohorn EI, Pescel RE, Schwartz PE. Uterine papillary serous carcinoma. *Obstet Gynecol* 1987; 69:109–113.

35. Carcangiu ML, Chambers JT. Uterine papillary serous carcinoma: a study of 108 cases with emphasis on the prognostic significance of associated endometrioid carcinoma, absence of invasion, and concomitant ovarian carcinoma. *Gynecol Oncol* 1992; 47:298–305.

36. Jeffrey JF, Krepart GV, Lotocki RJ. Papillary serous adenocarcinoma of the endometrium. *Obstet Gynecol* 1986; 67:670–674.

37. Matthews RP, Hutchinson-Colas J, Maiman M, Fruchter RG, Gates J, Gibbon D, Remy JC, Sedlis A. Papillary serous and clear cell type lead to poor prognosis of endometrial carcinoma in black women. *Gynecol Oncol* 1997; 65:206–212.

38. Christopherson WM, Alberhasky RC, Connelly PJ. Carcinoma of the endometrium II. Papillary adenocarcinoma: a clinical pathologic study of 46 cases. *Am J Clin Pathol* 1982; 77:534–540.

39. Nicklin JL, Copeland LJ. Endometrial papillary serous carcinoma: patterns of spread and treatment. *Clin Obstet Gynecol* 1996; 39:686–695.

40. Goff BA, Kato D, Schmidt RA, Ek M, Ferry JA, Muntz HG, Cain JM, Tamini HK, Figge DC, Greer BE. Uterine papillary serous carcinoma: patterns of metastatic spread. *Gynecol Oncol* 1994; 54:264–268.

41. Geisler JP, Geisler HE, Melton ME, Wiemann MC. What staging surgery should be performed on patients with uterine papillary serous carcinoma? *Gynecol Oncol* 1999; 74:465–467.

42. Gitsch G, Friedlander ML, Wain G, Hacker NF. Uterine papillary serous carcinoma. A clinical study. *Cancer* 1995; 75:2239–2243.

43. O'Hanlan KA, Levine PA, Harbatkin D, Feiner C, Goldberg GL, Jones JG, Rodriguez-Rodriguez L. Virulence of papillary endometrial carcinoma. *Gynecol Oncol* 1990; 37:12–19.

44. Bristow RE, Asrari F, Trimble EL, Montz FJ. Extended surgical staging for uterine papillary serous carcinoma: survival outcome of locoregional (Stage I-III) disease. *Gynecol Oncol* 2001; 81:279–286.

45. Bristow RE, Duska LR, Montz FJ. The role of cytoreductive surgery in the management of Stage IV uterine papillary serous carcinoma. *Gynecol Oncol* 2001; 81:92–99.

46. Tay EH, Ward BG. The treatment of uterine papillary serous carcinoma (UPSC): are we doing the right thing? *Int J Gynecol Cancer* 1999; 9:463–469.

47. Grice J, Ek M, Greer B, Koh WJ, Muntz HG, Cain J, Tamini H, Stelzer K, Figge D, Goff BA. Uterine papillary serous carcinoma: evaluation of long-term survival in surgically staged patients. *Gynecol Oncol* 1998; 69:69–73.

48. Turner BC, Knisely JPS, Kacinski BM, Haffty BG, Gumbs AA, Roberts KB, Frank AH, Peschel RE, Rutherford TJ, Edraki B, Kohorn EI, Chambers SK, Schwartz PE, Wilson LD. Effective treatment of Stage I uterine papillary serous carcinoma with high dose-rate vaginal apex radiation (192Ir) and chemotherapy. *Int J Radiat Oncol Biol Phys* 1998; 40:77–84.

49. Kato DT, Ferry JA, Goodman A, Sullinger J, Scully RE, Goff BA. Uterine papillary serous carcinoma (UPSC): a clinicopathologic study of 30 cases. *Gynecol Oncol* 1995; 59:384–389.

50. Ward BG, Wright RG, Free K. Papillary carcinomas of the endometrium. *Gynecol Oncol* 1990; 39:347–351.

51. Zanotti KM, Belinson JL, Kennedy AW, Webster KD, Markman M. The use of paclitaxel and platinum-based chemotherapy in uterine papillary serous carcinoma. *Gynecol Oncol* 1999; 74:272–277.

52. Craighead PS, Sait K, Stuart GC, Arthur K, Nation J, Duggan M, Guo D. Management of aggressive histologic variants of endometrial carcinoma at the Tom Baker Cancer Centre between 1984 and 1994. *Gynecol Oncol* 2000; 77:248–253.

53. Resnik E, Taxy JB. Neoadjuvant chemotherapy in uterine papillary serous carcinoma. *Gynecol Oncol* 1996; 62:123–127.

54. Le TD, Yamada SD, Rutgers JL, DiSaia PJ. Complete response of a stage IV uterine papillary serous carcinoma to neoadjuvant chemotherapy with Taxol and carboplatin. *Gynecol Oncol* 1999; 73:461–463.

12

Surgical Management of Recurrent Endometrial Cancer

NICHOLAS LAMBROU, LUIS MENDEZ, AND MANUEL PENALVER

University of Miami School of Medicine, Miami, Florida, U.S.A.

INTRODUCTION

In the United States, cancer of the endometrium is the most common female pelvic malignancy reported by the American Cancer Society, and the fourth most common cancer in women, ranking behind breast, bowel, and lung cancers (1). The diagnosis of endometrial cancer (EC) generally carries a favorable prognosis. At the time of diagnosis of EC the majority of patients have stage I disease based on the surgical-pathologic criteria of the International Federation of Gynecology and Obstetrics (FIGO) staging system (2). These patients can expect an overall 5-year survival rate of 80% to 90% (3). Primary treatment usually consists of surgical therapy, followed by radiotherapy, hormonal treatment, or chemotherapy in selected patients considered to be at risk for recurrent disease based on pathologic factors.

A generally accepted definition of recurrent EC is the histologic or cytologic confirmation of cancer 3 months after an apparently complete remission from primary therapy. Patients with residual cancer detected within 3 months of completing their initial treatment are considered to have persistent disease. The patterns of recurrence depend on initial disease distribution. Tumor recurrence is most common in women with high-risk features in their primary tumor and in women with advanced stage disease (4,5). Approximately two-thirds of recurrences are distant or multifocal; however, approximately one-third of recurrences seen in women whose primary tumor was confined to the uterus are limited to the pelvis. In a review published by Aalders et al. (6), 11% of 3,393 patients with EC treated at their institution were identified with recurrent disease. Of the patients with recurrent disease, 50% were found to have local recurrences only. Other published series have demonstrated a similar incidence of recurrence for clinical stage I disease (4); however, most demonstrate a predominance of distant or multifocal recurrences (4,7,8). The difference may be attributed to the more common use in the more recent series of adjuvant radiation therapy in patients considered to have high-risk factors for local recurrence.

Although EC has an overall low recurrence rate, when recurrences do occur and they are disseminated, treatment options are limited and mostly palliative. Treatment for metastatic recurrent EC includes progestational agents and/or chemotherapy, with response rates in general of approximately 25%. Surgical resection of recurrent EC does not offer any survival benefit when disease is disseminated. When recurrence is limited to the pelvis in patients who have not had previous pelvic irradiation, pelvic radiation therapy is very effective. The survival benefit in the setting of recurrence is still modest, however. In a report by Kuten et al. (9)

the 5-year progression free survival rate for patients with an isolated vaginal recurrence treated with radiation alone was 40%. When recurrence extended to the vagina and pelvis, survival decreased to 20%. Similar results have been reported by Poulsen and Roberts with a 45% 10-year survival for patients treated with radiation therapy of isolated vaginal vault recurrences (10). Only 24% of patients survived 10 years if there was pelvic extension of their recurrence prior to radiation treatment. The most favorable recurrence is the isolated vaginal recurrence less than 2 cm in diameter, occurring late (after 3 years since primary therapy) (11,12). However, the recurrence of tumor in a previously irradiated pelvis is ominous. The only subset of patients who are potentially curable are those whose pelvic recurrence is centrally located. For these patients, pelvic exenteration is a viable treatment option.

PELVIC EXENTERATION

Pelvic exenteration was developed by Dr. Alexander Brunschwig in the 1940s primarily for palliative treatment of large pelvic cancers (13). Advances in patient selection, surgical technique, and perioperative care have resulted in improvements in morbidity, mortality, and quality of life for these patients. Currently in patients undergoing pelvic exenteration for treatment of a gynecologic malignancy, the disease-free survival at 5 years approaches 50% (14–16). The vast majority of these patients are treated for pelvic recurrence of cancer of the uterine cervix. Although data are limited, recent reports have demonstrated that adequate long-term survival can be achieved in highly selected patients with recurrent EC (17,18).

Barber and Brunschwig were the first to report on the treatment of recurrent EC with pelvic exenteration (19). In their series of 36 patients between 1947 and 1963, the absolute 5-year survival rate was 14%. Only 5 of the 36 patients, however, had localized disease. More recently, Morris et al. (18) reported on 20 patients who underwent pelvic exenteration with curative intent for recurrent EC. The study was a retrospective review of data from four institutions. All of the patients received pelvic irradiation prior to exenteration either as part of their primary treatment or after initial recurrence. For this group, the 5-year disease free survival rate was 45%. Of eight patients who had known recurrences, the median time to recurrence was 17 months.

Barakat et al. (17) identified a total of 44 patients who underwent pelvic exenteration for recurrent EC at a single institution; 23% percent of these patients had never received radation therapy. The type of exenteration performed was total in 52%, anterior in 46%, and posterior in one patient. Median survival for the entire group of patients was 10.2 months; however, 9 patients (20%) achieved long-term survival (>5 years). Interestingly, two of the nine long-term survivors had positive pelvic lymph nodes at the time of exenteration. Major postoperative complications occurred in 80% of patients. Complications included urinary/intestinal fistulas, pelvic abscess, septicemia, pulmonary embolism, and cerebrovascular accident. The high morbidity and operative mortality in this group may reflect the fact that the majority of cases were performed between 1940 and 1980, with only three cases performed after 1980. The availability of modern antibiotics, surgical intensive care units, and improvements in surgical technique and reconstruction have decreased morbidity in patients undergoing pelvic exenteration and may improve overall survival in these patients (14–16,20,21).

Indications and Preoperative Evaluation

The indication for performing pelvic exenteration with curative intent in the setting of recurrent EC remains very specific to patients who have a histologically confirmed recurrence in the central pelvis after previous radiation therapy. Spread to the pelvic sidewall and/or metastatic disease are contraindications. As a general rule, unilateral obstructive uropathy, unilateral leg edema, and sciatic leg pain are suggestive of pelvic sidewall disease that is unresectable. That said, it is often difficult on physical exam to differentiate between tumor extent and radiation fibrosis. Preoperative assessment with pelvic MRI can be helpful in evaluating the extent of recurrent tumor within the pelvis and help predict the likelihood of surgical resection. Whenever in doubt, however, the ultimate determination of tumor resection must be made in the operating theater. Preoperatively, metastases outside of the pelvis should be ruled out using CT of the chest, pelvis, and abdomen. Although to-date there is little published data, the use of FDG-PET may prove helpful in the detection of distant metastases (22). Any suspicious findings such as hepatic lesions, enlarged lymph nodes, or pulmonary nodules need to be assessed with fine-needle aspiration to confirm metastases prior to exenteration.

If the preoperative workup is negative, the patient should then be counseled on the risks and benefits of undergoing this surgical procedure. The magnitude of physiologic stress and surgical risk associated with the surgery may be prohibitive for patients with major medical problems. In addition, the value of strong family or social support cannot be emphasized enough. The patient and her family must understand and accept all possible consequences of the surgery and be prepared for a prolonged hospitalization and home rehabilitation. At the University of Miami, we routinely arrange preoperative consultations for the patient and her family with our specialized team of social workers and ostomy nurses. They help educate the patient on management of a colostomy and urinary diversion, and review the potential psychological and emotional impact of exenterative surgery and any reconstructive procedures planned.

Surgical Exploration

The first step in pelvic exenteration is the exploratory laparotomy. A thorough evaluation of the pelvis and abdomen for evidence of disseminated disease is performed. The presence of metastatic implants to the small or large bowel is a contraindication to the procedure. However, direct involvement of the small or large bowel that is adherent in the pelvis may not represent systemic disease and is not considered a contraindication for pelvic exenteration. At our institution, approximately 40% to 50% of exploratory laparotomies for exenterations were abandoned because of extrapelvic disease (15,23). We routinely perform a pelvic lymphadenectomy as part of the initial surgical exploration. The presence of grossly positive pelvic lymph nodes is considered a contraindication to proceeding with exenteration. However, as mentioned earlier, long-term survival can been achieved in patients with microscopic positive pelvic lymph nodes (17). When possible, we routinely perform a lymph node sampling from the lower para-aortic chain with a frozen section evaluation as part of the exploratory procedure. When para-aortic lymph nodes are positive for metastatic disease, it is reflective of systemic disease and pelvic exenteration for curative purposes is abandoned.

The retroperitoneal spaces are then explored beginning with the pararectal and paravesical spaces to confirm the absence of sidewall involvement. For total pelvic exenterations, the space of Retzius, presacral, and retrorectal spaces are next dissected to ensure complete resection of the pelvic tumor. After dissection of the retroperitoneal spaces, confirming the absence of direct tumor extension to either of the bony boundaries including the sidewall, sacrum, or pubis, the surgeon is then ready to proceed with resection of pelvic organs.

Resection of Pelvic Organs

The ureters are mobilized as far into the pelvis as possible and are transected at least 2 cm from the tumor. Care is taken to preserve the vascularized adventitia surrounding the ureters during mobilization. The rectosigmoid colon is mobilized and transected using standard stapling techniques. After the tumor has been mobilized circumferentially, attention is turned to the lateral dissection down to the levator muscles. This resection can be performed using an Endo-GIA stapling device followed by large curved Heaney clamps. If an infralevator exenteration is required, the perineal phase is started at this point. If a supralevator exenteration is sufficient to adequately excise the tumor, then attention is turned to transection of the vagina and rectosigmoid individually using a roticulating TA-stapling device.

Although initially pelvic exenteration was synonymous with surgical removal of all pelvic organs including bladder, uterus, cervix, vagina, rectosigmoid, and possibly the vulva in an en bloc specimen, a more complete description includes subdivision into an anterior and posterior component and an infralevator and supralevator component (Table 1) (16). When disease is limited to the anterior lower genital tract, an anterior approach may be warranted, sparing the rectosigmoid and posterior vagina. Similarly, when disease is limited to the posterior lower genital tract, a posterior resection may be performed, sparing the bladder from resection. When performed with curative intent, it is of paramount importance to achieve negative surgical margins. Any tumor transection or incomplete tumor resection will result in prompt recurrence and death. Although anterior and posterior exenterations are beneficial in sparing either the rectosigmoid or the bladder, complete excision of the tumor must be ensured. It is also important to differentiate between infralevator and supralevator pelvic exenteration (Fig. 1) (16). The supralevator pelvic exenteration includes removal of the bladder, upper vagina, cervix, uterus, and rectosigmoid; however, the pelvic floor is preserved. When disease involves the lower part of the vagina, vulva, perineum or anus, an infralevator pelvic exenteration must be performed with removal of pelvic floor mus-

Table 1 Classification of Pelvic Exenteration

Group	Type
Anterior	I. Supralevator
Posterior	II. Infralevator
Total	III. With vulvectomy
Extended	

With permission from Magrina JF, Stanhope CR, Weaver AL: Pelvic exenterations: Supralevator, infralevator, and with vulvectomy. Gynecol Oncol 64: 130–135, 1997.

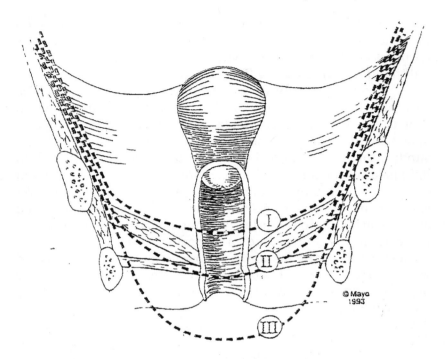

Figure 1 Extent and level of resection of pelvic tissues of the three different types of pelvic exenterations: (I) supralevator, (II) infralevator, and (III) infralevator with vulvectomy.

cles. Infralevator exenterations leave a large pelvic defect (Fig. 2) and reconstruction with myocutaneous flaps, omental flap, or dura mater have been described and is recommended (24–28).

Surgical Reconstruction

As described by Sevin and Koechli, the reconstructive phase of pelvic exenteration includes four parts: (1) construction of a urinary diversion, (2) colostomy or low coloanal anastamosis, (3) reconstruction of the pelvic floor, and (4) reconstruction of the vagina (29).

In general when choosing a urinary diversion, a choice is made between a conduit (non-continent urinary diversion),

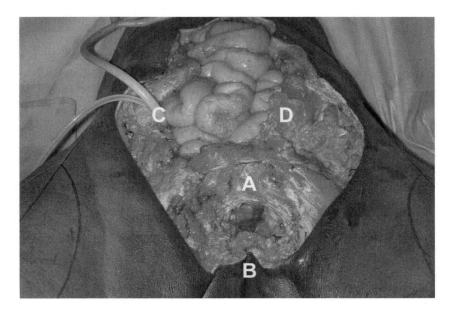

Figure 2 Anterior infralevator pelvic exenteration with vulvectomy. (A) Pubic symphisis; (B) intact rectum; (C) Foley catheter leading to Miami pouch; (D) rectus abdominis muscle.

which is faster and carries a smaller risk for complications, or a reservoir (continent urinary diversion), which is technically more challenging and associated with more frequent complications, but offers the benefit of urinary continence. Since 1988, at the University of Miami, we have used the continent ileocolonic reservoir, the Miami pouch, as the preferred method of continent urinary diversion (30). The Miami pouch offers an acceptable complication rate generally managed by conservative and non-invasive measures with a very reliable continent urinary mechanism (31). When the ileum is not available for reconstructive use because of severe radiation effects, the transverse colon is the preferred segment of bowel for the creation of a urinary conduit (32).

End-colostomy is currently the standard in patients undergoing total pelvic exenterations or posterior exenterations. However, recent attempts have been made to perform a low rectal anastamosis in patients who have undergone a supralevator exenteration (33). The rectal anastamosis is performed using standard circular stapling techniques and an omental pedicle flap should be placed around the anastamosis when available. Because of the high risk of fistula formation in patients with previous pelvic irradiation, a protective colostomy should always be performed and kept in place for approximately 3 months. Low rectal anastomosis is not an option for patients who undergo infralevator exenterations.

Pelvic floor reconstruction and/or the creation of a neovagina should be contemplated in all patients undergoing exenteration. Neovaginas offer the potential for improving the patient's quality of life as well as decreasing surgical morbidity by filling the large pelvic defect with well-vascularized tissue. Several options are available for pelvic reconstruction. Miller et al. (20) demonstrated a reduction in the incidence of intestinal fistula formation from 16% to less than 5% in those patients who had an omental pedicle graft or a gracilis myocutaneous flap at the time of exenteration. Jurado et al. (24) reported their results from a series of 16 patients who underwent vaginal reconstruction with a rectus abdominis myocutaneous flap, gracilis flap, or Singapore fasciocutaneous flap, and demonstrated a significant reduction in postoperative pelvic abscess compared with patients who had no vaginal reconstruction. Other types of vaginal reconstruction include various uses of colon, skin grafts, and local flaps. More recent data are emerging on the use of rectus flaps (25,34) and our preference at the University of Miami is to perform vaginal reconstruction with a rectus abdominis myocutaneous flap. The creation of a neovagina requires approximately 2–3 hours of additional operative time, a surgical team with the technical knowledge and experience to perform the reconstruction, and meticulous attention to postoperative care. However, not all patients are good candidates for vaginal reconstruction. Because of the large pelvic defect after an infralevator exenteration, the major risk has been the prolapse of pelvic organs such as the small bowel and of bowel fistulas. In these cases and especially when vaginal reconstruction is not an option, dura mater may be used to reconstruct the pelvic floor (26,35). It is advisable to drape an omental pedicle flap over the dura and denuded area in the pelvis when an omental flap is possible, and to place close-suctioned drains intraoperatively both above and below the reconstructed pelvic floor.

PALLIATION

Pelvic exenteration for recurrent EC should be performed with curative intent in the vast majority of cases. Because of advances in the non-invasive or minimally invasive management of genitourinary and gastrointestinal consequences of recurrent disease, the utility of pelvic exenteration as a palliative measure has been reduced. There remain however, specific groups of patients for whom palliative exenteration may be indicated. One group includes patients with advanced pelvic disease with extensive fistula caused by tumor involvement of the bladder or rectum in whom radiation is not initially safe or feasible. Urinary diversion or fecal diversion would be indicated initially. This might be followed by radiation and/or primary exenteration. In addition, there are patients in whom pelvic irradiation has resulted in severe chronic hemorrhagic radiation cystitis, proctitis, or extensive fistulae. If attempts at conservative and minimally invasive management fail, these patients are candidates for anterior or posterior exenteration as palliation for their symptoms. A final subset of patients includes those whose quality of life is so poor secondary to frank tumor extruding from the vagina or unbearable malodorous discharge and unmanageable hygiene, that pelvic exenteration may offer the only palliation for their symptoms. In a report by Magrina et al. (16), palliative exenterations did not have an increase in perioperative complications; however, survival, as expected, was lower than in patients undergoing exenteration for cure. Stanhope and Symmonds (36) retrospectively reviewed 59 patients at the Mayo Clinic who underwent pelvic exenteration for palliation between 1955 and 1981. Of these patients, four had EC. They demonstrated a 46% 2-year survival and 23% 5-year survival with pelvic nodal involvement. Median survival for the total group was 19 months, with 47% surviving more than 2 years and 17% surviving greater than 5 years. Pelvic exenteration for palliation of recurrent EC is reserved for a highly specific group of patients (as described above), but when performed appropriately, may offer a marked improvement in quality of life for these women.

REFERENCES

1. Greenlee RT, Murray T, Bolden S, et al. Cancer statistics, 2000. *CA Cancer J Clin* 2000; 50:7.

2. International Federation of Gynecology and Obstetrics: Corpus cancer staging. *Int J Gynaecol Obstet* 1989; 28:190.

3. Creasman WT, Morrow CP, Bundy BN, et al. Surgical pathologic spread patterns of endometrial cancer: Gynecologic Oncology Group study. *Cancer* 1987; 60:2035.

4. Reddoch JM, Burke TW, Morris M, Tornos C, Levenback C, Gershenson DM. surveillance for recurrent endometrial carcinoma: development of a follow-up scheme. *Gynecol Oncol* 1995; 59, 221–225.

5. Brown JM, Dockerty MB, Symmonds RE, Banner EA. Vaginal recurrence of endometrial carcinoma. *Am J Obstet Gynecol* 1968; 100(4):544–549.

6. Aalders JG, Abeler V, Kolstad P. Recurrent adenocarcinoma of the endometrium: a clinical and histopathological study of 379 patients. *Gynecol Oncol* 1984; 17:85.

7. Burke TW, Heller PB, Woodward JE, et al. Treatment failure in endometrial carcinoma. *Obstet Gynecol* 1990; 75:96.

8. Yoonessi M, Anderson DG, Morley GW. Endometrial carcinoma: causes of death and sites of treatment failure. *Cancer* 1979; 43:1944.

9. Kuten A, Grigsby PW, Perez CA, Fineberg B, Garcia DM, Simpson JR. Results of radiotherapy in recurrent endometrial carcinoma: a retrospective analysis. *Int J Radiat Oncol Biol Phys* 1989; 17:29.

10.   Poulsen MG, Roberts SJ. The salvage of recurrent endometrial carcinoma in the vagina and pelvis. *Int J Radiat Oncol Biol Phys* 1988; 15:809.

11.   Greven K, Olds W. Isolated vaginal recurrences of endometrial adenocarcinoma and their management. *Cancer* 1987; 60:419.

12.   Phillips GL, Konald AP, Adcock LL, Twiggs LB. Vaginal recurrence of adenocarcinoma of the endometrium. *Gynecol Oncol* 1982; 13:323–328.

13.   Brunschwig A. Complete excision of pelvic viscera for advanced carcinoma. *Cancer* 1948; 1:177–183.

14.   Rutledge FN, Smith JP, Wharton JT, O'Quinn AG. Pelvic exenteration: analysis of 296 patients. *Am J Obstet Gynecol* 1977; 129(8):881–890.

15.   Averette HE, Lichtinger M, Sevin BU, et al. Pelvic exenteration: a 15–year experience in a general metropolitan hospital. *Am J Obstet Gynecol* 1984; 150:179–184.

16.   Magrina JF, Stanhope CR, Weaver AL. Pelvic exenterations: supralevator, infralevator, and with vulvectomy. *Gynecol Oncol* 1997; 64:130–135.

17.   Barakat RB, Goldman NA, Patel DA, Venkatraman ES, Curtin JP. Pelvic exenteration for recurrent endometrial cancer. *Gynecol Oncol* 1999; 75:99–102.

18.   Morris M, Alvarez R, Kinney W, Wilson T. Treatment of recurrent adenocarcinoma of the endometrium with pelvic exenteration. *Gynecol Oncol* 1996; 60:288.

19.   Barber HRK, Brunschwig A. Treatment and results of recurrent cancer of corpus uteri in patients receiving anterior and total pelvic exenteration. *Cancer* 1968; 22(5):949–955.

20.   Miller B, Morris M, Gershenson DM, Levenbeck CL, Burke TW. Intestinal fistulae formation following pelvic exenteration: a review of the University of Texas M.D. Anderson Cancer Center Experience, 1957–1990. *Gynecol Oncol* 1995; 56:207–210.

21.   Morgan LS, Daly JW, Monif GR. Infectious morbidity associated with pelvic exenteration. *Gynecol Oncol* 1980; 10:318–328.

22. Nakahara T, Fujii H, Ide M, Mochizuki Y, Takahashi W, Yasuda S, Shohtsu A, Kubo A. F-18 FDG uptake in endometrial cancer. *Clin Nucl Med* 2001; Jan 26(1):82–83.

23. Penalver MA, Barreau G, Sevin BU, et al. Surgery for the treatment of locally recurrent disease. *J Natl Cancer Inst Monogr* 1996; 21:117–122.

24. Jurado M, Bazan A, Elejageitia J, Paloma V, Martinez-Monge R, Alcazar JL. Primary vaginal and pelvic floor reconstruction following pelvic exenteration: a study of morbidity. *Gynecol Oncol* 2000; 77(2):293–297.

25. Smith HO, Genesen MC, Runowicz CD, Goldberg GL. The rectus abdominis myocutaneous flap: modifications, complications, and sexual function. *Cancer* 1998; 83(3):510–520.

26. Angioli R, Sevin B, Penalver M, et al. Pelvic floor reconstruction with dura mater allograft after pelvic exenteration: the University of Miami experience. *J Pelvic Surg* 1996; 2:58–62.

27. Wheeless CR, Neovagina constructed from an omental "J" flap and a split thickness skin graft. *Gynecol Oncol* 1989; 35:24.

28. Kusiak JF, Rosenblum NG. Neovaginal reconstruction after exenteration using an omental flap and split-thickness skin graft. *Plast Reconstr Surg* 1996; 97:775–783.

29. Sevin BU, Koechli OR. Pelvic exenteration In Penalver M, Mendez L, Angioli R. The Surgical Clinics of North America: *Gynecol Oncol* 2001; 81(4):771–779.

30. Penalver MA, Benjany DE, Averette, et al. Continent urinary diversion in gynecologic oncology. *Gynecol Oncol* 1989; 34:274–288.

31. Angioli R, Estape R, Cantuaria G, et al. Urinary complications of Miami pouch: trend of conservative management. *Am J Obstet Gynecol* 1998; 179:343–348.

32. Hohenfellner R, Muller SC, Riedmiller H, et al. Continent urinary diversion: The Mainz pouch technique. In Knapstein PG, Friedberg V, Sevin B (eds): Reconstructive Surgery in Gynecology. New York, Thieme Medical Publishers, 1990, pp. 231–247.

33. Mirhashemi R, Averette HE, Estape R, Angioli R, Mahran R, Mendez L, Cantuaria G, Penalver M. Low colorectal anasta-

mosis after radical pelvic surgery: a risk factor analysis. *Am J Obstet Gynecol* 183(6):1375–1380.

34. Carlson JW, Soisson AP, Fowler JM, Carter JR, Twiggs LB, Carson LR. Rectus abdominis myocutaneous flap for primary vaginal reconstruction. *Gynecol Oncol* 1993; 51:323–329.

35. Sevin B, Malinin T. Dura mater allograft in gynecologic reconstruction. In Knapstein PG, Friedberg V, Sevin B (eds): *Reconstructive Surgery in Gynecology*. New York, Thieme Medical Publishers, 1990, pp. 151–167.

36. Stanhope CR, Symmonds RE. Palliative exenteration—what, when and why? *Am J Obstet Gynecol* 1985; 152(1):12–16.

13

Radiation Treatment for Early Stage Endometrial Cancer and Uterine Sarcoma

PERRY W. GRIGSBY

Washington University Medical Center,
St. Louis, Missouri, U.S.A.

INTRODUCTION

Carcinoma of the endometrium is the most common invasive gynecologic neoplasm in women in the United States. Over 30,000 new cases will be diagnosed this year. One of the most controversial topics in the field of gynecologic oncology is the postoperative management of patients with edometrial cancer (EC) and uterine sarcoma (US). The majority of patients with EC present with stage I or II disease. The survival of these patients, when treated with surgery only, ranges from 70% to 80%. Identifying the subset of patients at risk for recurrent disease and the appropriate treatment of these patients often elicits strong opinions from oncologists. Patients with uterine sarcomas often present with advanced pathologically staged disease that puts the patients at high risk for developing distant metastatic disease for which there is no good prophylactic treatment. The Radiation Therapy Oncology Group (RTOG) and the Gynecologic Oncology Group (GOG) have initiated several clinical trials for patients with EC and US. Unfortunately, many of these clinical trials failed to accrue a sufficient number of patients to permit completion of the study and data analysis.

After surgery, adjuvant irradiation may be indicated based on surgical–pathological staging information. The irradiation may be given locally in the vagina or to the pelvis. Local irradiation to the vagina may be performed as an inpatient using low-dose rate brachytherapy or as an outpatient using high-dose rate brachytherapy. Pelvic irradiation may be given with external irradiation alone or with the addition of vaginal brachytherapy.

For occasional patients with serious medical conditions, radiation therapy is used as an alternative to surgery. Severe cardiopulmonary disease and morbid obesity are the primary reasons a patient with EC does not undergo surgery. Patients not undergoing surgery are clinically staged. Irradiation may be internal, external, or a combination, depending on patient and tumor characteristics.

Despite the current recommendations for surgical staging for EC, not all of the required specimens are obtained for all patients. It is therefore difficult to compare the results of therapy for patients from one report to another because there is no consistent definition of the patient populations.

Few, successfully completed, prospective randomized studies have been performed for patients with EC and uterine sarcomas. However, in recent years, randomized studies have been performed in an attempt to answer questions regarding the best management for these patients.

Outlined below are treatment recommendations for patients who are surgically staged and for those who have incomplete surgical staging. Recommendations are based upon the results of prospective randomized studies, to the extent that they exist, and upon the results of retrospective studies. Also described is the use of irradiation alone for medically inoperable patients. The techniques for both external irradiation and high-dose rate (HDR) brachytherapy are given.

ENDOMETRIAL CANCER

Stages I and II: Postoperative Management

Numerous risk factors have been identified for patients with EC. In general, patients can be divided into one of three categories of risk for developing locally recurrent and metastatic disease: low risk, intermediate risk, and high risk. When the patient's tumor is confined to the uterus, the primary risk factors for developing recurrent disease are tumor histology, tumor grade, depth of myometrial invasion, lymphovascular space involvement by tumor, and patient age. Depending on the individual patient risk factors, the patients with tumor confined to the uterus are classified to either the low-risk or the intermediate-risk groups for developing recurrent disease. Patients with tumor outside the uterus (stages III or IV) are considered to be at a high risk of developing recurrent disease.

Patients with surgical stage IA, grade 1 and 2 endometrial adenocarcinomas are at low risk for developing recurrent disease when no adjuvant postoperative therapy is administered. This treatment issue has not been tested in a prospective randomized study because the risk of recurrence is less than 10% and a phase III study of this patient population would require a prohibitively large number of patients to be entered into the study. However, from the results of the numerous retrospective studies and pathologic models of survival, it is evident that postoperative adjuvant irradiation should not be routinely administered to most patients in this category.

Patients with surgical stages IA, IB, and IIC disease, grades 1, 2, and 3, can be considered to be at intermediate risk for developing recurrent disease postoperatively if no adjuvant therapy is administered. Only one (successfully completed) prospective randomized study has specifically addressed the issue of postoperative adjuvant irradiation for this patient population, the GOG's phase III study, GOG-99 (1). Patients entered onto this study were randomized to receive surgery alone or surgery and adjuvant postoperative pelvic irradiation. The surgery consisted of a TAH-BSO, pelvic and para-aortic lymph node sampling, and peritoneal cytology in all patients. All patients entered onto the study had surgical stages I or IIA disease and negative lymph nodes. When administered, postoperative pelvic irradiation consisted of 50.4 Gy to the pelvis delivered by a four-field box technique given at 1.8 Gy per day. Vaginal cuff brachytherapy was not administered. A total of 392 patients were entered into the study. The stage distribution of patients was IA in 9%, IB in 58%, and IC in 32%. The grades of the tumor were grades 1 or 2 in 82% and grade 3 in 18%. The median follow-up of patients at the time of data analysis was 56 months. The results of the study demonstrated that the overall survival was 94% for the irradiated patients and 89% for the surgery only patients ($p = 0.09$). However, there was a statistically significant difference in recurrence-free survivals in the two treatment groups. Irradiated patients had a 96% recurrence-free survival compared to 88% for the unirradiated patients ($p = 0.004$). The failure rate in the pelvis was 2% for the irradiated patients compared to 12% for those not receiving irradiation ($p = 0.001$). Death from EC occurred in 5% of the irradiated patients compared to 7% in the unirradiated patients (not significant). However, the severe complication rate (grades 3 and 4) was greater in the patients receiving irradiation. The complication rate was 15% for the group receiving pelvic irradiation and 6% for the surgery only group ($p = 0.007$).

Most of the patients entered onto GOG-99 had either stage IB disease or tumors that were grade 1 or 2. These patients are at a rather low risk for developing recurrent disease. A subgroup analysis of GOG-99 indicated that significant risk factors for developing recurrent disease were advancing patient age, grades 2 and 3 histology, greater than one-third myometrial invasion, or the presence of lymphovascular space involvement by tumor. When patient survival was analyzed by prognostic factors (grades 2 or 3, greater than one-third myometrial invasion, and lymphovascular space invasion) and stratified by patient age, significant differences in overall and recurrence-free survival were observed. If patients were more than 70 years old with one of the prognostic factors, more than 50 years old with any two of the prognostic factors, or any age with all three of the prognostic factors, then the recurrence-free survival was 87% for the irradiated patients compared to 73% for the unirradiated patients ($p < 0.01$).

A currently open study being performed by the national Cancer Institute of Canada–Clinical Trials Group (NCIC) is similar to GOG-99. In the NCIC study, patients undergo a laparoscopically assisted vaginal hysterectomy or total abdominal hysterectomy and bilateral salpingo-oophorectomy. Patients cannot have pathologically involved lymph nodes if that surgical staging procedure is performed. Patients eligible for the study are those with grade 3 disease with either no myometrial invasion or any degree of myometrial invasion. Patients with grade 2 tumors must have greater than 50% myometrial invasion. Patients with more than 50% myometrial (grades 1 or 2) or less than 50% myometrial invasion (grade 3) but with positive peritoneal cytology are also eligible. Postoperatively patients are randomized to be treated with pelvic irradiation versus observation. All patients randomized to the treatment arm receive external pelvic irradiation. Vaginal brachytherapy is allowed but not required. Approximately 400 patients will be accrued to this study. This NCIC study and further follow-up of GOG-99 will aid in making appropriate therapeutic decisions for this patient population.

The RTOG performed a phase II clinical trial to assess the safety and toxicity of combined pelvic irradiation and chemotherapy for patients with grades 2 and 3 endometrial adenocarcinoma with either greater than 50% myometrial invasion, stromal invasion of the cervix, or pelvic confined extrauterine disease (2). The single arm study was designed to administer 45 Gy to the pelvis and concurrent cisplatin chemotherapy on days 1 and 28. Vaginal cuff brachytherapy was given with either low-dose rate or high-dose rate. Four courses of combined cisplatin and paclitaxel were given at 4-week intervals following the completion of irradiation. Forty-six patients were entered into the study. Acute grade 3 toxicity occurred in 33% of patients and acute grade 4 toxicity occurred in 2%. Chronic grade 3 toxicity occurred in 14% and chronic grade 4 toxicity occurred in 2%. The overall survival rate at 12 months was 95%. The authors concluded that the toxicity of this treatment regimen was acceptable (2). Therefore, the RTOG has proceeded with performing a currently open phase III randomized clinical trial (RTOG 99–05) to evaluate the use of chemotherapy in this patient population. In RTOG 99–05, patients undergo a total abdominal hysterectomy, vaginal hysterectomy, or laparoscopic assisted vaginal hysterectomy and bilateral salpingo-oophorectomy with or without additional surgical staging. Patients eligible for the study must have grade 2 or 3 adenocarcinoma with greater than 50% myometrial invasion, cervical glandular involvement, or cervical stromal invasion. There can be no known disease outside the uterus. Following surgery, patients are randomized to one of two study arms. In arm one of the study, the patients receive 50.4 Gy to the pelvis at 1.8 Gy per day. In arm two of the study the patients receive the same pelvic irradiation as in arm one and they also receive concurrent cisplatin (50 mg/m^2) on days 1 and 28 and paclitaxel (160 mg/m^2) on days 56, 84, 112, and 140 from the start of irradiation. This study is currently open for patient accrual.

The Nordic Society for Gynecologic Oncology (NSGO) is currently performing a phase III study (NSG 9501) in patients with surgical stage I EC with the following histologic types: papillary serous carcinoma, clear cell carcinoma, undifferentiated carcinoma, and poorly differentiated (grade 3) adenocarcinoma. The objectives of NSGO 9501 are to evaluate the survival, toxicity, and relapse patterns in patients treated with adjuvant irradiation alone or adjuvant sequential pelvic irradiation and chemotherapy. All patients receive pelvic irradiation to 50.4 Gy (1.8 Gy per day). Those randomized to receive chemotherapy are prescribed four courses of cisplatin plus doxorubicin (or epirubicin) every 3 weeks. This study is currently open to patient accrual.

Before the adoption by FIGO of the surgical staging system for patients with EC, routine lymph node sampling was rarely performed. The majority of published retrospective studies report the results of patients who did not undergo a lymph node sampling. The value of lymph node sampling is currently being tested in a clinical trial performed by the Medical Research Council (MRC-UK). The objective of the MRC study is to compare the effects of conventional surgery alone and conventional surgery plus lymph adenectomy in patients with stage I EC who are thought preoperatively to have tumor confined to the uterine corpus.

Patients without a lymph node sampling can be divided into low-, intermediate-, or high-risk groups for developing recurrent disease based upon the grade of the tumor, the depth of myometrial invasion, the presence of lymphovascular space invasion by tumor, lower uterine segment involvement, and cervical involvement.

Patients with grades 1 and 2 endometrial adenocarcinoma with no myometrial invasion or less than 50% myometrial invasion have a greater than 90% 5-year disease-free survival if the initial disease is confined to the uterus. The survival rates correlate with the incidence of lymph node metastasis found by Creasman and colleagues in a GOG surgical staging study (3). The results of the GOG surgical staging study revealed that patients with grades 1 and 2 disease and no myometrial invasion, or less than 50% myometrial invasion, had less than a 10% chance of having positive pelvic or para-aortic lymph nodes. These patients usually require no adjuvant postoperative therapy.

Patients who are at an intermediate risk of developing recurrent disease following surgery are those with grade 3 disease and no myometrial invasion or less than 50% myometrial invasion, and those with grades 1 and 2 disease with greater than 50% myometrial invasion. These patients have 5-year survival rates ranging from 70% to 85%.

A recent prospective randomized phase III study performed by Creutzberg and associates (4) from the Dutch Postoperative Radiation Therapy in Endometrial Cancer (PORTEC) study group addressed the use of postoperative irradiation as adjuvant therapy in this group of patients (i.e., those at intermediate risk) (4). In the PORTEC study, patients underwent a TAH/BSO and no lymph node sampling or dissection. Postoperatively, patients who were eligible for this study were those with grade 1 disease with more than 50% myometrial invasion, patients with grade 2 disease and any degree of myometrial invasion, and patients with grade 3 disease and less than 50% myometrial invasion. Patients with grade 3 disease and greater than 50% myometrial invasion were not eligible for the study. Patients were randomized to receive postoperative pelvic irradiation to 46 Gy or no further therapy after surgery. The study enrolled 715 patients; the median follow-up was 52 months. The results of the study demonstrated that the 5-year actuarial pelvic failure rates were 4% in the irradiated group and 14% in the control group ($p < 0.001$). The actuarial 5-year overall survival rates were 81% for the irradiated patients and 85% for the control group ($p = 0.31$). Deaths due to EC occurred in 9% of the patients treated with irradiation and in 6% of the control group ($p = 0.37$). Complications of any severity were reported to be 25% for those receiving irradiation and 6% for those in the control group ($p < 0.001$). Grades 3 and 4 complications occurred in only 7 patients (7 of 715), with 6 of the 7 complications occurring in irradiated patients. The authors performed a Cox multivariate regression analysis and found that the three significant prognostic factors for death from EC or pelvic recurrence of the disease were patient age greater than 60 years old, greater than 50% myometrial invasion, and grade 3 differentiation of the tumor. Lymphovascular space invasion was not evaluated in their analysis. The investigators found that patients with grade 3 histology with less than 50% myometrial invasion were associated with a risk of locoregional recurrence similar to patients with grades 1 and 2 tumors with greater than 50% myometrial invasion, and the risk of death was greatest for those with grade 3 tumors.

The results of the PORTEC study are similar to the findings of Grigsby and colleagues in their retrospective study of

858 patients with clinical stage I endometrial adenocarcinoma (5). These investigators found that the 5-year survival
results for clinical stage I patients (no lymph node sampling
or dissection) were greater than 90% for patients with grades
1 and 2 histology with no myometrial invasion or less than
50% myometrial invasion. Patients with grade 3 disease and
no myometrial invasion or less than 50% myometrial invasion, and those with grades 1 and 2 histology with greater
than 50% myometrial invasion, had 5-year survival rates
ranging from 69% to 85%. In addition, patients with deep
myometrial invasion and grade 3 histology had only a 42% 5-
year survival.

Stages I and II: Irradiation Alone

The hallmark of the therapeutic management of patients
with EC is hysterectomy. In contradistinction to carcinoma of
the uterine cervix, empirical studies in patients with EC indicated that irradiation alone was not optimal therapy. The best
clinical outcomes for patients with EC seem to be achieved
with either surgery alone or a combination of surgery and
adjuvant postoperative irradiation. However, some patients
with clinical stages I and II EC present with advanced age
and severe co-morbidities that preclude surgical staging or
hysterectomy. These patients may have an expected survival
of several years despite their severe illnesses. Most of these
patients should be treated with irradiation alone with a curative intent, which can be achieved.

   Patients with stage I disease may be treated with
brachytherapy alone or with combined external irradiation
and brachytherapy based upon tumor grade, depth of myometrial invasion, and lymph node status. Tumor grade is determined from the results of the endometrial biopsy or dilation
and curettage (D&C). Depth of myometrial invasion can be
determined from an MRI of the pelvis. Lymph node status of
the pelvis and para-aortic lymph node is ascertained from a
CT scan of the abdomen and pelvis. No clinical trials have
been performed for patients with stage I, medically inoperable EC. This is because of the limited number of patients

available for study in this patient population. However, several retrospective studies have been performed to evaluate the results of therapy for these patients. These studies indicate that overall survivals are in the range of 70% to 80% for this elderly, medically inoperable group of patients. Grigsby and colleagues (6) demonstrated that the 5-year progression-free survival rates for clinical stage I disease was 94% for patients with grade 1 tumors, 92% for grade 2, and 78% for grade 3 if patients received both external irradiation and intracavitary brachytherapy. A current update of these data indicate that the 5-year overall and disease-free survivals for 143 patients with clinical stage I, medically inoperable EC are 65% and 85%. The poor overall survival reflects the advanced age and co-morbidity of the patients.

Patients with clinical stage II disease who are medically inoperable are usually treated with combined external irradiation and intracavitary brachytherapy. Retrospective studies report the 5-year survival for these patients to range from 50% to 60%. A current update of the database from the Mallinckrodt Institute of Radiology indicates that the 5-year overall and disease-free survivals for 62 patients with clinical stage II, medically inoperable EC was 36% and 47%, respectively.

Stages I and II: Summary

The treatment of patients with EC has evolved over the past several years. Most patients with early stage disease undergo extrafascial hysterectomy. Complete surgical staging is performed in a minority of patients within the United States. Recommendations for adjuvant irradiation are based upon the individual patient's risk factors, which must take into account whether or not the patient had complete surgical staging.

For patients who have had complete surgical staging, no postoperative adjuvant irradiation is recommended for those with stages IA, grades 1 and 2, and stages IB, grades 1 and 2 disease. Postoperative vaginal cuff brachytherapy is recommended for those with stages IA, grade 3; IB, grade 3; IC, grades 1 and 2; and stages IIA, all disease grades with less than 50% myometrial invasion. Vaginal cuff brachytherapy should be considered for those with stages IA and IB, grade 2, with lower uterine segment involvement by tumor. Postoperative external pelvic irradiation and vaginal cuff brachytherapy are recommended for patients with stages IC, grade 2; IIA, grades 1, 2, and 3 with greater than 50% myometrial invasion, and most patients with stage IIB disease. Patients with stage IIB, grades 1 and 2 disease with less than 50% myometrial invasion may be considered for vaginal cuff brachytherapy alone. Prognostic factors, in addition to tumor grade and depth of myometrial invasion, that should be considered when developing a therapeutic strategy for the individual patient are patient age and the presence of lymphovascular space invasion. Patient age greater than 70 years and the presence of lymphovascular space invasion by tumor are two independent poor prognostic factors.

Treatment recommendations for patients who undergo incomplete surgical staging (i.e., unknown lymph node status) would include no adjuvant postoperative irradiation for patients with stage I, grades 1 and 2 disease with less than 50% myometrial invasion. Patients with grade 3 disease with no myometrial invasion should receive postoperative vaginal cuff brachytherapy. Patients with less than 50% myometrial invasion with tumor of any grade should receive postoperative pelvic irradiation and vaginal cuff brachytherapy. All patients with stage II disease should receive postoperative vaginal cuff brachytherapy and external pelvic irradiation.

Irradiation alone is utilized for clinical stage I patients who are medically inoperable. Patients with negative lymph nodes by radiographic imaging and less than 50% myometrial invasion as determined by pelvic MRI, and grades 1 and 2, can be treated by intracavitary brachytherapy alone. Patients with greater than 50% myometrial invasion by MRI and of any tumor grade, and all patients with grade 3 disease, should receive external pelvic irradiation and intracavitary brachytherapy. All patients with clinical stage II disease who are medically inoperable should receive external pelvic irradiation and intracavitary brachytherapy.

UTERINE SARCOMA

Stages I and II: Postoperative management

The pathologic classification and terminology to describe uterine sarcomas has varied over time. The three most common groups of uterine sarcomas are the mixed mesodermal tumor, leiomyosarcomas, and endometrial stromal sarcomas. Other types of uterine sarcomas may occur but are very uncommon. The prognostic factors for uterine sarcomas are similar to those for EC; that is, histologic types, depth of myometrial invasion, and lymph node status.

Mixed mesodermal tumors represent about 50% of all uterine sarcomas. Carcinosarcomas (malignant mixed müllerian tumor, homologous type) is the most common type. The GOG performed a clinicopathologic evaluation of clinical stages I and II uterine sarcomas from 1979 through 1988. The significant prognostic factors, as determined by multivariate analysis for progression-free interval, were grade of sarcoma, histologic cell type (homologous versus heterologous), adnexal spread of tumor, and lymph node metastases (7). Univariate analysis of progression-free intervals for these patients also identified tumor size, lymphovascular space invasion, and depth of myometrial invasion as significant prognostic factors.

Leiomyosarcomas represent about 2.5% of all uterine sarcomas. In their GOG study, Major and colleagues (7) also evaluated clinicopathologic prognostic factors for uterine leiomyosarcomas. Univariate and multivariate analysis of prognostic factors yielded only one surgicopathologic factor that correlated significantly with the progression-free interval—the mitotic index. Their study described no failures in women with less than 10 mitoses/10 high-power fields (hpf), 61% failures at 3 years in those with 10 to 20 mitoses/10 hpf, and 79% failures in these with greater than 20 mitoses/10 hpf.

Endometrial stromal sarcomas occur in about 15% to 20% of patients with uterine sarcomas. As with other uterine sarcomas, endometrial stromal sarcomas have a tendency to spread locally and to develop distant metastasis. Although this tumor type is uncommon, several investigators have evaluated prognostic factors for this patient population. No prospective studies have been performed. However, the recurring theme that is evident from several retrospective studies is that the most significant prognostic factor for survival is the mitotic index of the tumor (8–12).

There is a paucity of prospective randomized studies for the management of patients with uterine sarcomas. There are two studies by the GOG that were performed to evaluate the utility of adjuvant chemotherapy in patients with uterine sarcomas, but the use of adjuvant irradiation was uncontrolled (13,14). The RTOG and the GOG attempted to perform an intergroup study in 1984 on the use of postoperative pelvic irradiation for stages I and II malignant mixed mesodermal sarcomas of the uterus. The design of the study was to randomize patients to postoperative pelvic irradiation versus no further therapy. The study was closed prematurely due to lack of patient accrual. The EORTC is currently evaluating, in an open study, the use of postoperative pelvic irradiation in patients with stages I and II, high-grade uterine sarcomas (leiomyosarcomas, malignant mixed mesodermal sarcomas, or endometrial stromal sarcomas) randomized to receive either postoperative pelvic irradiation or observation. This study is currently ongoing. A second currently active study is GOG 150 in which patients with optimally debulked stages I to IV carcinosarcomas of the uterus are randomized, postoperatively, to receive either whole abdominal irradiation or chemotherapy. The chemotherapy consists of cisplatin and ifosfamide every 3 weeks for three courses. This GOG study is nearing completion of patient accrual.

In the absence of phase III, prospective randomized studies, treatment recommendations for patients with uterine sarcomas must be based on the results of retrospective reviews. One of the first, and most often cited, reviews of the treatment of patients with uterine sarcomas is a study by Salazar and colleagues (15). This was a retrospective review of 73 patients with uterine sarcomas treated with surgery only, surgery plus postoperative pelvic irradiation, or irradiation alone. The conclusions of the investigators on this limited number of patients continue to hold true; that is, patients treated with surgery alone or irradiation alone have inferior survival results to those patients treated with surgery and postoperative pelvic irradiation. Postoperative pelvic irradiation reduced the incidence of pelvic recurrences, but did not seem to influence a prolongation in overall survival. Outlined below are the findings of other, more recent retrospective reviews of patients with uterine sarcomas.

Mixed Mesodermal Tumors

Mixed mesodermal tumors are the most common type of uterine sarcoma. Major and associates performed a prospective surgical staging study and evaluated the survival and sites of failure in their patients who received postoperative adjuvant therapy in an uncontrolled setting (7). The authors found that the pelvic failure rate for patients with mixed mesodermal tumors was 24% for those treated with surgery alone and was reduced to 11% for those receiving postoperative adjuvant pelvic irradiation. The disease-free survival was 46% for those treated with surgery alone and 50% for those receiving adjuvant irradiation. The Major study included patients with surgical stages I to IV disease. More recent studies have begun to report the results of treatment by early stage disease and advanced stage disease. Yamada and colleagues evaluated the survival of 62 patients with carcinoma of the uterus (16). They found that the 5-year survival rate was 74% for patients whose tumor was confined to the uterus, but the 5-year survival rate decreased to 24% ($p = 0.0013$) for patients with tumor outside the uterus. Knocke and associates reported on 63 patients with mixed müllerian tumors (17). The disease-free survivals at 5 years were 75% for stage I, 50% for stage II, 34% for stage III, and 33% for stage IV. A retrospective review of 60 patients receiving definitive therapy for carcinosarcoma was performed by Gerszten and colleagues (18). All patients were treated with a TAH/BSO and a lymph node sampling was performed in 74%. Twenty-nine patients received adjuvant postoperative radiotherapy. The investigators noted that the relative risk of local recurrence of unirradiated patients versus irradiated patients was 17.5% (p

= 0.055). They also reported that for patients with stages I and II disease, the 5-year overall survival rates were 83% for patients receiving pelvic irradiation compared to 50% for unirradiated patients (p = 0.02). Similar results were found by Malpus and associates (19). In the Malpus study, there was also a statistically significant improvement in cause-specific survival for patients with stages I and II disease who received pelvic irradiation compared to unirradiated patients (p = 0.001). Manolitsas and colleagues (20) expanded the concept of postoperative pelvic irradiation in patients with surgical stages I and II disease. They performed a pilot study on 38 patients with surgical stages I and II malignant mixed müllerian tumors. The patients were treated with adjuvant irradiation and four to six cycles of cisplatin (75 mg/m^2) and epirubicin (75 mg/m^2). The overall survival rate for all patients was 74% with a mean follow-up of 55 months. The overall survival rate for 21 patients who completed treatment per protocol was 95% compared to 47% for 17 patients who did not complete treatment per protocol.

Prospective randomized studies for patients with mixed mesodermal tumors are difficult to perform because of the low incidence of the disease. The RTOG and the GOG began an intergroup study of patients with surgical stages I and II mixed mesodermal tumors (INT-0019). Following TAH/BSO, patients were randomized to receive pelvic irradiation (50.4 Gy) versus no further therapy. The study was terminated early due to lack of patient accrual.

Since many patients with mixed mesodermal tumors will fail in the upper abdomen, the GOG is currently performing a phase III randomized study of whole abdominal irradiation versus ifosfamide and cisplatin in patients with optimally debulked stages I to IV carcinosarcoma of the uterus. This study is currently ongoing and no preliminary results are available.

Leiomyosarcoma

In the GOG study by Major and associates, there were 59 patients with leiomyosarcoma (7). The patients had stages I to IV disease. Pelvic irradiation was administered at the discretion of the treating physician. The disease-free survival was 23% for the irradiated patients and 30% for those not receiving irradiation. The most common site of failure for these patients was the lung followed by other extrapelvic failures. The results of therapy for patients with leiomyosarcoma are difficult to ascertain because of the low incidence of the disease and the tendency of investigators to combine all histologic types of uterine sarcomas when reporting their results. Knocke and colleagues (21) treated 30 patients with stages I to IV uterine leiomyosarcoma with surgery and postoperative pelvic irradiation. They reported on a 76% pelvic control rate at 5 years and the disease-free survival at 5 years was 52%. Pellenda and associates have reported on the largest group of patients with leiomyosarcomas (22). Their study consisted of 80 patients. There were 56 patients with stage I disease, 8 with stage II, 8 with stage III, 4 with stage IV, and in 4 patients the stage of the disease could not be determined. All patients underwent a TAH/BSO. Postoperatively, 54 patients received adjuvant pelvic irradiation. Twelve patients received adjuvant chemotherapy. The 5-year overall and disease-free survival rates were 51% and 37%, respectively. About 50% of patients developed distant metastatic disease. The authors reported that their data indicated that adjuvant irradiation did not appear to affect either overall survival nor local or locoregional control.

ENDOMETRIAL STROMAL SARCOMA

Most investigators report that the primary prognostic factor for patients with endometrial stromal sarcoma is the number of mitoses per 10 hpf. Those patients whose tumor has less than 10 mitoses/10 hpf have a better outcome than those with greater than 10 mitoses/10 hpf. Nonetheless, all patients with endometrial stromal sarcoma are at a high risk for developing local recurrences and distant metastasis after initial surgery. Weitman and associates (23) reviewed the results of therapy for 21 patients with endometrial stromal sarcoma. All patients underwent a TAH/BSO and 15 received postoperative pelvic irradiation. The overall local control rate was 94% at 5 years and the overall survival was 63%. The authors concluded from this small series of patients that the most effective treatment was surgery followed by adjuvant pelvic irradiation. Bodner and colleagues (12) evaluated 31 patients with endometrial stromal sarcoma. A TAH/BSO was performed in all patients. Twenty patients received adjuvant irradiation and 5 received adjuvant chemotherapy. In the irradiated patients, 20% developed a local recurrence and 50% developed recurrent disease at any site. The authors concluded that adjuvant therapy appeared to offer no survival advantage in their patient population.

Stages I and II: Irradiation Alone

There is a true paucity of data on the use of irradiation alone for patients with uterine sarcomas. Medically inoperable patients often have severe co-morbidity and a large tumor burden. The survival outcome in these patients is poor. However, there are reports of long-term survivors with uterine sarcoma treated with irradiation alone. Knocke and colleagues (17) reported the results of therapy in 13 patients treated with irradiation alone for mixed müllerian tumors of the uterus. Only 6 out of 13 patients were treated with a full course of combined external irradiation and brachytherapy. One patient had no evidence of disease at 18 months, one patient died at 48 months of intercurrent disease without evidence of cancer (autopsy proven), one patient developed distant metastasis and died at 14 months without evidence of local recurrence, and three patients developed local recurrences at 6 to 19 months after therapy. Similarly poor results in limited numbers of patients have been reported by other investigators (24–27).

Summary

Patients with uterine sarcomas are a heterogeneous group. In general, patients with mixed mesodermal tumors have a better survival outcome than do patients with leiomyosarcoma or endometrial stromal sarcoma. However, there are some patients with early stage, low-grade leiomyosarcoma who have an excellent prognosis. Patients should be treated with a TAH/BSO and tumor debulking when possible. Irradiation alone is clearly an inferior treatment strategy, but is necessary in some medically inoperable patients. A benefit to postoperative pelvic irradiation has been demonstrated in stage I and II patients in retrospective studies. This finding is best summarized for all three major sarcoma types in a combined group of patients with uterine sarcomas of these three types in a retrospective review by Ferrer and associates (28) who evaluated 103 patients with leiomyosarcoma (43 patients), mixed müllerian tumors (40 patients), endometrial stromal sarcomas (17 patients), and other types (3 patients). In their study, 101 patients underwent TAH/BSO. The stages of disease were I to IVA. Adjuvant pelvic irradiation was administered in 54 cases. Thirty-three patients received chemotherapy. The authors reported on three end points: locoregional disease-free interval, disease-free interval, and overall survival. The locoregional disease-free interval at 5 years was 76% for those receiving pelvic irradiation and 36% for those not receiving pelvic irradiation. The disease-free interval was 53% at 5 years for those receiving pelvic irradiation and 33% for those not receiving pelvic irradiation. Finally, the authors reported the overall survivals at 5 years to be 73% for irradiated patients and 37% in unirradiated patients. A multivariate analysis was performed which demonstrated that pelvic irradiation was the only significant independent prognostic factor for locoregional failure, disease-free interval, and overall survival. In conclusion, it is recommended that postoperative pelvic irradiation be administered to patients with uterine sarcomas of all types with stages I and II disease. Some patients with low-grade leiomyosarcomas may not require irradiation. The role of whole abdominal irradiation and chemotherapy remains undefined.

TECHNIQUE OF EXTERNAL IRRADIATION

The anatomy of the uterus and its draining lymphatics form the basis for the administration of external pelvic irradiation.

Lymphatics from the body of the uterus may drain to the pelvic lymph nodes and subsequently to the para-aortic lymph nodes and upper abdomen. These lymphatics may also drain directly to the para-aortic lymph nodes and upper abdomen without coursing through the pelvic lymph nodes. The lymphatics from the lower uterine segment and cervix usually drain to the parametrial and pelvic lymph nodes. The lymphatics of the distal vagina drain directly to the inguinal lymph nodes.

External whole pelvic irradiation is usually administered to the pelvis in 1.8 Gy to 2.0 Gy per daily fractions to a total dose of 46 Gy to 50.4 Gy. External irradiation should be delivered to the pelvis with greater than or equal to 4 MV photons. Pelvic fields should be treated with a four-field "box" technique. Parallel opposed anterior–posterior (AP) fields can be used if photons of 15 MV or greater are utilized. However, if the patients AP separation is greater than 30 cm, then a four-field "box" technique should be utilized even if the photon energy is as high as 18 MV. The pelvic should extend from the L4–5 interspace superiorly to encompass the common iliac lymph nodes to the lower border of the obturator foramen or 4 cm inferior to the distal vaginal disease. The lateral border of the pelvic field should be 1 cm lateral to the widest diameter of the true pelvis. The anterior border of the lateral pelvic field should be at the level of the pubic symphysis. The posterior border of the lateral field should extend posteriorly to the sacrum to cover the pre-sacral lymph nodes.

TECHNIQUES FOR HDR BRACHYTHERAPY

HDR vaginal cuff brachytherapy is now one of the most common methods of administering postoperative cuff irradiation for patients with EC and uterine sarcomas. HDR vaginal cuff brachytherapy is administered with HDR vaginal cylinders placed in the entire length of the vagina. Only the upper one-third of the vagina is treated with the HDR vaginal cylinder (usually a 2.5 cm diameter cylinder).

The irradiation dose for the HDR vaginal cuff implant depends on whether the patient is also receiving external irradiation. By convention, the prescription point for HDR therapy is at a depth of 0.5 cm from the surface of the cylinder (the vaginal mucosa). The irradiation dose that is most frequently prescribed when only brachytherapy is performed is 7 Gy at 0.5 cm every 1 to 2 weeks for a total of three administrations (21 Gy). When external irradiation is also administered with whole pelvic doses of 46 Gy to 50.4 Gy, then the HDR brachytherapy dose is consequently decreased. When combined with external irradiation, the HDR dose is often 4 Gy at 0.5 cm for 3 treatments (12 Gy total) or 2 Gy at 0.5 cm for 6 weekly treatments (12 Gy total) during external irradiation.

REFERENCES

1. Roberts JA, Brunetto VL, Keys HM, Zaino R, Spirtos NM, Bloss JD, Pearlman A, Maiman MA, Bell JG. A phase III randomized study of surgery vs. surgery plus adjunctive radiation therapy in intermediate risk endometrial adenocarcinoma (GOG 99) (abstract). *Gynecol Oncol* 1998; 68:135.

2. Greven K, Winger K, Underhill K, Moorthy C, Cooper J, Burke T. Preliminary analysis of RTOG 9708: adjuvant postoperative irradiation combined with cisplatin/taxol chemotheray following surgery for patients with high-risk endometrial cancer (abstract). *Int J Radiat Oncol Biol Phys* 2001;1:34.

3. Creasman WT, Morrow CP, Bundy BN. Surgical pathologic spread patterns of endometrial cancer. A Gynecologic Oncology Group study. *Cancer* 1987; 60:2035–2041.

4. Creutzberg CL, van Putten WL, Koper PC, Lybeert ML, Jobsen JJ, Warlam-Rodenhuis CC, De Winter KA, Lutgens LC, van den Bergh AC, van de Steen-Banasik E, Beerman H, van Lent M. Surgery and postoperative radiotherapy versus surgery alone for patients with stage-1 endometrial carcinoma: multicentre randomised trial. PORTEC Study Group. Post Operative Radiation Therapy in Endometrial Carcinoma. *Lancet* 2000; 355:1404–1411.

5. Grigsby PW, Perez CA, Kuten A, Simpson JR, Garcia DM, Camel HM, Kao MS, Galakatos AE. Clinical stage I endometrial cancer: prognostic factors for local control and distant

metastasis and implications of the new FIGO surgical staging system. *Int J Radiat Oncol Biol Phys* 1992; 22:905–911.

6.   Grigsby PW, Kuske RR, Perez CA, Walz BJ, Camel MH, Kao MS, Galakatos AE. Medically inoperable stage I adenocarcinoma of the endometrium treated with radiotherapy alone. *Int J Radiat Oncol Biol Phys* 1987;13:483–488.

7.   Major FJ, Blessing JA, Silverberg SG, Morrow CP, Creasman WT, Currie JL, Yordan E, Brady MF. Prognostic factors in early-stage uterine sarcoma. A Gynecologic Oncology Group study. *Cancer* 1993; 71:1702–1709.

8.   Chang KL, Crabtree GS, Lim-Tan SK, Kempson RL, Hendrickson MR. Primary uterine endometrial stromal neoplasms. *Am J Surg Pathol* 1990; 14:415–438.

9.   Nordal RN, Kjorstad KE, Stenwig AE, Trope CG. Leiomyosarcoma (LMS) and endometrial stromal sarcoma (ES) of the uterus. A survey of patients treated in the Norwegian Radium Hospital 1976–1085. *Int J Gynecol Can* 1993; 3:110–115.

10.   Gadducci A, Sartori E, Landoni F, Zola P, Maggino T, Urgesi A, Lissoni A, Losa G, Fanucchi A. Endometrial stromal sarcoma: analysis of treatment failures and survival. *Gynecol Oncol* 1996; 63:247–253.

11.   Huang K-T, Chen C-A, Tseng G-C, Chen T-M, Cheng W-F, Hsieh C-Y. Endometrial stromal sracoma of twenty cases. *Acta Obstet Gynecol Scand* 1996; 75:551–555.

12.   Bodner K, Bodner-Adler B, Obermair A, Windbichler G, Petru E, Mayerhofer S, Czerwenka K, Leodolter S, Kainz C, Mayerhofer K. Prognostic parameters in endometrial stromal sarcoma: a clinicopathologic study in 31 patients. *Gynecol Oncol* 2001; 81:160–165.

13.   Omura GA, Major FJ, Blessing JA, Sedlacek TV, Thigpen JT, Creasman WT, Zaino RJ. A randomized study of adriamycin with and without dimethyl triazenoimidazole carboxamide in advanced uterine sarcomas. *Cancer* 1983; 52:626–632.

14.   Omura GA, Blessing JA, Major F, Lifshitz S, Ehrlich CE, Mangen C, Beecham J, Park R, Silverberg S. A randomized clinical trial of adjuvant adriamycin in uterine sarcomas: a

364 Grigsby

Gynecologic Oncology Group Study. *J Clin Oncol* 1985; 3:1240–1245.

15. Salazar OM, Bonfiglio TA, Patten SF, Keller BE, Feldstein ML, Dunne ME, Rudolph JH. Uterine sarcomas: Analysis of failures with special emphasis on the use of adjuvant radiation therapy. *Cancer* 1978; 42:1161–1170.

16. Yamada SD, Burger RA, Brewster WR, Anton D, Kohler MF, Monk BJ. Pathologic variables and adjuvant therapy as predictors of recurrence and survival for patients with surgically evaluated carcinosarcoma of the uterus. *Cancer* 2000; 88:2782–2786.

17. Knocke TH, Weitmann HD, Kucera H, Kolbl H, Pokrajac B, Potter R. Results of primary and adjuvant radiotherapy in the treatment of mixed mullerian tumors of the corpus uteri. *Gynecol Oncol* 1999; 73:389–395.

18. Gerszten K, Faul C, Kounelis S, Huang Q, Kelley J, Jones MW. The impact of adjuvant radiotherapy on carcinosarcoma of the uterus. *Gynecol Oncol* 1998; 68:8–13.

19. Malpus KL, Redlin-Frazier S, Reed G, Burnett LS, Jones HW. Postoperative pelvic irradition in early stage uterine mixed müllerian tumors. *Eur J Gynaecol Oncol* 1998; 19:541–546.

20. Manolitsas TP, Wain GV, Williams KE, Freidlander M, Hacker NF. Multimodality therapy for patients with clinical stage I and II malignant mixed müllerian tumors of the uterus. *Cancer* 2001; 91:1437–1443.

21. Knocke TH, Kucera H, Dorfler D, Pokrajac B, Potter R. Results of postoperative radiotherapy in the treatment of sarcoma of the corpus uteri. *Cancer* 1998; 83:1972–1979.

22. Pellenda AF, Ozsahin M, Deniaud-Alexandre E, Krengli M, VanHoutte P, Richetti A, Villa S, Kuten A, Jassem J, Bolla M, Hoogenraad WJ. Primary uterine leiomyosarcoma: outcome and prognostic factors in eighty consecutive patients. a rare cancer network study (abstract). *Int J Radiat Oncol Biol Phys* 2001; 51:336.

23. Weitman HD, Knocke TH, Kucera H, Potter R. Radiation therapy in the treatment of endometrial stromal sarcoma. *Int J Radiat Oncol Biol Phys* 2001; 49:739–748.

24. Vongtama V, Karlen JR, Piver SM, Tsukada Y, Moore RH. Treatment, results and prognostic factors in stage I and II sarcomas of the corpus uteri. *AJR* 1976; 126:139–147.

25. Callister M, Jhingran A, Ramondetta L, Burke T, Eifel P. Malignant mixed mullerian tumors of the uterus: analysis pf patterns of failure, prognostic factors, and tratment outcome (abstract). *Int J Radiat Oncol Biol Phys* 2001; 51:37–38.

26. Tinkler SD, Cowie VJ. Uterine sarcomas: a review of the Edinburgh experience from 1974–1992. *Br J Radiol* 1993; 66:998–1001.

27. Olah KS, Dunn JA, Gee H. Leiomyosarcomas have a poorer prognosis than mixed mesodermal tumours when adjusting for known prognostic factors: the result of a retrospective study of 423 cases of uterine sarcoma. *Br J Obstet Gynaecol* 1992; 99:590–594.

28. Ferrer F, Sabater S, Barrus B, Guedea F, Rovirosa A, Anglada L, Delannes M, Marin S, DuBois J-B, Daly-Schveitzer N. Impact of radiotherapy on local control and survival in uterine sarcomas: a retrospective study from the Grup Oncologic Catala-Occita. *Int J Radiat Oncol Biol Phys* 1999; 44:47–52.

14

Radiation Treatment of Advanced or Recurrent Endometrial Cancer

ELEANOR E. R. HARRIS

University of Pennsylvania,
Philadelphia, Pennsylvania, U.S.A

While the majority of patients diagnosed with endometrial cancer (EC) present with early stage disease, 10–15% have advanced (stage III–IV) disease at presentation. This includes patients with positive pelvic and para-aortic lymph nodes, local invasion into other pelvic organs, inoperable cancers, pelvic recurrence at the vaginal cuff or in pelvic lymph nodes, and distant metastases. The International Federation of Gynecology and Obstetrics (FIGO) revised the staging system for EC in 1989 from a clinical staging system to one based on surgical pathologic staging (1). Since that time, the definition of subgroups of pathologically staged patients and the prognostic importance of patterns of microscopic pelvic and nodal spread has been ongoing. Radiation therapy is

367

often used to reduce the risk of local recurrence, to treat areas of residual disease, or to palliate symptoms related to recurrent cancer. It may also be used preoperatively in technically inoperable patients, or even as the primary therapy in patients with medically inoperable disease. While radiation therapy has not been shown to improve overall survival in these situations, it is very effective therapy for both local-regional control and palliation. Adjuvant radiation has a particularly important role in EC, given relatively low response rates to chemotherapeutic agents.

ROLE OF RADIATION THERAPY FOR STAGE III–IV EC

Results of therapy for stage III disease depend upon whether patients have pathologic stage III diagnosed after surgical staging, or whether they present with clinical stage III disease. Surgically staged III disease includes those with stage IIIA due to positive washings alone or microscopic extension to the serosa or adnexae, or IIIC due to microscopic lymph node involvement. Clinical stage III disease involves gross extrauterine extension, pelvic adenopathy detectable on preoperative scans, or clinically evident vaginal extension. Thus, clinical stage III disease comprises bulkier tumors by definition, and often includes patients requiring radical surgery, such as an exenteration, or those that are technically inoperable. Inevitably, outcomes are poorer for these patients.

Pathologic Stage III

Positive Peritoneal Cytology Alone

The most favorable subgroup of stage III patients are those with positive peritoneal washings as their sole criterion of advanced disease, which occurs in about 5% of patients. The selection of adjuvant treatment of these patients is controversial. The likelihood of positive washings may be related to the type of surgical procedure, the timing of the pelvic fluid sampling during the procedure, and the use of preoperative irradiation, as well as subjectivity in the pathologic interpretation of cytologic specimens. Assuming accuracy of the sampling procedure, the prognostic significance of this finding remains uncertain. Over half of patients with positive pelvic washings will have adnexal or other areas of pelvic spread of disease. McLellan et al. reported that 11% of patients with FIGO stage I EC had positive peritoneal washings, and that this finding was associated with depth of invasion, high grade, and positive nodes. They concluded that these patients were at high risk for recurrence (2). In a series of 270 patients with stage I disease, 5% demonstrated positive washings, correlated with tumor grade and depth of invasion, and positive cytology was predictive of survival (3). However, peritoneal cytology failed to identify any additional patients who were candidates for postoperative therapy that were not also indicated by grade and depth of invasion.

In a series from Roswell Park, ten patients with stage I disease and positive washings and no adjuvant therapy were followed for at least 10 years, and only one recurred (4). Other series also failed to show any difference in outcomes based on positive peritoneal cytology (5,6). Conversely, Zuna and Behrens reported on long-term follow-up of 135 patients of whom 13% had malignant peritoneal cytology, including 6% of stage I patients (7). Disease free survival was 87% for stage I patients with negative cytology compared to only 17% for those with positive washings. These authors concluded that positive cytology was a poor prognostic factor even if it were the only indicator of extrauterine disease. A series of 28 patients with stage I cancers and malignant cytology from M.D. Anderson Cancer Center were compared to those with negative washings (8). Recurrence was significantly increased in patients with positive cytology (32%) compared to the negative cytology group (7%), and progression free survival was worse. In another group of 41 clinical stage I patients with positive peritoneal cytology, recurrences were seen in 29%, and 75% experienced an abdominal relapse, compared to 3% of patients with negative cytology (9). Adjuvant radiation, both pre- and postoperative, was given to some patients, but was not considered in the analysis of risk factors for recurrence. Two series reporting the results of surgery alone with no adjuvant therapy for isolated positive

peritoneal cytology have noted diverse recurrence rates of 7%
(10) and 46% (11).

Despite data suggesting a poorer prognosis for these
patients, only a few series have reported exclusively on outcomes in pathologic stage IIIA patients, as outlined in Table 1.
A classic series by Creasman et al. reported that 26 patients
with stage I disease and positive peritoneal washings had a
34% recurrence rate compared to 9% among women with negative washings (12). Of thirteen patients with no extrauterine
disease and positive cytology, 46% died of disseminated
intraperitoneal recurrence. These investigators subsequently
treated 23 patients with malignant washings with intraab-

Table 1   Results for Stage IIIA with Positive Peritoneal Washings Only

Author (Ref.)	No. of Patients	Adjuvant Treatment	Recurrence Rate	Disease-Free Survival
Turner (8)	28	None	32%	84% (5Y OS)
Yazigi (4)	10	None	10%	87% (5Y OS)
Zuna (7)	8	None	—	17%
Morrow (10)	14	None	7%	76% (5Y RFI)
	18	Pelvic RT	28%	(all patients)
Creasman (12)	13	None	46%	—
	23	IP P-32	13%	—
Soper (13)	43	IP P-32 (all) Pelvic RT-3; ICRT	8%	89%
Lurain (6)	30	Pelvic RT; ICRT; CT or hormones	17%	—
Konski (15)	11	Pelvic RT	9%	100%
	8	WART	25%	75%
Martinez (16)	18	WART	11%	73%
Mazurka (17)	16	Hormones or CT ($n = 13$)	25%	—
Piver (18)	25	Progestins	0%	100%
Kennedy (3)	14	Various (CT, P-32, hormones)	—	67%
Harouny (9)	41	Various (Pre-op RT, Pelvic RT, CT, hormones)	29%	71%

RT = Radiation therapy; WART = Whole Abdominal Radiation Therapy; IP =
Intraperitoneal; CT = Chemotherapy; ICRT = Intracavitary Radiation Therapy;
OS = Overall Survival; RFI = Recurrence Free Interval.

dominal P-32 colloid postoperatively. They concluded that P-32 therapy was efficacious as none of these patients had any pelvic or abdominal recurrence, although three developed distant disease. A report by Soper et al. on 65 women with clinical stage I–III EC with malignant cytology treated with intraperitoneal radioactive P-32 suspension, demonstrated an 8% intraperitoneal recurrence rate, most with simultaneous extraperitoneal metastases (13). Chronic bowel problems were not seen in patients receiving P-32 alone, but occurred in 29% of women who also received external irradiation to the pelvis, including two deaths. Potish described 5-year relapse free survival of 77% of women with microscopic peritoneal spread treated with whole abdominal radiation, and an overall 4% rate of bowel obstructions (14). In another group of 19 patients with positive washings treated with postoperative radiation, 9% of patients receiving pelvic irradiation developed a pelvic recurrence, compared to 25% of patients treated with whole abdominal radiation (15). When compared to patients who had negative cytology, there was no statistical difference in survival noted in this series of 134 patients. No comparison of these approaches to no postoperative therapy has been performed. Postoperative therapy is recommended for women with other extrauterine disease. A study by Martinez et al. included 43 high risk patients with cytology performed, 34 of whom had positive peritoneal washings, and some may have had other extrauterine disease, although this is not specified (16). All were treated with whole abdominal radiation therapy. Relapse free survival was 100% for those with negative cytology versus 73% for positive, which was not statistically different. While total failures were reduced from a predicted 39% to 11% with adjuvant therapy, no comparison group was available in this series, as all patients were treated uniformly. Thus, the use of adjuvant radiation in patients with positive peritoneal washings, particularly as the only evidence of extrauterine spread, remains controversial, and should be considered in the setting of a clinical trial.

Hormonal therapy with progestins or systemic chemotherapy has also been used adjuvantly in small groups of patients with isolated positive washings. These studies report relapse rates of 0–25% (17,18) and disease free survival of 67%, compared to 85% (3), although the numbers of patients were small. Piver conducted a pilot study of 25 patients with surgical stage I disease and malignant pelvic washings who were treated with progesterone (18). Twenty-two underwent a second look laparoscopy and 95% had no evidence of disease with negative washings. One patient with persistent positive washings was treated with an additional year of progestins and remained free of disease. While these data are intriguing, there are too few patients treated exclusively with hormonal therapy to assess the efficacy of this therapy compared to adjuvant radiation, although either treatment appears superior to no adjuvant therapy. Most patients will have other risk factors for pelvic or distant recurrence that guide treatment decisions, including grade, depth of invasion, and lymph vascular space invasion.

Isolated Adnexal Invasion

Patients with pathologic stage III disease due to isolated adnexal involvement also comprise a more favorable subset among stage III patients. Invasion may occur directly transtubally, or may be due to lymphatic spread. Some of these patients may have concurrent early stage ovarian cancers as well, thus careful pathologic assessment is warranted. The Gynecologic Oncology Group (GOG) reported that 5% of surgically staged patients with clinical stage I disease had adnexal involvement (19). This pathologic finding was associated with a 32% risk of pelvic lymph node metastases, and 23% had para-aortic lymph node spread. Table 2 summarizes the findings from several small series. In the largest reported subgroup of 42 patients with isolated adnexal involvement, Greven et al. noted a 5-year survival rate of 60%, compared to 54% for the entire group of pathologic stage III patients (20). The grade and depth of myometrial invasion further defined the prognosis for these patients, in whom the high grade reduced the survival to 40%, and invasion through greater than one-third of the myometrium resulted in a 47% survival rate. Most patients had received postoperative pelvic irradia-

Table 2   Results for Stage III with Isolated Adnexal Involvement

Author (Ref.)	No. of Patients	Adjuvant Treatment	Outcome
Greven (20)	42	Pelvic RT +/– ICRT	60% (5Y OS)
Nori (21)	21 (microscopic)	Pelvic RT + ICRT	80% (5Y OS)
	12 (gross)	Pelvic RT + ICRT	40% (5Y OS)
Mackillop (26)	12	Pelvic RT	83% (5Y OS)
	6	None	
Bruckman (22)	15	Pelvic RT	80% (5Y RFS)
Antoniades (23)	7	Pelvic RT	71% (RFS)
Potish (24)	9	WART	90% (5Y RFS)
Greer (25)	9	WART	88% (5Y OS)

RT = Radiation therapy; ICRT = intracavitary radiation therapy; WART = whole abdominal radiation therapy; OS = overall survival; RFS = relapse free survival.

tion with or without a boost. Isolated abdominal failure in this series was uncommon (7%). Nori et al. analyzed a group of patients treated with surgery and either pre- or postoperative pelvic irradiation with an intravaginal boost, which included 21 patients with microscopic involvement of the adnexa, and 12 patients with gross adnexal involvement (21). The 5-year survival was better for those with microscopic invasion (80%) than with gross invasion of the adnexa (40%) even though this was the only extrauterine disease. Several other smaller series that analyzed this subset of patients have reported 5-year relapse-free survival rates from 60–90% in patient treated postoperatively with either pelvic (22,23) or whole abdominopelvic radiation (24,25). In a series from Princess Margaret Hospital of 18 patients with isolated adnexal disease, 6 received no postoperative radiation, and 5 of these were disease free at 5 years (26). Overall, small reported patient numbers preclude any conclusion as to the relative efficacy of pelvic versus whole abdominal radiation in this subset.

Optimally Debulked Stage III

For surgically treated pathologic stage III patients overall treated with hysterectomy and postoperative radiation, 5-

year disease free survival or 64%, and 21% pelvic recurrence rates have been reported (27). Predictors of survival include grade, depth of invasion, number of extrauterine sites of disease, and papillary serous or clear cell histology. Grade was the strongest predictor of pelvic recurrence; histology and number of extrauterine sites predicted for abdominal recurrence. A retrospective series from Stanford University examined results in 22 patients with optimally debulked stage III–IV endometrial adenocarcinoma treated with whole abdominoplevic irradiation, who demonstrated a 3-year disease free survival and overall survival of 79% and 89%, respectively, and a 7% rate of major complications (28). The University of Pittsburgh reported on 32 patients with stage IIIA–C endometrial adenocarcinoma who underwent abdominal hysterectomy, 78% of whom had surgical lymph node sampling (29). All patients received postoperative pelvic irradiation with or without a brachytherapy boost to the vaginal vault. Forty-five percent of stage IIIC patients developed recurrence, usually distant metastases, while there were only three local recurrences overall.

Lymph Node Positive Stage IIIC

Patients at highest risk for recurrence are those with positive pelvic or para-aortic lymph nodes. The GOG examined pathologic factors in clinical stage I–II EC patients (10). In their series of 1180 women, 13% (3% grossly positive) overall had positive pelvic nodes, with about one-third of patients with positive pelvic nodes also documented to have para-aortic nodal metastases. Lymph nodes were involved in 51% of women with extrauterine disease, 32% with adnexal invasion, and 25% with deep myometrial invasion. Patients with positive pelvic nodes treated with postoperative pelvic irradiation had a 5-year disease free survival of 72%. In addition, 47 patients had positive para-aortic nodes, all of whom had grossly positive pelvic nodes ($n = 17$), adnexal involvement ($n = 15$), or deep myometrial invasion ($n = 38$). Of these, 77% received postoperative radiation with a 5-year disease free survival of 36%. In this series, 75% of patients who had posi-

tive pelvic nodes as a sole risk factor and received pelvic irradiation were free of disease at 5 years (10). Better survivals
have been reported for patients presenting with microscopically positive lymph nodes versus grossly involved nodes. One
series reported a mean survival of greater than 60 months if
nodes were microscopically involved compared to 35 months
for macroscopically involved nodes (30).

The presence of positive pelvic lymph nodes only is more
favorable than involvement of the para-aortic nodes as well.
Morrow et al. noted a recurrence rate of 28% for those with
positive pelvic nodes compared to 40% for those with positive
aortic nodes (10). A small study of 17 patients with nodal
spread confined to the pelvic nodes exhibited a 5-year overall
survival of 72% (31). All patients had postoperative radiation,
13 to the pelvis only and 4 to the whole abdomen with a pelvic
boost. There were no pelvic or upper abdominal failures at a
median follow-up of 4.3 years, but 2 patients failed distantly,
and 2 in para-aortic nodes.

Outcomes with adjuvant radiation (with or without systemic therapy) have been retrospectively reviewed, although
treatment techniques have varied significantly. Table 3
reviews the results of various series. In a recent study of 47
patients with stage IIIC disease, 38% of patients had pelvic
lymph node involvement only, and 58% had para-aortic nodal
disease with (41%) or without (17%) positive pelvic nodes. In
this group, 36% had whole abdominal radiation, 19% had
extended pelvic and para-aortic nodal irradiation, and 17%
had pelvic irradiation alone (32). In addition, 17% were
treated with chemotherapy and 11% with progestins. Five-
year overall survival was 65%, with distant metastases seen
in 21% and pelvic recurrence in 9%, with only 1 abdominal
failure. Predictors of failure included depth of invasion and
positive cytology or adnexal involvement. The role of the various adjuvant treatments used, however, could not be clearly
defined. Patients whose nodal disease is confined to the pelvic
lymph nodes but who have negative para-aortic lymph node
sampling were still at risk for para-aortic recurrence. Mundt
et al. reported on 30 stage IIIC patients, all with positive
pelvic nodes and 54% with positive para-aortic lymph nodes,

Table 3 Results for Stage IIIC Patients with Positive Pelvic or Para-aortic Lymph Nodes

Author (Ref.)	No. of Patients	Treatment	Relapse Rate		5-Year Survival
Nelson (31)	17 (+ pelvic LNs only)	PRT or WART	PA LNs:	12%	72%
			DM:	12%	
McMeekin (32)	47	WART; EFRT;	Pelvic:	9%	65%
		PRT; +/–CT or progestins	DM:	21%	
Martinez (16)	8	WART; PA + Pelvic boost	NS		70% (RFS)
Mundt (33)	30	PRT or EFRT	Pelvic:	23%	34% (DFS)
			DM:	40%	
			PA LNs:	13%	
			Abdomen:	13%	
Rose (36)	17	EFRT + Megace	DM:	29%	53%
Onda (37)	20	CT + EFRT	NS		75% (+PA LNs)
					100% (+ Pelvic LNs only)

PRT = Pelvic radiation therapy; EFRT = extended field radiation therapy; WART = Wwhole abdominal radiation therapy;
PA LN = paraaortic lymph nodes; DM = distant metastases; DFS = disease free survival; RFS = relapse free survival; NS = not stated.

and all treated with TAH-BSO followed by pelvic or extended field radiation (33). They noted a 5-year disease free survival of 34%, with 23% of patients experiencing pelvic failure (including four vaginal failures), 13% abdominal, and 13% para-aortic failures; 40% developed distant metastases. No patient treated with extended field irradiation developed a para-aortic nodal recurrence, although 8 of 10 had positive para-aortic nodes at the time of surgery. Treatment was well tolerated, with only two late sequelae (one chronic enteritis and one bowel obstruction).

For patients with positive para-aortic nodes and no other abdominal disease, the optimal radiation field arrangement remains uncertain. Two series report the use of extended fields to encompass the para-aortic nodal region in patients with either surgical or clinical staging. Potish et al. reported on 48 women treated with extended para-aortic fields, half of whom had abnormal lymphangiograms and half had pathologically documented nodal metastases. They found that 88% of recurrences were outside the radiation fields, including 44% of first failures in the abdomen (34). In this series, survival was better in clinically staged patients than surgically staged (57% versus 47%), suggesting an uncertainty in clinical staging of nodal disease. Corn et al. examined outcomes in 50 women, 26 with pathologically staged para-aortic nodal involvement and 24 diagnosed with lymphangiography, treated pre- and postoperatively or primarily with extended field radiation. Para-aortic lymph node dissection significantly decreased the para-aortic failures, and the authors noted only three abdominal failures (35).

Two other series looked at the impact of extended field irradiation in patients all with pathologically documented para-aortic nodal spread. In one group of 26 patients, 17 received extended field radiation treatment, most with adjuvant Megace, and the remaining 9 patients received Megace or chemotherapy alone (36). Six of the 17 irradiated patients died of disease, 5 with distant metastases, although 2 patients died of bowel complications, one of whom was disease free. Overall survival was significantly improved in the irradiated group (53% versus 22%). In the second series, 20 patients with para-aortic metastases received 3 cycles of postoperative chemotherapy followed by extended field irradiation (37). Five-year survival was 75% for positive para-aortic nodes, compared to 100% if only the pelvic nodes were positive. Patterns of failure were not discussed.

Reported series of patients treated with whole abdominal radiation have represented heterogeneous stage and histologic groups, and generally included small numbers of patients with para-aortic metastases as the primary reason for whole abdominal radiation fields. In a set of 22 patients with adenocarcinoma who received whole abdominal radiation, four failures were noted and all were extra-abdominal (28). Another group of 30 diversely staged patients, including 8 with stage IIIC disease, all receiving whole abdominal fields, demonstrated a 7% rate of para-aortic failures and upper abdominal failures, respectively (38). Martinez et al. reported on a group of 47 patients with risk factors for abdominopelvic failure, including high grade, deep myometrial invasion, surgical stage III–IV, positive peritoneal cytology, or residual disease after surgery of up to 2 cm or positive nodes (16). All were treated with hysterectomy and staging, followed by whole abdominal radiation to the entire peritoneal cavity, then a boost to the diaphragm, para-aortic nodes, pelvis, and vagina. No patients received adjuvant systemic therapy unless they relapsed. At a mean follow-up of 40 months, patients with residual nodal disease in the pelvic or para-aortic regions, who had all received a boost dose of radiation to the gross disease, had a relapse-free survival of 70%.

When extended field or whole abdominal irradiation are given, the treatment technique must minimize the exposure to normal tissues, and in particular to the small bowel, liver, and kidneys. The most common acute effects of large abdominopelvic radiation fields are acute gastrointestinal symptoms including nausea, vomiting, diarrhea, and cramping. Loss of fluid and electrolytes through vomiting and diarrhea may lead to acute dehydration, so antiemetics and antidiarrheals should be prescribed early in therapy, and patients monitored closely. Myelosuppression through exposure of the bone marrow may also occur, therefore blood counts should be monitored and supportive therapy given accordingly. Four-field pelvic arrangements including anterior, posterior, and lateral fields often allow for blocking of anterior segments of the small bowel. When the para-aortic nodes or whole abdomen is treated, larger volumes of small bowel are inevitably included, leading to a greater likelihood of acute enteritis. Typically the whole abdomen dose is limited to a range of 25–30 Gy, keeping the exposure of the kidneys to less than 20 Gy and the whole liver is usually limited to 22–25 Gy. Doses beyond 45–50 Gy to large volumes of small bowel will significantly increase the risk of late complications. Series using these dose parameters and techniques report late bowel complications, primarily small bowel obstruction, in 3–12% for extended field irradiation (33,37), and in 0–9% for whole abdominal irradiation (14,16,28,38).

Clinical Stage III and IV Disease

The original FIGO staging system from 1971 was based on findings on clinical exam (39). In that era fewer patients were treated with surgery, and primary irradiation was often used. Clinical stage III EC was defined as carcinoma extending outside the uterus but not outside of the true pelvis. Stage IV disease included invasion of the bladder or rectum, or disease beyond the true pelvis.

Clinical Stage III

Treatment for clinical stage III EC has included radiation alone or surgery and radiation. Grigsby et al. reported on a series of patients including 27 with clinical stage III disease treated with total hysterectomy and salpingo-oophorectomy combined with pre- or postoperative irradiation (40). The 5-year disease-free survival was 33%, with a distant metastatic rate of 48% and pelvic recurrence in 33% of patients. Aalders et al. compared outcomes in 108 clinical stage III patients to 67 patients with pathologic stage III disease (41). Radical surgery was possible in 70% of pathologic stage III patients compared to only 13% of those with clinical stage III; thus, 66 patients were treated with radiation alone. Surgical debulking was an important prognostic factor. The 5-year overall survival was 16% versus 40% for clinical and pathologic stage III, respectively. In the series by Greven et al. 52 patients had clinical stage III disease, 20 of whom had radiation alone after biopsy (20). Overall survival for this stage was 36%, with a median survival of 9 months for patients treated with radiation alone, compared to 60 months for patients treated with surgery and radiation. The radiation-only group also demonstrated very poor pelvic control, with 89% pelvic failures among 18 evaluable patients. In the combined treatment group, 5-year survival was 48%, with 40% pelvic failures. Isolated abdominal failure was much less common at 6%, but 38% overall had a component of abdominal failure, and 16% developed distant metastases alone. Thus, while a combined treatment approach of surgery and adjuvant irradiation results in far superior outcomes to radiation alone for clinical stage III patients, they still experience a high rate of pelvic and abdominal failures. Further clinical trials studying the efficacy of systemic therapy or intraperitoneal therapies are warranted.

Bulky Residual Disease After Surgery

Bulky residual disease has been defined as greater than 2 cm of residual tumor after primary surgery. This may include pelvic implants, residual nodal disease, or other intraperitoneal sites. There appears to be a benefit with respect to recurrence and survival if tumor is debulked to as small a volume as feasible. Surgery is then followed by adjuvant irradiation to the pelvis, pelvis and para-aortic nodes, or whole abdomen as indicated by the location of residual disease. In a study of surgical cytoreduction in 65 stage IVB patients, optimal debulking to less than 1 cm residual was accomplished in 55% (42). Those patients had a significantly improved median survival of 34 months versus 11 months for those with bulkier residual disease. Among those with optimal cytoreduction, adjuvant chemotherapy or radiation was associated with improved survival. A second series of 55 patients with stage IV disease were reviewed for outcomes, and included 24 patients who had optimal debulking to less than 2 cm of residual disease, 21 patients with bulkier residual disease, and 10 patients with unresectable peritoneal carcinomatosis (43). Median survivals were 31, 12, and 3 months, respectively.

Whole abdominal radiation for bulky residual disease appears to be inadequate, and such patients with greater than 2 cm of residual disease are seldom controlled (25). This may be due to the lower radiation doses that are required in whole abdominal treatment, due to limitations of dose tolerance for the small bowel, liver, and kidneys. Limited field boosts to areas of bulky residual disease should be considered, particularly for para-aortic nodes, which can be treated to higher doses without exposing the liver or kidneys to excessive radiation. For patients with bulky disease confined to the pelvis, preoperative radiation may be considered to improve the likelihood of optimal surgical resection.

Clinical Stage IV

Patients with stage IVA disease, presenting with invasion of the bladder or rectum, with or without lymph node metastases, should be treated similarly to stage III disease with combined surgery and radiation with or without systemic therapy. Pre-operative radiation may be considered in patients who are marginally operable or inoperable but with disease confined to the pelvis. Although little data exist for this approach in EC, it has been used successfully in a variety of other pelvic malignancies. Patients presenting with stage IVB disease are rare, and most often treated palliatively. Residual or progressive pelvic disease can be a major source of symptomatology for these patients. Five-year survivors are uncommon, with rates of 0–10% (44,45). As with less advanced disease, surgical debulking may be of benefit or may be considered for palliation of symptoms. Surgical extirpation in these patients may require exenteration.

In inoperable patients with advanced disease, palliative radiation therapy should be considered. All stage IV patients are also candidates for systemic chemotherapy or hormonal therapy. Bulky disease requires high dose irradiation, even for palliation. Unfortunately, due to poor tolerance of the bowel to high dose fractions of radiation, palliative treatment may require several weeks of daily therapy. Conventional doses of

50–60 Gy of external irradiation may be followed by low-dose
rate or high-dose rate brachytherapy depending upon the location and extent of disease. Palliation of bleeding may also be
accomplished with brachytherapy alone, which is useful for
debilitated patients. Alternate fractionation schemes have
been investigated. In one group of 27 patients with EC who
were not surgical candidates, primarily due to age or co-morbidities, 1–3 doses of 10 Gy fractions to the pelvis were delivered (46). Bleeding resolved in 90%, malodorous discharge was
reduced in 38%, and 22% had a complete tumor response with
a median survival of 9 months. Only 3 patients had significant
bowel effects. The Radiation Therapy Oncology Group (RTOG)
reported a phase II trial in patients with advanced pelvic
malignancies treated with accelerated split course irradiation,
consisting of 44.4 Gy in three courses over 6 days and 12 fractions with 2- or 4-week breaks between each 2 fractions (47).
Patients completing all three courses had a 42% response rate
and therapy was well tolerated. This or other accelerated or
hypofractionated schemes may be considered, especially if limited volumes are to be irradiated.

For patients presenting with distant metastases or with
distant relapses after primary therapy, chemotherapy or hormonal therapy are the mainstay of initial treatment. The most
common sites of distant metastases are lung (35%), liver (29%),
omentum or peritoneum (25%), gastrointestinal tract (21%),
and bone (15%), with rare instances of adrenal (10%) or brain
(6%) involvement (48). Radiation is rarely used for visceral disease, however, palliative irradiation is indicated for specific situations, including painful bony metastases, symptomatic brain
metastases, spinal cord compression, and airway obstruction.
Short courses of hypofractionated radiation are most commonly employed over 1 to 2 weeks. Therapy is delivered to the
whole brain or painful portion of involved bone.

RADIATION THERAPY FOR PELVIC RECURRENCE

Incidence of Pelvic Recurrence

Recurrence in the pelvis after hysterectomy is a common site
of relapse in patients with EC. Most locoregional recurrences

are diagnosed in the first 2 to 3 years after initial treatment. For patients presenting with pathologic stage I–II disease, the main risk factors for pelvic recurrence are high grade and myometrial invasion greater than one-third to one-half of the myometrial width. With no postoperative adjuvant therapy, the pelvic recurrence risk for these patients has been reported at 10–40%, which is reduced to less than 5% with adjuvant pelvic irradiation, with or without a vaginal brachytherapy boost (10,49–51). Distant metastatic rates of 15–20% and overall survival rates are not altered by the addition of adjuvant pelvic irradiation. Most series have reported failures as all pelvic recurrences, including the vaginal cuff, pelvic lymph nodes, or other limited pelvic sites. High risk stage I patients (i.e., those with high grade or deep invasion), appear to have a 15% risk of vaginal recurrence at 10 years when treated with initial surgery alone (52). The GOG conducted a randomized study comparing surgery alone to surgery and postoperative pelvic irradiation for "intermediate risk" patients, including stage IB, IC, and occult II (GOG-99) (53). Early results showed a 2-year progression-free interval of 88% for surgery alone and 96% for surgery with postoperative irradiation ($p = 0.004$). When patterns of recurrence were examined, there were 13 vaginal recurrences among 202 women randomized to surgery alone (6%), compared to 3 vaginal recurrences in 190 women (1.6%) randomized to adjuvant irradiation. There were also 4 pelvic and vaginal recurrences in the surgery alone arm compared to none in the adjuvant radiation arm. Patients with extrauterine disease have a higher risk of pelvic recurrence, which depends upon the type and number of extrauterine sites.

A group of Dutch institutions conducted the PORTEC randomized trial comparing surgery alone (without lymphadenectomy) versus surgery and postoperative pelvic radiation for selected patients with stage I disease (grade 1 and >50% myometrial invasion; grade 2 and any invasion; grade 3 and <50% invasion) (54). Cancer-related deaths at 5 years were seen in 6% in the surgery-only arm and 9% in the adjuvant-radiation arm. However, locoregional recurrences were significantly reduced in the adjuvant-radiation arm.

Locoregional relapses were seen in 14% after surgery alone and 4% after adjuvant radiation at 5 years, 73% of which were confined to the vagina. Adjuvant pelvic radiation reduced both vaginal vault and pelvic recurrences compared to surgery alone. This study also found that salvage treatment for vaginal relapse was associated with a 3-year survival of 69%, compared to 13% after pelvic or distant relapse. This salvage rate was better in the surgery arm, presumably because high dose radiation could more readily be delivered for salvage therapy when none was given postoperatively.

Treatment of Pelvic Recurrence

Exenteration

Surgical treatment for pelvic relapse often requires partial or total exenteration. Barakat et al. has reported on 44 patients treated with exenteration for recurrent EC in the pelvis (location not otherwise described), 77% of whom had received prior irradiation (55). The median interval to recurrence in this series was 28 months, and one-half of the patients required a total exenteration. The median survival after salvage surgery was 10 months, with 0 patients (20%) alive at more than 5 years. However, 80% had major postoperative complications.

Radical Radiation

Radical irradiation is usually the treatment of choice for patients initially treated with surgery alone. High dose pelvic radiation with intravaginal brachytherapy is effective salvage therapy. Isolated vaginal recurrences are more successfully treated than pelvic side wall or pelvic lymph node recurrences, but the latter may still require high dose palliation. Factors associated with treatment outcome for recurrence include tumor size, grade, location in the vagina (distal versus apical), and disease free interval (56)

Pelvic Recurrence

Prognostic factors and outcomes in patients experiencing pelvic recurrences have been examined. Methods of salvage therapy have varied depending upon the presentation and extent of recurrent disease and the type of prior therapy. A series of 42 women with recurrent EC after surgery alone were treated at Princess Margaret Hospital, all with combined external beam and intracavitary therapy to a median total dose of 81.5 Gy (57). The median time to recurrence postoperatively was 1.3 years. Five-and 10-year survivals after salvage treatment were 53% and 41%, respectively. Local control was 65%, influenced by vaginal stage and size of the recurrence. These authors also noted that local control was better for vaginal location (66% for apex and 100% for distal) compared to central pelvic sites (44%). Only one patient had a pelvic side wall recurrence. While local control was better with a total dose > 80 Gy (72% vs. 54% for < 80 Gy), this was not statistically significant. Sears et al. reported on 45 patients who had not received postoperative pelvic radiotherapy who then developed vaginal (85%) or pelvic (15%) recurrence of EC; recurrences were analyzed by the corresponding vaginal cancer stage (58). The median time to recurrence was 12 months, and long-term median follow-up had elapsed. Salvage treatment consisted of external beam alone in 40%, external beam and brachytherapy in 56%, and brachytherapy alone in 4%, with a median dose of 50 Gy. Five-year disease specific survival was 51%, overall survival was 44%, and locoregional control was 54%. Factors associated with local control were vaginal stage of recurrent disease, tumor size, radiation boost technique, time to recurrence, and age. Disease specific survival was influenced by local control (74% for local control vs. 23% without local control).

An Austrian series of 56 patients with pelvic relapse after hysterectomy included 41% having received adjuvant irradiation, and 71% of recurrences were vaginal (59). A re-irradiation dose of approximately two-thirds of the initial dose was used in previously irradiated patients (30–40 Gy) and was increased as the interval from prior radiation increased. Almost one half of the patients were treated with pelvic radiation and brachytherapy, 25% with brachytherapy alone, and 16% with external irradiation only, while 12% had no radiotherapy. Better 3-year survival was seen in patients who had no prior irradiation (59% vs. 25%), low grade disease (48% vs. 22%), a relapse-free interval exceeding 2 years (55% vs. 35%), and recurrence only in the vagina (54% vs. 19%). A series of 26 patients treated with external radiotherapy and/or brachytherapy for locoregional recurrence of EC reported a 5-year overall survival of 44% (60). These authors also noted that the size of recurrent disease affected the success of salvage therapy. Locoregional control was achieved in 100% of patients with recurrent tumors <2 cm, in 83% with tumors 2–4 cm, and 67% of those with tumors >4 cm. Also, the use of combined external irradiation and brachytherapy resulted in 100% locoregional control, while use of either treatment mode alone resulted in second relapse in 4 out of 10 patients.

Other series have had less promising results. More extensive pelvic recurrence may account for the poorer results. Kuten et al. reviewed a group of patients with recurrent disease, only 33% of whom had isolated vaginal recurrence, while another third had pelvic and distant recurrence simultaneously (61). For the entire group, locoregional control was only 35%, and 5-year survival was 18%. The overall vaginal control rate was 82%, and patients with isolated vaginal recurrence had a 5-year progression free survival of 40%. No patients with pelvic recurrence were alive beyond 1.5 years. In a study of 73 women undergoing salvage radiotherapy for pelvic recurrence after surgery alone, 60% received combined external and brachytherapy, 23% brachytherapy alone, and 17% external radiation alone, to a mean physical dose of 76 Gy (62). The majority of patients in this study had vaginal stage II (60%) or III (34%) disease. The 5-year survival was 25%, and a 73% response rate, with 67% experiencing progressive disease, just over half of whom had local progression.

Isolated Vaginal Recurrence

Salvage therapy for isolated vaginal recurrence may include treatment with external beam irradiation plus a vaginal brachytherapy boost, or intravaginal brachytherapy alone. Several series have examined the prognosis and out-comes for this selected group of patients, and are summarized in Table 4. Overall survivals after salvage therapy for vaginal recurrence range from 25–60%. Curran et al. reported 55 women with isolated vaginal recurrence post-hysterectomy (63). Nearly one-half received pelvic radiation and vaginal brachytherapy, 30% had external radiation alone, and 7% had brachytherapy alone, to a median dose of 60 Gy. Five-year survival was 31% and 5-year pelvic control rate was 42%. The outcome was highly dependent upon the radiation dose, with a 68% pelvic control rate at 5 years if ≥60 Gy was delivered, compared to 10% for those receiving <60 Gy (including some patients who received no radiation). The 5-year survival was also worse for patients being re-irradiated, 16% at 5 years versus 48% for those receiving a first course of radiotherapy. Using the vaginal carcinoma staging criteria as a descriptor of the extent of disease, this study found that survival rates diminished as the "stage" of recurrent disease increased. In addition, better pelvic control rates were seen in recurrences located in the vaginal apex than in the suburethral area (56% versus 20%). Greven and Olds treated 18 patients with iso-lated vaginal recurrence with a combination of external pelvis radiation and intravaginal ovoids (64). They achieved a 44% 3-year local control rate and an overall survival of 33% at a follow-up range of 3 to 10 years. Morgan et al. used pelvic fields and either intracavitary or interstitial brachytherapy to treat 34 patients with isolated vaginal recurrence, resulting in an 85% pelvic control rate, 5-year survival of 68%, and 60% disease free survival (65). Better control rates were seen in patients with <2 cm of disease and in those treated with radi-ation doses greater than 60 Gy.

A group of patients from the University of Milan who presented with isolated vaginal recurrence after surgery alone were treated with low-dose rate intravaginal ovoids or cylinders to a dose of 60–70 Gy at the vaginal surface (66). The median time to relapse was 14 months and vaginal recur-rences were located in the upper third of the vagina in 69%, the middle third in 9%, the lower third in 11%, and diffusely in 11%. All patients exhibited a complete response to therapy

Table 4 Results For Treatment of Isolated Vaginal Recurrence

Author (Ref.)	No. of Patients	Treatment	Pelvic Control	5-Year Survival
Curran (63)	55	Pelvic RT and/or Brachy	Stage[a] I: 100% Stage IIA: 53% Stage IIB: 35%	85% 59% 26%
Wylie (57)	46	Pelvic RT +/- ICRT	Stage I: 94% Stage IIA: 65% Stage IIB: 45%	71% 61% 27%
Sears (58)	39	Pelvic RT and/or Brachy	Stage I: 77% Stage II: 51%	44% (entire group)
Greven (64)	18	Pelvic RT and ICRT	44%	33%
Kuten (61)	17	Pelvic RT and/or Brachy	82% (vaginal control)	40% (PFS)
Colombo (66)	35	ICRT (LDR)	86%	57%
Morgan(65)	34	Pelvic RT and/or Brachy	85%	68%
Tewari (68)	30	Interstitial (LDR) +/- Pelvic RT	83%	65%
Charra (70)	37	Interstitial (LDR) +/- Pelvic RT	70%	56%
Nag (69)	10	Interstitial (LDR)	64%	42%
	5	Pelvic RT + Interstitial (LDR)	100%	
Pai (67)	20	IC RT (HDR) +/- Pelvic RT	74% (10 year)	71% (CSS)

[a]Stage refers to extent of recurrent vaginal disease.
RT = Radiation therapy; Brachy = brachytherapy (various); ICRT = Iintracavitary radiation therapy; LDR = low-dose rate;
HDR = high-dose rate; CSS = cause specific survival; PFS = progression free survival.

and 12% subsequently failed, for an overall local control rate of 86%.

Low-dose rate brachytherapy, as described in the previous studies, is thought to provide equivalent tumor control rates compared to high-dose rate. Both methods have been widely used in the adjuvant postoperative setting to deliver a vaginal cuff boost, with or without external pelvic irradiation. Pai et al. have reported on the use of HDR intracavitary brachytherapy for isolated vaginal recurrence (67). Thirteen of 20 patients received external pelvic radiation (44 Gy) and an high-dose rate vaginal boost (24 Gy), while the other were treated with high-dose rate intracavitary therapy alone (35 Gy). Complete response was noted in 90%, with second local relapses in 22% within 30 months, for a 10-year local control rate of 74%. Ten-year disease-free survival was 46% and the complication rate was 15% with no grade 3 or 4 late complications. This study suggests that high-dose rate intravaginal therapy is also an effective treatment for vaginal recurrence and is well tolerated.

Interstitial brachytherapy has also been used for treatment of vaginal wall recurrences. Tewari et al. reported on 30 patients who presented with isolated vaginal relapse who were treated with external irradiation followed by an interstitial implant, after initial surgery alone (18 patients), or implant alone for previously irradiated patients (12 patients) (68). The method used was the Syed-Neblett vaginal template, placed transperineally and given a prescribed mean maximal tumor dose of 25.5 Gy, for a cumulative dose of 86 Gy in the postoperative relapses, and 98.5 Gy in the re-irradiation group. All of the recurrent tumors were >2 cm in size, with a median time to relapse of 29 months from initial diagnosis. Complete clinical reponses were noted in 93%, with 18% second local relapses at a median interval of 16 months. The median survival after recurrence was 60 months, with a 5-year survival of 65%. Only 5 patients experienced major morbidity, including fistula ($n = 2$), stricture ($n = 1$), and proctitis ($n = 2$). A perineal interstitial template was also used by Nag et al. for vaginal recurrences, combining external beam with a 30-Gy boost for postoperative relapses, and 50–55 Gy

interstitial therapy alone for previously irradiated patients
(69). They reported an overall local control rate of 66% and a
5-year survival of 42%. A French group utilized an intravaginal template with imbedded needles to treat vaginal vault
recurrences, and achieved a 70% local control and overall survival of 56% (70). Thus, interstitial brachytherapy provides a
reasonable chance of local control, and may be used to treat
more extensive tumors not amenable to simple intravaginal
brachytherapy.

RADIATION THERAPY FOR MEDICALLY
INOPERABLE PATIENTS

EC is associated with risk factors including older age, obesity, hypertension, and diabetes. As a result, a significant
number of patients present with multiple medical problems
and are not candidates for radical surgery due to intercurrent disease. Typical illnesses preventing surgical intervention include morbid obesity, hypertension, diabetes mellitus,
pulmonary insufficiency, congestive heart failure or coronary artery disease, history of stroke, or myocardial infarction. As surgical and anesthesia techniques have improved
over the years, a higher percentage of patients with co-morbidities have been deemed operable. Series dating from the
1970s report over 20% of patients presenting with medical
contraindications to surgery who were treated with radiation alone. Since the 1980s, 3–13% of patients presenting
with endometrial cancer have medical conditions precluding
surgical treatment (71–73). Radiation therapy alone is a reasonable treatment approach for this group of patients, the
majority of whom will die of intercurrent disease rather
than EC when treated. Several institutional series have
reported their retrospective experience using radiation therapy alone in medically inoperable patients. Treatment techniques have varied and include external pelvic irradiation
alone, intracavitary or interstitial therapy alone, or a combination of external irradiation and brachytherapy.
Pathologic response rates assessed by post-treatment dila-

tion and currettage (D&C) with currettings at 3–6 months after radiation have documented complete responses in 74–93% (73,81).

Results of Primary Radiation Treatment

Clinical tumor stage and grade are the primary prognostic factors for medically inoperable patients treated only with radiation. Table 5 outlines the local control, disease specific survival, overall survival, and rate of death from intercurrent disease noted in this patient group. While radiation techniques vary among series, local control for stage I disease ranges from 61–93%, and for stage II from 41–87%. Most series consist primarily of stage I–II patients, therefore data for pelvic control in stage III–IVA patients are limited, but are reported as 62–73%. Radiation technique may impact outcomes. Landgren et al. noted that high dose intracavitary therapy alone or in combination with external irradiation was superior to external beam therapy alone (74). Patanaphan et al. used intracavitary therapy alone for stage I patients with low grade tumors and achieved a 75% 5-year survival, but noted that combined therapy resulted in the best control rates for their overall group (75). Rouanet et al. treated all patients with pelvic irradiation and uterovaginal brachytherapy to achieve 75–85 Gy to point A, and reported local control rates of 72%–90%, depending upon the tumor stage (76). Abayomi achieved local control in 74% of patients treated with external pelvic irradiation and intrauterine applications, with a disease free survival of 78% (77). Taghian et al. found a trend toward better survival when a combination of external radiotherapy and intrauterine applications was used (71). Other studies show no significant impact of the use of external pelvic irradiation in addition to intracavitary therapy. Varia et al. noted no difference in local or pelvic failures among a cohort of stage I and II patients whether they received intracavitary only (42%), external irradiation only (42%), or both (39%) (78). Grigsby et al. reported exclusively on clinical stage I patients who all received intrauterine Heyman capsules and colpostats, and some patients also received pelvic irradiation (79). They found no difference in patterns of failure among the different treatment groups. Kupelian et al. reported on a series of 152 patients, 79% of whom presented as stage I, and 91% of stage I patients were treated with brachytherapy alone (80). So while these authors noted no impact of the addition of pelvic treatment, few patients in this series received the combined techniques.

Table 5 further illustrates that intercurrent disease is a major cause of mortality, ranging from 22–88%. The wide range reflects the variability by which patients were determined to be medically inoperable, and few series specify the criteria by which the decision was made. In the series from Fishman et al., patients were evaluated by the American Society of Anesthesiologists (ASA) physical status classification, the Eastern Cooperative Oncology Group (ECOG) performance status, and medical profile (72). The majority of these patients had severe cardiac or hypertensive disease. These authors compared outcomes for similarly staged operable and medically inoperable patients. The mean ASA score for the inoperable group was 3; their mean ECOG score was also 3. Among the inoperable group, 88% with stage I and 70% with stage II cancers died of intercurrent disease, compared with 20% and 33% of operable patients, respectively.

Disease specific survivals in most studies were significantly higher than overall survivals due to the high rate of death from non-cancer related causes, ranging from 57–87% for stage I patients and from 26–88% for stage II patients. Thus, despite the presence of significant co-morbidities, definitive radiation therapy is clearly an effective treatment for medically inoperable patients, and very reasonable to consider.

Operable Compared with Medically Inoperable

Two studies have performed case-control series between inoperable and operable patients of comparable stage. Rose et al. performed a case control study of 64 patients treated with primary radiation, matched 2-to-1 with surgical controls of com-

Table 5 Results of Radiation Alone for Medically Inoperable Patients

Author (Ref.)	No. Treated	Radiation Technique	Local Control	DFS/DSS	5 Yr OS	10 Yr OS	DID
Landgren (74)	124	EBRT and/or ICRT	Ia: 89% Ib: 78% II: 82% III: 62%	—	68%	57%	45%
Abayomi (77)	66	EBRT and ICRT	74%	—	78% (3 year)	—	—
Patanaphan (75)	54	EBRT and/or ICRT	—	I: 72% II: 40% III–IV: 20%	46%	—	—
Varia (78)	73		I: 61% II: 41%	I: 57% II: 26%	78% (crude)	—	26%
Grigsby (79)	69	EBRT and/or ICRT	I: 93%	88%	77%	43%	
Taghian (71)	104	EBRT and/or ICRT	I–IV: 88%	72%	52%	22%[a]	36%
Rose (73)	64	EBRT and/or ICRT	—	—	I: 71% II: 35% III: 0% IV: 0%	—	
Rouanet (76)	250	EBRT and ICRT	76%	—	58%	46%	32%
Kupelian (80)	152	EBRT and/or ICRT	I: 84% II: 87% III–IV: 68%	I: 87% II: 88% III–IV: 49%	55%	28%	62%
Fishman (72)	54	ICRT	—	I: 80% II: 85%	I: 30% II: 24%	—	I: 88% II: 70%

[a] Estimated from curves.

EBRT = External beam radiaton therapy; ICRT = intracavitary radiation therapy; DFS = disease free survival; OS = overall survival; DSS = disease specific survival; DID = dead of intercurrent disease.

parable clinical stage, grade, and time of diagnosis (73). Radiation-alone patients were treated with pelvic irradiation followed by intracavitary Simon capsules, although a few patients received brachytherapy alone or were unable to undergo the implant procedure. Overall survival corrected for death from intercurrent disease was compared between stage I and II patients treated with surgery versus radiation, and no survival difference was noted. Fishman et al. compared outcomes in 54 medically inoperable patients with stage I and II EC with 108 operable patients matched for age, treatment year, clinical stage, and grade (72). Stage I patients were typically treated with intracavitaary radiation alone, usually placed under regional anesthesia or sedation. Stage II patients had intracavitary therapy followed by pelvic irradiation. Most surgical patients received preoperative brachytherapy, followed by abdominal hysterectomy. For stage I patients, inoperable patients had a mean disease free-interval of 36 months, and 5-year cancer specific survival of 80%, compared to 74 months and 98% for operable patients, respectively. Inoperable stage II patients had a mean DFI of 50 months and a cancer-free survival of 85%, compared to 68 months and 85%, respectively, for the operable group. Overall the operable patients had a significantly longer survival and better disease-free survival. In this series 87% of stage I and 70% of stage II medically inoperable patients died of intercurrent disease. When deaths from intercurrent disease were excluded, inoperable patients had a similar median 5-year survival as the operable group (stage I, 62 months; stage II, 72 months).

High-Dose Rate Brachytherapy

While the majority of series reporting on treatment of medically inoperable patients who have received low-dose rate brachytherapy, there are several studies reporting their experience with high-dose rate brachytherapy as well. Sorbe et al. treated 366 patients with stage I patients with high-dose rate brachytherapy using remote afterloading cobolt-60 sources, and a fraction size of 5–10 Gy (81). Abdominal hysterectomy was performed 6 weeks later in 275 cases. Complete pathologic response was noted in 58% of surgical specimens. In the remaining patients not undergoing surgery, currettings were obtained 3 months after treatment, and 74% revealed no residual carcinoma. The best tumor responses were seen in the 10-Gy per fraction group. Five-year survivals were 88% in the preoperative radiation group and 72% in the radiation-alone group. Nguyen et al. treated 27 patients with stage I or II EC and medical contraindications to surgery with high-dose rate intracavitary therapy; 8 also received external pelvic radiation, usually for stage II disease (82). The median high-dose rate was 20 Gy in 2 or 3 fractions (range, 4.4–34 Gy) using either a tandem alone, or tandem and vaginal colpostats. Disease specific survival was 76%, but much better for stage I (95%) than stage II (21%) patients. As expected, high grade was a poor prognostic factor. Four patients (15%) had pelvic failures, and three of these had received less than 20 Gy. Salvage hysterectomy was successful in all three patients. There were no acute complications, and 11% late reactions including bowel obstruction, and anal or sigmoid stenosis. A series from University of Wisconsin reported on 36 clinical stage I patients treated with high-dose rate brachytherapy alone, using a remote afterloading iridium source, mostly with an intrauterine tandem alone, although a few cases incorporated a vaginal ring or ovoids (83). Five fractions of 8.2 Gy to the vaginal mucosa were given. Three-year disease-free survival was 85% and the uterine control rate was 88%. Forty percent of patients died in the study period, 15% from recurrence and 25% from intercurrent disease, and there was a 30-day mortality rate of 6%. These authors report a late complication rate of 21%, which they postulated was related to prescription points that exposed the bowel and ureters to excessive dose. Kucera et al. also reviewed treatment results for 228 patients with clinical stage I disease who received high-dose rate iridium therapy alone (84). Most patients were treated with 8.5 Gy per fraction intrauterine dose to a total uterine dose of 34 Gy. Overall survival was 60% at 5 years and 30% at 10 years; disease specific survival was 85% and 75% at 5 and 10 years respectively. Local control was achieved in 74%, with no significant difference by grade. Late complications (grade 3, 4, or 5) were seen in 5%, and there was one treatment-related death (small bowel obstruction complicated by peritonitis).

Treatment Sequelae

For this group of patients, treatment sequelae must be considered. While brachytherapy is likely the most important component of therapy when definitive radiation is used, intracavitary or interstitial implants may require general anesthesia to perform. The M.D. Anderson series examined their acute complications associated with intracavitary treatment and anesthesia (80). Procedure-related complications were noted in 8% of patients, with 8 of the 12 patients undergoing general anesthesia. While none of the complications were fatal, they included a resuscitated cardiac arrest, cardiac arrhythmia, labile blood pressure, possible myocardial infarction, and acute respiratory distress, and therefore were potentially life-threatening. The authors note that no such complications were observed during applications that were performed under regional anesthesia or monitored sedation. Chao et al. noted that for patients requiring intrauterine implants performed under general anesthesia, the median duration of anesthesia was 60 min (range, 30–120 min), and a median application duration of 46 hr (range, 11–96 hr) (85). Four patients (5%) developed life-threatening complications, including myocardial infarction, congestive heart failure, and pulmonary embolism, resulting in two treatment-related deaths (2%). Patients undergoing even brief anesthesia for radiation implants should be monitored closely. Postoperatively they require frequent nursing evaluations while immobilized, and prophylaxis against deep vein thromboses with low dose heparin and pneumatic compression stockings should be administered to appropriate patients. Therefore, thorough training of house staff and nursing staff responsible for the care of inpatient brachytherapy patients is crucial. Late complications in these studies occurred in 2-17% of patients, primarily affecting the rectum and bladder, including proctitis, bladder contracture, fistula, and stricture. Complications tend to be increased by combined external and intracavitary therapy, higher total radiation doses, or hypofractionation schemes, and are more likely in patients with more advanced disease.

REFERENCES

1. International Federation of Gynecology and Obstetrics: Corpus cancer staging. *Int J Gynecol Obstet* 1989; 28:190.

2. McLellan R, Dillon MB, Currie JL, Rosenshein NB. Peritoneal cytology in endometrial cancer: a review. *Obstet Gynecol Surv* 1989; 44(10)711-719.

3. Kennedy AW, Webster KD, Nunez C, Bauer LJ. Pelvic washings for cytologic analysis in endometrial adenocarcinoma. *J Reprod Med* 1993; 38(8):637-642.

4. Yazigi R, Piver MS, Blumenson L. Malignant peritoneal cytology as prognostic indicator in stage I endometrial cancer. *Obstet Gynecol* 1983; 62(3):359-362.

5. Macdonald RR, Thorogood J, Mason MK. A randomized trial of progestogens in the primary treatment of endometrial carcinoma. *Br J Obstet Gynaecol* 1988;95(2):166-174.

6. Lurain JR, Rumsey NK, Schink JC, Wallemark CB, Chmiel JS. Prognostic significance of positive peritoneal cytology in clinical stage I adenocarcinoma of the endometrium. *Obstet Gynecol* 1989; 74(2):175-179.

7. Zuna RE, Behrens A. Peritoneal washing cytology in gynecologic cancers: long-term follow-up of 355 patients. *J Natl Cancer Inst* 1996; 88(14):980-987.

8. Turner DA, Gershenson DM, Atkinson N, Sneige N, Wharton AT. The prognostic significance of peritoneal cytology for stage I endometrial cancer. *Obstet Gynecol* 1989; 74(5):775-780.

9. Harouny VR, Sutton GP, Clark SA, Geisler HE, Stehman FB, Ehrlich CE. The importance of peritoneal cytology in endometrial carcinoma. *Obstet Gynecol* 1988; 72(3 Pt 1):394-398.

10. Morrow CP, Bundy BN, Kurman RJ, Creasman WT, Heller P, Homesley HD, Graham JE.Relationship between surgical-pathological risk factors and outcome in clinical stage I and II

carcinoma of the endometrium: a Gynecologic Oncology Group study. *Gynecol Oncol* 1991; 40(1):55–65.

11. Creasman WT, Rutledge F. The prognostic value of peritoneal cytology in gynecologic malignant disease. *Am J Obstet Gynecol* 1971; 110(6):773–781.

12. Creasman WT, Disaia PJ, Blessing J, Wilkinson RH Jr, Johnston W, Weed JC Jr. Prognostic significance of peritoneal cytology in patients with endometrial cancer and preliminary data concerning therapy with intraperitoneal radiopharma-ceuticals. *Am J Obstet Gynecol* 1981; 141(8):921–929.

13. Soper JT, Creasman WT, Clarke-Pearson DL, Sullivan DC, Vergadoro F, Johnston WW. Intraperitoneal chromic phosphate P-32 suspension therapy of malignant peritoneal cytology in endometrial carcinoma. *Am J Obstet Gynecol* 1985; 153(2):191-196.

14. Potish RA. Abdominal radiotherapy for cancer of the uterine cervix and endometrium. *Int J Radiat Oncol Biol Phys* 1989; 16(6):1453–1458.

15. Konski A, Poulter C, Keys H, Rubin P, Beecham J, Doane K. Absence of prognostic significance, peritoneal dissemination and treatment advantage in endometrial cancer patients with positive peritoneal cytology. *Int J Radiat Oncol Biol Phys* 1988; 14(1):49–55

16. Martinez A, Podratz K, Schray M, Malkasian G. Results of whole abdominopelvic irradiation with nodal boost for patients with endometrial cancer at high risk of failure in the peritoneal cavity. A prospective clinical trial at the Mayo Clinic. *Hematol Oncol Clin North Am* 1988; 2(3):431–446.

17. Mazurka JL, Krepart GV, Lotocki RJ. Prognostic significance of positive peritoneal cytology in endometrial carcinoma. *Am J Obstet Gynecol* 1988; 158(2):303–306.

18. Piver MS. Progesterone therapy for malignant peritoneal cytology surgical stage I endometrial adenocarcinoma. *Seminars in Oncology* 1988; 15(2 Suppl 1):50–52.

19. Creasman WT, Morrow CP, Bundy BN, Homesley HD, Graham JE, Heller PB. Surgical pathologic spread patterns of endometrial cancer. A Gynecologic Oncology Group study. *Cancer* 1987; 60(8 suppl):2035–2041.

20. Greven KM, Curran WJ Jr, Whittington R, Fanning J, Randall ME, Wilder J, Peters AJ. Analysis of failure patterns in stage III endometrial carcinoma and therapeutic implications. *Int J Radiat Oncol Biol Phys* 1989; 17(1):35–39.

21. Nori D, Hilaris BS, Tome M, Lewis JL Jr, Birnbaum S, Fuks Z. Combined surgery and radiation in endometrial carcinoma: an analysis of prognostic factors. *Int J Radiat Oncol Biol Phys* 1987; 13(4):489–497.

22. Bruckman JE, Bloomer WD, Marck A, Ehrmann RL, Knapp RC. Stage III adenocarcinoma of the endometrium: two prognostic groups. *Gynecol Oncol* 1980; 9(1)12-17.

23. Antoniades J, Brady LW, Lewis GC. The management of stage III carcinoma of the endometrium. *Cancer* 1976; 38(4):1838–1842.

24. Potish RA, Twiggs LB, Adcock LL, Prem KA. Role of whole abdominal radiation therapy in the management of endometrial cancer; prognostic importance of factors indicating peritoneal metastases. *Gynecol Oncol* 1985; 21(1):80–86

25. Greer BE, Hamberger AD. Treatment of intraperitoneal metastatic adenocarcinoma of the endometrium by the whole-abdomen moving-strip technique and pelvic boost irradiation. *Gynecol Oncol* 1983; 16(3):365–373.

26. Mackillop WJ, Pringle JF. Stage III endometrial carcinoma. A review of 90 cases. *Cancer* 1985; 56(10):2519–2523.

27. Greven KM, Lanciano RM, Corn B, Case D, Randall ME. Pathologic stage III endometrial carcinoma. Prognostic factors and patterns of recurrence. *Cancer* 1993; 71(11):3697–3702.

28. Smith RS, Kapp DS, Chen Q, Teng NN. Treatment of high-risk uterine cancer with whole abdominopelvic radiation therapy. *Int J Radiat Oncol Biol Phys* 2000; 48(3):767–778.

29. Gerszten K, Faul C, Huang Q. Pathologic stage III endometrial cancer treated with adjuvant radiation therapy. *Int J Gynecol Cancer* 1999; 9(3):243–246.

30. Katz LA, Andrews SJ, Fanning J. Survival after multimodality treatment for stage IIIC endometrial cancer. *Am J Obstet Gynecol* 2001; 184(6):1071–1073.

31. Nelson G, Randall M, Sutton G, Moore D, Hurteau J, Look K. FIGO stage IIIC endometrial carcinoma with metastases con-

fined to pelvic lymph nodes: analysis of treatment outcomes, prognostic variables, and failure patterns following adjuvant radiation therapy. *Gynecol Oncol* 1999; 75(2):211–214.

32. McMeekin DS, Lashbrook D, Gold M, Johnson G, Walker JL, Mannel R. Analysis of FIGO stage IIIc endometrial cancer patients. *Gynecol Oncol* 2001; 81(2):273–278.

33. Mundt AJ, Murphy KT, Rotmensch J, Waggoner SE, Yamada SD, Connell PP. Surgery and postoperative radiation therapy in FIGO Stage IIIC endometrial carcinoma. *Int J Radiat Oncol Biol Phys* 2001; 50(5):1154-1160.

34. Potish RA, Twiggs LB, Adcock LL, Savage JE, Levitt SH, Prem KA. Paraaortic lymph node radiotherapy in cancer of the uterine corpus. *Obstet Gynecol* 1985; 65(2)251–256.

35. Corn BW, Lanciano RM, Greven KM, Schultz DJ, Reisinger SA, Stafford PM, Hanks GE. Endometrial cancer with para-aortic adenopathy: patterns of failure and opportunities for cure. *Int J Radiat Oncol Biol Phys* 24(2):223–227.

36. Rose PG, Cha SD, Tak WK, Fitzgerald T, Reale F, Hunter RE. Radiation therapy for surgically proven para-aortic node metastasis in endometrial carcinoma. *Int J Radiat Oncol Biol Phys* 1992; 24(2):229–233.

37. Onda T, Yoshikawa H, Mizutani K, Mishima M, Yokota H, Nagano H, Ozaki Y, Murakami A, Ueda K, Taketani Y. Treatment of node-positive endometrial cancer with complete node dissection, chemotherapy and radiation therapy. *Br J Cancer* 1997; 75(12):1836–1841.

38. Small W Jr, Mahadevan A, Roland P, Vallow L, Zusag T, Fishman D, Massad S, Rademaker A, Kalapurakal JA, Chang S, Lurain J. Whole-abdominal radiation in endometrial carcinoma: an analysis of toxicity, patterns of recurrence, and survival. *Cancer* J 2000; 6(6):394–400.

39. International Federation of Gynecology and Obstetrics: Classification and staging of malignant tumors in the female pelvis. *Int J Gynaecol Obstet* 1971; 9:172.

40. Grigsby PW, Perez CA, Kuske RR, Kao MS, Galakatos AE. Results of therapy, analysis of failures, and prognostic factors for clinical and pathologic stage III adenocarcinoma of the endometrium. *Gynecol Oncol* 1987; 27(1):44–57.

41. Aalders JG, Abeler V, Kolstad P. Clinical (stage III) as compared to subclinical intrapelvic extrauterine tumor spread in endometrial carcinoma: a clinical and histopathological study of 175 patients. *Gynecol Oncol* 1984; 17(1):64–74.

42. Bristow RE, Zerbe MJ, Rosenshein NB, Grumbine FC, Montz FJ. Stage IVB endometrial carcinoma: the role of cytoreductive surgery and determinants of survival. *Gynecol Oncol* 2000; 78(2):85–91.

43. Chi DS, Welshinger M, Venkatraman ES, Barakat RR. The role of surgical cytoreduction in stage IV endometrial carcinoma. *Gynecol Oncol* 1997; 67(1):56–60.

44. Pliskow S, Penalver M, Averette HE. Stage III and stage IV endometrial carcinoma: a review of 41 cases. *Gynecol Oncol* 1990; 38(2):210–215.

45. Burke TW, Heller PB, Woodward JE, Davidson SA, Hoskins WJ, Park RC. Treatment failure in endometrial carcinoma. *Obstet Gynecol* 1990; 75(1):96–101.

46. Onsrud M, Hagen B, Strickert T. 10–Gy single-fraction pelvic irradiation for palliation and life prolongation in patients with cancer of the cervix and corpus uteri. *Gynecol Oncol* 2001; 82(1):167–171.

47. Spanos WJ Jr, Perez CA, Marcus S, Poulter CA, Doggett RL, Steinfeld AD, Grigsby PW. Effect of rest interval on tumor and normal tissue response—a report of phase III study of accelerated split course palliative radiation for advanced pelvic malignancies (RTOG-8502). *Int J Radiat Oncol Biol Phys* 1993; 25(3):399–403.

48. Salazar OM, Feldstein ML, DePapp EW, Bonfiglio TA, Keller BE, Rubin P, Rudolph JH. Endometrial carcinoma: analysis of failures with special emphasis on the use of initial preoperative external pelvic radiation. *Int J Radiat Oncol Biol Phys* 1977; 2(11–12):1101–1107.

49. Kadar N, Malfetano JH, Homesley HD. Determinants of survival of surgically staged patients with endometrial carcinoma histologically confined to the uterus: implications for therapy. *Obstet Gynecol* 1992; 80(4):655–659.

50. Carey MS, O'Connell GJ, Johanson CR, Goodyear MD Murphy KJ, Daya DM, Schepansky A, Peloquin A, Lumsden BJ. Good

outcome associated with a standardized treatment protocol using selective postoperative radiation in patients with clinical stage I adenocarcinoma of the endometrium. *Gynecol Oncol* 1995; 57(2):138–144.

51. Aalders J, Abeler V, Kolstad P, Onsrud M. Postoperative external irradiation and prognostic parameters in stage I endometrial carcinoma: clinical and histopathologic study of 540 patients. *Obstet Gynecol* 1980; 56(4):419–427.

52. Elliott P, Green D, Coates A, Krieger M, Russell P, Coppleson M, Solomon J, Tattersall. The efficacy of postoperative vaginal irradiation in preventing vaginal recurrence in endometrial cancer. *Cancer* 1994; 4(2):84–89.

53. Roberts JA, Brunetto VL, Keyes HM, et al. A phase II randomized study of surgery vs. surgery plus adjuvant radiation therapy in intermediate risk endometrial cancer. *Gynecol Oncol* 1998; 68:135.

54. Creutzberg CL, van Putten WL, Koper PC, Lybeert ML, Jobsen JJ, Warlam-Rodenhuis CC, De Winter KA, Lutgens LC, van den Bergh AC, van de Steen-Banasik E, Beerman H, van Lent M. Surgery and postoperative radiotherapy versus surgery alone for patients with stage-I endometrial carcinoma: multicentre randomised trial. PORTEC Study Group. Post Operative Radiation Therapy in Endometrial Carcinoma. *Lancet* 2000; 355(9213):1404–1411.

55. Barakat RR, Goldman NA, Patel DA, Venkatraman ES, Curtin JP. Pelvic exenteration for recurrent endometrial cancer. *Gynecol Oncol* 1999; 75(1):99–102.

56. Ingersoll FM. Vaginal recurrence of carcinoma of the corpus. Management and prevention. *Am J Surg* 1971; 121(4):473–477.

57. Wylie J, Irwin C, Pintilie M, Levin W, Manchul L, Milosevic M, Fyles A. Results of radical radiotherapy for recurrent endometrial cancer. *Gynecol Oncol* 2000; 77(1):66–72.

58. Sears JD, Greven KM, Hoen HM, Randall ME. Prognostic factors and treatment outcome for patients with locally recurrent endometrial cancer. *Cancer* 1994; 74(4):1303–1308.

59. Vavra N, Denison U, Kucera H, Barrada M, Kurz C, Salzer H, Sevelda P. Prognostic factors related to recurrent endometrial

carcinoma following initial surgery. *Acta Obstet Gynecol Scand* 1993; 72:205–209.

60. Hoekstra CJ, Koper PC, van Putten WL. Recurrent endometrial adenocarcinoma after surgery alone: prognostic factors and treatment. *Radiother Oncol* 1993; 27(2):164–166.

61. Kuten , Grigsby PW, Perez CA, Fineberg B, Garcia DM, Simpson JR. Results of radiotherapy in recurrent endometrial carcinoma: a retrospective analysis of 51 patients. *Int J Radiat Oncol Biol Phys* 1989; 17(1):29–34.

62. Jereczek-Foss, Badzio A, Jassem J. Recurrent endometrial cancer after surgery alone: results of salvage radiotherapy. *Int J Radiat Oncol Biol Phys* 2000; 48(2):405–413.

63. Curran WJ Jr, Whittington R, Peters AJ, Fanning J. Vaginal recurrences of endometrial carcinoma: the prognostic value of staging by a primary vaginal carcinoma system. *Int J Radiat Oncol Biol Phys* 1988; 15(4):803–808.

64. Greven K, Olds W. Isolated recurrences of endometrial adenocarcinoma and their management. *Cancer* 1987; 60(3):419–421.

65. Morgan JD, Reddy S, Sarin P, Yordan E, Geest K, Hendrickson F. Isolated vaginal recurrences of endometrail cancer. *Radiology* 1993; 189(2):609–613.

66. Colombo, Cormio G, Placa F, Landoni F, Ardizzoia A, Gabriele A, Lissoni A. Brachytherapy for isolated vaginal recurrences from endometrial carcinoma. *Tumori* 1998; 84(6):649–651.

67. Pai HH, Souhami L, Clark BG, Roman T. Isolated vaginal recurrences in endometrial carcinoma: treatment results using high-dose-rate intracavitary brachytherapy and external beam radiotherapy. *Gynecol Oncol* 1997; 66(2):300–307.

68. Tewari K, Cappuccini F, Syed AM, Puthawala A, DiSaia PJ, Berman ML, Manetta A, Monk BJ. Interstitial brachytherapy in the treatment of advanced and recurrent vulvar cancer. *Am J Obstet Gynecol* 1999; 181(1):91–98.

69. Nag S, Martinez-Monge R, Copeland LJ, Vacarello L, Lewandowski GS. Perineal template interstitial brachytherapy salvage for recurrent endometrial adenocarcinoma metastatic to the vagina. *Gynecol Oncol* 1997; 66(1):16–19.

70. Charra , Roy P, Coquard R, Romestaing P, Ardiet JM, Gerard JP. Outcome of treatment of upper third vaginal recurrences of cervical and endometrial carcinomas with interstitial brachytherapy. *Int J Radiat Oncol Biol Phys* 1998; 40(2) 421–426.

71. Taghian A, Pernot M, Hoffstetter S, Luporsi E, Bey P. Radiation therapy alone for medically inoperable patients with adenocarcinoma of the endometrium. *Int J Radiat Oncol Biol Phys* 1988; 15(5):1135–1140.

72. Fishman DA, Roberts KB, Chambers JT, Kohorn EI, Schwartz PE. Chambers SK. Radiation therapy as exclusive treatment for medically inoperable patients with stage I and II endometrioid carcinoma with endometrium. *Gynecol Oncol* 1996; 61(2):189–196.

73. Rose PG, Baker S, Kern M, Fitzgerald TJ, Tak WK, Reale FR, Nelson BE, Hunter RE. Primary radiation therapy for endometrial carcinoma: a case controlled study. *Int J Radiat Oncol Biol Phys* 1993; 27(3):585–590.

74. Landgren RC, Fletcher GH, Delclos L, Wharton JT. Irradiation of endometrial cancer in patients with medical contraindication to surgery or with unresectable lesions. *Am J Roentgen* 1976; 126(1):148–154.

75. Patanaphan V, Salazar OM, Chougule P. What can be expected when radiation therapy becomes the only curative alternative for endometrial cancer? *Cancer* 1985; 55(7):1462–1467.

76. Rouanet P, Dubois JB, Gely S, Pourquier H. Exclusive radiation therapy in endometrial cancer. *Int J Radiat Oncol Biol Phys* 1993; 26(2):223–228.

77. Abayomi O, Tak W, Emami B, Anderson B. Treatment of endometrial cancer with radiation therapy alone. *Cancer* 1982; 49(12):2466–2469.

78. Varia M, Rosenman J, Halle J, Walton L, Currie J, Fowler W. Primary radiation therapy for medically inoperable patients with endometrial carcinoma—stages I-II. *Int J Radiat Oncol Biol Phys* 1987; 13(1):11–15.

79. Grigsby PW, Kuske RR, Perez CA, Walz BJ, Camel MH, Kao MS, Galakatos A. Medically inoperable stage I adenocarcinoma of the endometrium treated with radiotherapy alone. *Int J Radiat Oncol Biol Phys* 1987; 13(4):483–488.

80   Kupelian PA, Eifel PJ, Tornos C, Burke TW, Delclos L, Oswald MJ. Treatment of endometrial carcinoma with radiation therapy alone. *Int J Radiat Oncol Biol Phys* 1993; 27(4):817–824.

81.   Sorbe B, Frankendal B, Risberg B. Intracavitary irradiation of endometrial carcinoma stage I by a high dose-rate afterloading technique. *Gynecol Oncol* 1989; 33(2):135–145.

82.   Nguyen C, Souhami L, Roman TN, Clark BG. High-dose-rate brachytherapy as the primary treatment of medically inoperable stage I–II endometrial carcinoma. *Gynecol Oncol* 1995; 59(3):370–375.

83.   Nguyen TV, Petereit DG. High-dose-rate brachytherapy for medically inoperable stage I endometrial cancer. *Gynecol Oncol* 1998; 71(2):196–203.

84.   Kucera, Knocke TH, Kucera E, Potter R. Treatment of endometrial carcinoma with high-dose-rate brachytherapy alone in medically inoperable stage I patients. *Acta Obstet Gynecol Scand* 1998; 77(10):1008–1012.

85.   Chao CKS, Grigsby PW, Perez CA, Camel HM, Kao M, Galaktos AE, Boyle WA. Brachytherapy-related complications for medically inoperable stage I endometrial carcinoma. *Int J Radiat Oncol Biol Phy* 1994; 31(1):37–42.

15

Systemic Therapies for Endometrial Carcinoma

BRIAN M. SLOMOVITZ AND KAREN H. LU
University of Texas, M.D. Anderson Cancer
Center, Houston,Texas, U.S.A.

Because of the hematogenous and lymphatic spread of endometrial cancer (EC), patients with recurrent or advanced disease often present with tumor outside of the pelvis. Systemic therapy, therefore, plays an important role in the management of these patients. Both hormonal and cytotoxic agents have activity in patients with advanced or recurrent EC. However, neither of these types of therapies is considered curative in patients with distant, metastatic disease.

EC represents a heterogeneous disease. The most important difference in disease outcomes arises between the endometrioid and non-endometrioid histologic subtypes. In particular, patients with uterine papillary serous carcinoma

(UPSC) have a distinct clinical course. In this chapter we
review systemic treatment options for endometrioid endometrial carcinoma (EEC) and UPSC separately. Newer molecular based therapeutic options are reviewed briefly at the end
of the chapter.

ENDOMETRIOID ENDOMETRIAL CARCINOMA (EEC)

Chemotherapy for Advanced and Recurrent EEC

Several chemotherapeutic agents or combinations of agents
have demonstrated activity in patients with EEC.
Combination therapy is more effective than single agent therapy in treating this disease. The challenge has been to combine agents to maximize efficacy while attempting to limit
toxicity. Because there are only a few randomized control trials of cytotoxic therapies in EC, treatment decisions often use
information obtained in smaller phase II studies.

Doxorubicin was one of the first drugs identified with
good activity against EC. Single-agent doxorubicin has a
response rate of approximately 25% (1–3), with a median
duration of response less than 1 year (1,3). Cyclophosphamide
also demonstrated modest activity in earlier studies (2). In a
randomized Gynecologic Oncology Group (GOG) study comparing doxorubicin alone to doxorubicin and cyclophosphamide, no significant difference was seen in the response
rate, the median progression-free interval, or the median
overall survival.

During the same time period, single-agent cisplatin
demonstrated response rates between 20% and 42% when
used as a first line agent (4–6). The duration of response was
again very short (3–5 months) (4,5). In several phase II studies, adding cisplatin to doxorubicin resulted in response rates
between 45% and 60% (7–9). In a GOG randomized phase III
study, cisplatin and doxorubicin in combination had a higher
response rate as compared to single-agent doxorubicin (45%
vs. 27%). There was no difference in overall survival (10). The
EORTC performed a similar trial comparing the same two
regimens. Again, the combination arm had a higher response
rate than the doxorubicin-alone treatment group (11). In this

study there was a modest survival advantage in those patients who received the combination regimen. The median overall survival in cisplatin- and doxorubicin-treated patients was 9 months compared to 7 months in the patients who received doxorubicin alone (p = 0.065). Burke et al. evaluated triple therapy with cyclophosphamide, doxorubicin, and cisplatin (CAP) and found a 45% response rate to this regimen (12). The response rates in this trial and in other phase II trials of CAP (6,13,14) were similar to the response rates of doxorubicin and cisplatin without cyclophosphamide. Therefore, doxorubicin in combination with cisplatin was viewed as the standard systemic chemotherapy in women with advanced or recurrent endometrial adenocarcinoma at this time.

More recently, phase II studies of paclitaxel found significant activity in chemo-naive patients with recurrent EC with a response rate of 36% (15). In patients who failed prior chemotherapy, paclitaxel also demonstrated activity with a response rates up to 43% (16–19). The anti-tumor effect of single-agent paclitaxel led to the incorporation of paclitaxel into combination therapy regimens. In a phase II study, the combination of cisplatin and paclitaxel demonstrated a 67% response rate (20). In a phase III study, the GOG found similar activity between the combination of cisplatin and doxorubicin versus doxorubicin and paclitaxel (21). Following this study, the GOG performed a phase III trial evaluating doxorubicin and cisplatin compared to doxorubicin, cisplatin, and paclitaxel with granulocyte colony stimulating factor (22). Preliminary findings suggest a survival advantage in patients receiving the triple therapy.

In an attempt to decrease the toxicity related to cisplatin therapy, carboplatin has been investigated. Single-agent carboplatin demonstrates modest activity in chemo-naive patients (23–27) with little or no activity in patients pretreated with chemotherapy (27). In a phase II study, the combination of paclitaxel and carboplatin was evaluated in patients with advanced and recurrent disease (28). In patients with advanced EEC, there was a 78% response rate to this combination. The median failure free survival time was 23 months and the 3-year overall survival rate was 62%.

In patients with recurrent disease, the response rate was 56% and the median failure-free interval was 6 months.

The combination of carboplatin and paclitaxel has a more favorable toxicity profile than cisplatin and paclitaxel. For this reason, many community physicians prefer this combination in the setting of advanced or recurrent EC. The GOG has recently opened a phase III randomized study to evaluate doxorubicin, cisplatin, and paclitaxel compared to carboplatin and paclitaxel to address this question.

Table 1 summarizes the randomized, phase III chemotherapeutic trials for advanced and recurrent EC.

Despite higher response rates, more effective cytotoxic agents with longer durations of response are needed. A number of phase II studies have been conducted in women with recurrent EC. The antiproliferative activity of topotecan is being investigated in patients with advanced EC cancer. Both single-agent topotecan and topotecan in combination with cisplatin have demonstrated early, promising results (29–31). Although doxorubicin-based treatment demonstrates good efficacy, it is associated with considerable toxicity, including irreversible cardiotoxicity, congestive heart failure, and necrotizing colitis. Because of this, peglyated liposomal doxorubicin, which has a more favorable toxicity profile, is being investigated. In phase II studies, response rates between 10% and 20% were achieved (32,33). Most of the patients in these studies had failed prior cytotoxic agents. The GOG is currently evaluating liposomal doxorubicin as a first-line chemotherapy for patients with recurrent EC. Based on the results of this study, pegylated liposomal doxorubicin may be a more suitable alternative to doxorubicin as a component of combination therapy.

Several other agents have modest effectiveness in treating patients with advanced or recurrent endometrial cancer. The alkylating agent, ifosfamide, demonstrated a response rate of 24% in chemo-naive patients (34,35) and a 0–15% response rate in patients pretreated with platinum agents (34,35). 5–fluorouracil (5–FU) has demonstrated activity both as a single agent and in combination with melphalan in the phase II setting (36–39). Oral etoposide has been shown to

Table 1 Phase III Randomized Control Studies for Advanced and Recurrent EC

Group/Author/ Date Published	Agents	Response (overall)	p-value	PFI	p-value	MOS	p-value
GOG (3) Thigpen et al., 1994	doxo	22%	$p = ns$	3.2 mo	$p = ns$	6.7 mo	$p = ns$
	doxo/cyclo	30%		3.9 mo		7.3 mo	
GOG (10) Thigpen et al., 1993[a]	doxo	27%	$p < 0.05$	NA		NA	
	doxo/cisplatin	45%		NA		NA	
EORTC (11) Aapr., 2003	doxo	17%	$p < 0.001$	7 mo	$p = ns$	7 mo	$p = 0.07$
	doxo/cisplatin	43%		8 mo		9 mo	
GOG (21) Fleming et al., 2000[a]	doxo/cisplatin	40%	$p = ns$	7.2 mo	$p = ns$	12.4 mo	$p = ns$
	doxo/tax	44%		6.0 mo		13.6 mo	
GOG (22) Fleming et al., 2002[a]	doxo/cisplatin	33%	$p < 0.001$	NA		NA	
	doxo/cisplatin/tax	57%		NA		NA	

[a]Published in abstract form only.
PFI = Progression-free interval; MOS = median overall survival; GOG = Gynecologic Oncology Group; EORTC = European Organization for Research and Treatment of Cancer; doxo = doxorubicin; cyclo = cyclophosphamide; tax = paclitaxel.

have some activity against chemo-naive patients with a tolerable toxicity profile (40), but was not seen in patients who had received prior chemotherapy (41).

Prognosis is very poor for patients who fail first-line chemotherapy. The response rates for second and third-line agents are often less than 10% and the overall survival is less than 9 months. Paclitaxel may have better activity than other agents in this setting. In patients who have failed prior chemotherapy, paclitaxel has response rates up to 43% (16–19). In particular, in a cohort of patients who were refractory to platinum, paclitaxel was shown to have a 22% response rate (16). Preliminary data suggest that re-treatment with a platinum/paclitaxel-based regimen may be effective in patients who previously responded to these agents (42).

Adjuvant Chemotherapy for Early Stage EEC

Adjuvant therapeutic options for patients with EC and high-risk features include radiation, progestins, and cytotoxic chemotherapy. Though the addition of postoperative radiation to high-risk patients does reduce the local recurrence rate (43), distant metastasis continues to be problematic. In approximately 25% of patients with low-stage, grade 3 lesions, the disease will recur at a distant site (44,45). In addition, in 20% of clinical stage II patients (46–48) and at least 30% of patients who present with extrauterine disease (49–51), there is recurrence at distant sites even after patients have received adjuvant pelvic radiation.

However, no studies have demonstrated a survival advantage of chemotherapy given in the adjuvant setting. In a GOG study of high-risk patients who received postoperative whole pelvic radiation alone or with doxorubicin, there was no statistical difference in survival rates or progression-free interval rates (52). In a phase II study, Burke et al. documented an excellent disease-free survival in high-risk patients without extrauterine disease who received six cycles of cisplatin, doxorubicin, and cyclophosphamide (53). In those patients with disease limited to the uterus, the 3-year survival rate was 82%. In patients with disease outside of the uterus, the 3-year survival rate was 46%.

Radiation and Chemotherapy

Chemotherapy given in combination with radiation may enhance the effect of the radiotherapy and reduce the incidence of failures both outside and within the treated field. Weekly cisplatin in combination with whole abdominal radiation has been reported to have no greater toxicity than radiation alone (54,55). The GOG is currently evaluating the role of adjuvant chemotherapy as a component of combination therapy in the management of primary advanced EC. By adding adjuvant chemotherapy prior to the completion of radiotherapy, this study design may address the concerns of distant metastasis.

HORMONAL THERAPY

Progestins for Advanced or Recurrent Disease

For the past 50 years, progestational agents have been valuable in the armamentarium against EC, particularly in patients with recurrent disease (56,57). Progestins are generally well tolerated. Side effects are usually minor and include weight gain, edema, thrombophlebitis, headache, and occasional hypertension. In patients with medical co-morbidities, use of hormonal agents may be preferable over cytotoxic chemotherapy. Initial clinical trials in patients with advanced or recurrent EC demonstrated response rates of 30–50% (58,59). Larger studies with more specific response criteria demonstrate more modest response rates, usually between 11% and 24% (60–62). Podratz et al. (60) treated 155 patients with advanced or recurrent endometrial cancer with progestational agents. The objective response rate was 11%. Overall, survival after initiation of hormone therapy was 40% at 1 year, 19% at 2 years, and 8% at 5 years. In a GOG phase II study (62), patients who had no prior exposure to chemotherapy or hormonal agents were treated with megesterol acetate (800 mg/day). The overall response rate was 24%. The progression-free survival and overall survival were 2.5 months and 7.6 months, respectively.

Current recommendations for progestin therapy include oral medroxyprogesterone acetate (MPA, Provera®), intramuscular MPA (Depo-Provera®), and megesterol acetate (Megace®). Although there are no randomized studies that have directly compared different formulations of progestins, response rates are similar (60,63). In addition, although a dose-response effect of progestin therapy has been reported in breast cancer (64), there is no evidence of this effect in patients with EC. In a randomized trial of oral MPA, patients receiving the low-dose regimen (200 mg/day) had a higher response to therapy than those receiving the high-dose regimen (1000 mg/day) (65).

There are a number of tumor characteristics that increase the likelihood of response to hormonal therapy. These include low-grade tumors, presence of steroid hormone receptors (i.e., PR and ER positive), and a longer disease-free interval (62,65,66). The GOG demonstrated a response rate of 8% in women whose tumors were PR negative and 37% for women whose tumors were PR positive. In addition, there was a 7% response rate in women with ER-negative tumors compared to a 26% response rate in women with ER-positive tumors (65). Patients with poorly differentiated tumors or hormone-receptor negative tumors have significantly lower response rates to progestin therapy (62,65).

Because of the low toxicity profile and modest efficacy, progestins should be considered in patients with recurrent EC. In particular, all patients not eligible for clinical trials with well-differentiated, hormone-receptor positive recurrent or advanced disease can be given a trial of progestin therapy. If the patient has an objective response, the progestin may be continued indefinitely until there is disease progression.

Selective Estrogen Receptor Modulators

Selective estrogen receptor modulators (SERMs) with anti-estrogenic effects in the uterus have been used to treat women with recurrent EC. First-generation SERMs such as tamoxifen have mixed estrogenic agonist and antagonist activity. Early response rates for tamoxifen in advanced or recurrent EC were between 20%–36% and (67,68). However, in a GOG phase II study of tamoxifen given at a dose of 20 mg twice daily, only 10% of patients demonstrated an objective response (69). Grade 1 and 2 tumors are more likely to respond to tamoxifen than grade 3 tumors (69).

Short-term administration of tamoxifen can cause an increase in the progesterone receptor levels in postmenopausal women with EC cancer (70,71). Studies with alternating tamoxifen and progestins have been performed to determine if this upregulation increases the response to progestin therapy. Phase II trials of tamoxifen plus alternating cycles of progestin demonstrated a 27–33% response rate (72,73). The Eastern Cooperative Oncology Group found no difference in response rates between patients treated with progestin alone and those treated with progestin in combination with tamoxifen (74).

Second- and third-generation SERMs, such as raloxifene and arzoxifene, have more selective estrogen antagonism in the uterus. The third-generation agent arzoxifene has enhanced bioavailability and potent estrogen antagonist activity in the uterus. Arzoxifene is 30–100 times more potent than raloxifene in antagonizing the effects of estrogen in the uterus (75). In a phase II GOG study, the response rate in patients with advanced or recurrent EC was 31% (9 of 29) with one complete response and 8 partial responses (76). All patients in this study had tumors that were either ER or PR positive or were low grade. These findings suggest that SERMS are an effective alternative to progestins.

Other Hormonal Agents

Anastrozole, an oral nonsteroidal aromatase inhibitor, is approved by the FDA for postmenopausal women with progressive breast cancer following tamoxifen therapy. Aromatase is elevated in the stroma of EC (77). In a phase II trial by the GOG, anastrozole was found to have minimal activity (9% response rate) in an unselected population of patients with advanced or recurrent EC (78). Over 25% of the patients in this study had non-endometrioid histologic subtypes and only 22% of the patients had ER- and PR-positive tumors or demonstrated a response to prior therapy. In the subset of women with FIGO grade 1 and 2 tumors with endometrioid histology, the response rate was 30%.

Danazol is a synthetic steroid with mixed agonist-antagonist activity on androgen, glucocorticoid, and progesterone receptors. Danazol is effective in converting endometrial hyperplasia to atrophic endometrium (79,80). In a phase II GOG study evaluating 22 patients with advanced, recurrent, or persistent EC with 400 mg/day of danazol, none of the patients demonstrated a response (81).

Because gonadotropin-releasing hormone receptors are present in approximately one-third of EC (82), the use of gonadotropin-releasing hormone agonists (leuprolide, goserelin, and triptorelin) has been investigated in EC. In phase II studies, a response was seen in 0–13% of patients (83–87).

Adjuvant Hormonal Therapy

Several studies have been performed evaluating the use of progestins as an adjuvant therapy for patients with EC. In trials that have recruited over 2500 patients (56,88–90), no difference in survival was demonstrated. A meta-analysis of randomized trials of progestins as an adjuvant therapy for patients with early stage EC failed to demonstrate any decrease in EC-related deaths (91). These earlier trials, however, were limited by including patients with low-risk prognostic features or by including only stage I patients. Recently, a large prospective randomized trial evaluated adjuvant progestin therapy in patients who were at high risk for recurrence (92). The study enrolled 1012 patients with grade 3 tumors, tumors with high-risk histologic subtypes, or tumors with greater than one-third myometrial invasion. There was a significant decrease in recurrences among the progestin-treated patients. There was, however, no difference in survival. The 5-year survival in the progestin-treated arm was 75% and 72% in the control arm. The use of progestins in the adjuvant treatment of EC is currently not standard.

Similar to progestins, there is no benefit from tamoxifen as an adjuvant therapy after primary surgery (93).

Fertility Preservation

Premenopausal women with well-differentiated, clinical stage
I EC may be given a trial of progestins alone in order to preserve their childbearing potential. Over 70% of patients with
who opt for conservative therapy respond to progestins and
many of these women are able to conceive and carry normal
pregnancies (94). Because the predisposing conditions that
led to developing the cancer (i.e., obesity, hypertension, diabetes) are usually still present after childbearing, a hysterectomy in these patients may be indicated once preservation of
fertility is no longer desired.

UTERINE PAPILLARY SEROUS CARCINOMA (UPSC)

Clinical, pathologic, and molecular features of UPSC differ
from typical EEC. Therefore, when evaluating treatment
options, patients with UPSC should be distinguished from
patients with other types of EC. UPSC comprises less than
10% of EC, but accounts for over 50% of deaths or recurrences
from this disease. Few effective therapies are available for
patients with this disease. This disease is histologically similar to serous carcinoma of the ovary, and is characterized by
distant metastasis and a high mortality rate, even in the setting of minimal uterine disease (95). Unlike endometrioid
endometrial adenocarcinoma, pathologic criteria cannot predict which patients are likely to recur. Chemotherapy is currently used for patients with advanced disease. The role of
adjuvant chemotherapy has yet to be determined. UPSC
rarely demonstrate ER or PR positivity (96), and these
tumors do not respond to hormonal therapy (97).

Chemotherapy for Advanced and Recurrent UPSC

The majority of information available for patients with UPSC
is from retrospective, nonrandomized case series. In addition,
response rates to therapy often come from subset analysis of
studies of all types of advanced or recurrent EC. Fitzgerald
and Rosenthal reported the first response to chemotherapy in

Table 2 Chemotherapy Trials for Patients with UPSC

Author (Year Published) (Ref.)	Adjuvant, Advanced, or Recurrent	Chemotherapy	N	RR (%)			Follow-up
				CR	PR	TR	
Price (1993) (100)	adjuvant	CAP	19				OS: 31 mo
	recurrent	CAP	11	13	13	27	OS: 21 mo
Levenback (1992) (99)	advanced or recurrent	CAP	11	18	0	18	5YS: 23%[a]
Hoskins (2001) (28)	advanced	CP	15	20	40	60	OS: 26 mo
	recurrent	CP	4	25	25	50	
Zanotti (1999) (101)	adjuvant	CP	9	78	11	89	PFI: 30 mo
	advanced	CP	9	36	27	64	PFI: 13 mo.
	recurrent	CP	11				PFI: 9 mo
Ramondetta (2001) (102)	adjuvant	paclitaxel	5				R: 60%; MTR: 7.2 mo
	recurrent	paclitaxel	13	31	46	77	PFI: 7.3 mo

[a]Includes 6 patients treated in the adjuvant setting.
CAP = cyclophosphamide, doxorubicin, cisplatin; CP = carboplatin (or cisplatin) and paclitaxel; N = number of patients; RR = Response rate; CR = complete response; PR = partial response; TR = total response; OS = overall survival; 5YS = 5-year survival; PFI = progression-free interval; R = % recurrence; MTR = median time to recurrence.

a patient with UPSC in 1985 (98). This patient was treated with cyclophosphamide, doxorubicin, and cisplatin (CAP). Levenback et al. reported 20 patients with recurrent or advanced UPSC treated with CAP (99). Fifty-eight percent of the patients were alive without disease after 24 months. However, this regimen was highly toxic. Price et al. also evaluated CAP in 19 patients with advanced disease and 11 patients with recurrent disease (100). Of the patients treated in the adjuvant setting for advanced disease, 58% were alive without evidence of disease with a median follow-up of 24 months. In the patients with recurrent disease, the response rate was 27%. In addition, all of the patients developed treatment-related toxicities. Most of these toxicities were hematological. One treatment-related death was from cardiotoxicity.

Recently, more favorable results using paclitaxel with and without carboplatin have been demonstrated. In a phase II study evaluating carboplatin and paclitaxel, the response rate was 60% in 20 patients with high stage UPSC (28). The failure-free survival time was 18 months and the 3-year overall survival was 39%. Two of four patients with recurrent UPSC demonstrated a response to carboplatin and paclitaxel. Zanotti et al. evaluated 24 patients with measurable disease (either progressive disease after initial surgery or recurrent disease) (101). There was an 89% response rate in patients treated after initial surgery, and a 64% response rate for patients with recurrent disease. At M.D. Anderson, single agent paclitaxel demonstrated a 77% response rate in patients with recurrent disease (102). Despite this activity, the duration of response in these studies is less than 1 year (101,102). Other agents are under investigation for the treatment of UPSC. In a pilot study, topotecan has shown activity against UPSC (103).

Adjuvant Therapy for UPSC

Over the last few years, several academic centers have tried to determine the best treatment for patients with early stage UPSC. Even with minimal uterine disease limited to the uterus, patients with UPSC often have recurrent disease.

Unlike the more common EEC, no prognostic features exist which would help identify which patients may benefit from adjuvant therapy. At this time, the use of chemotherapy in the adjuvant setting for patients with UPSC and with disease confined to the endometrium is investigational.

Combined chemotherapy and radiation therapy may play a role in the management of patients with early stage disease. Turner et al. reported the application of vaginal radiation at a high-dose rate in combination with chemotherapy in surgical stage I patients (104). The 5-year survival rate was 94%, which is higher than most other studies for patients with stage I disease. At M.D. Anderson Cancer Center, whole pelvic radiation therapy in combination with paclitaxel for the treatment of patients with early stage UPSC is currently being investigated.

MOLECULAR THERAPIES

Molecular characterization of EC may lead to the discovery of novel therapeutic agents. Increased understanding of the intracellular molecular pathways involved in cell function and proliferation may be accompanied by the development of novel therapeutic strategies. The identification of novel targets in malignant tumors has led to the development of inhibitors for the treatment of a wide range of cancers. Since the rapid approval of Gleevec® (imatinib mesylate) for the treatment of chronic myelogenous leukemia and gastrointestinal stromal tumors, the rationale for targeting dysregulated pathways has led to the development and testing of several targeted agents. The challenges of developing rational targets for therapeutic intervention in specific solid tumors remain an area of intense research.

The epidermal growth factor receptor (EGFR) has been implicated in cancer development. EGFR has been shown to be overexpressed in EC, where it is associated with a worse prognosis (105,106). Blockade of this receptor in patients with persistent or recurrent EC is currently being studied in a phase II GOG study. In addition, a subset of patients with EC overexpresses HER-2/neu (106–108). In breast cancer, blockade of this receptor with trastuzumab (Herceptin®) has been shown to be effective in patients who overexpress HER-2/neu by immunohistochemistry or who have amplification of this gene (109). The GOG is currently evaluating trastuzumab for the treatment of recurrent or advanced EC in patients with HER-2/neu overexpression. At M.D. Anderson, we recently evaluated the expression of Gleevec-targeted kinases (abl, c-Kit, PDGFR) in primary and recurrent UPSC. In this study, we found that over 80% of these tumors express at least one of these kinases (110). Based on these data, a clinical trial evaluating paclitaxel in combination with imatinib mesylate is underway.

SUMMARY

Treatment options for advanced and recurrent EC are limited. Because of the propensity for distant spread, systemic agents are necessary. Combination cytotoxic therapy with platinum-based therapy offers a survival advantage in patients with advanced or recurrent disease. In addition, hormonal agents have a clear role in the management of these patients. Because patients with metastatic or recurrent disease make up a small subset of all women with EC, multi-centered, collaborative studies are needed to better evaluate therapeutic options. Since clinical, pathologic, and molecular features of UPSC differ from typical EEC, patients with UPSC should be distinguished from patients with other types of EC in clinical trials. Given the aggressiveness of UPSC, even in the early stages, multi-center efforts to develop effective therapies are necessary. Finally, with continued understanding of the molecular pathogenesis of EC, novel, biologic therapeutic agents may provide more effective treatment options.

REFERENCES

1. Thigpen JT, Buchsbaum HJ, Mangan C, Blessing JA. Phase II trial of adriamycin in the treatment of advanced or recurrent endometrial carcinoma: a Gynecologic Oncology Group study. *Cancer Treat Rep* 1979; 63(1):21–27.

2. Horton J, Begg CB, Arseneault J, Bruckner H, Creech R, Hahn RG. Comparison of adriamycin with cyclophosphamide in patients with advanced endometrial cancer. *Cancer Treat Rep* 1978; 62(1):159–161.

3. Thigpen JT, Blessing JA, DiSaia PJ, Yordan E, Carson LF, Evers C. A randomized comparison of doxorubicin alone versus doxorubicin plus cyclophosphamide in the management of advanced or recurrent endometrial carcinoma: A Gynecologic Oncology Group study. *J Clin Oncol* 1994; 12(7):1408–1414.

4. Thigpen JT, Blessing JA, Homesley H, Creasman WT, Sutton G. Phase II trial of cisplatin as first-line chemotherapy in patients with advanced or recurrent endometrial carcinoma: a Gynecologic Oncology Group Study. *Gynecol Oncol* 1989; 33(1):68–70.

5. Seski JC, Edwards CL, Herson J, Rutledge FN. Cisplatin chemotherapy for disseminated endometrial cancer. *Obstet Gynecol* 1982; 59(2):225–228.

6. Edmonson JH, Krook JE, Hilton JF, Malkasian GD, Everson LK, Jefferies JA, Mailliard JA. Randomized phase II studies of cisplatin and a combination of cyclophosphamide-doxorubicin-cisplatin (CAP) in patients with progestin-refractory advanced endometrial carcinoma. *Gynecol Oncol* 1987; 28(1):20–24.

7. Barrett RJ, Blessing JA, Homesley HD, Twiggs L, Webster KD. Circadian-timed combination doxorubicin-cisplatin chemotherapy for advanced endometrial carcinoma. A phase II study of the Gynecologic Oncology Group. *Am J Clin Oncol* 1993; 16(6):494–496.

8. Trope C, Johnsson JE, Simonsen E, Christiansen H, Cavallin-Stahl E, Horvath G. Treatment of recurrent endometrial adenocarcinoma with a combination of doxorubicin and cisplatin. *Am J Obstet Gynecol* 1984; 149(4):379–381.

9. Pasmantier MW, Coleman M, Silver RT, Mamaril AP, Quiguyan CC, Galindo A, Jr, Treatment of advanced endometrial carcinoma with doxorubicin and cisplatin: effects on both untreated and previously treated patients. *Cancer Treat Rep* 1985; 69(5):539–542.

10. Thigpen JT, Blessing J, Homesley H, Malfetano J, DiSaia P, Yordan E. Phase III trial of doxorubicin +/- cisplatin in

advanced or recurrent endometrial carcinoma: a Gynecologic Oncology Group (GOG) study. *Proc Am Soc Clin Oncol* 1993; 12:261.

11. Aapro MS, Van Wijk FH, Bolis G, Chevallier B, Van Der Burg ME, Poveda A, De Oliveira CF, Tumolo S, Scotto Di Palumbo V, Piccart M, Franchi M, Zanaboni F, Lacave AJ, Fontanelli R, Favalli G, Zola P, Guastalla JP, Rosso R, Marth C, Nooij M, Presti M, Scarabelli C, Splinter TA, Ploch E, Beex LV, Ten Bokkel Huinink W, Forni M, Melpignano M, Blake P, Kerbrat P, Mendiola C, Cervantes A, Goupil A, Harper PG, Madronal C, Namer M, Scarfone G, Stoot JE, Teodorovic I, Coens C, Vergote I, Vermorken JB. Doxorubicin versus doxorubicin and cisplatin in endometrial carcinoma: definitive results of a randomised study (55872) by the EORTC Gynaecological Cancer Group. *Ann Oncol* 2003; 14(3):441–448.

12. Burke TW, Stringer CA, Morris M, Freedman RS, Gershenson DM, Kavanagh JJ, Edwards CL. Prospective treatment of advanced or recurrent endometrial carcinoma with cisplatin, doxorubicin, and cyclophosphamide. *Gynecol Oncol* 1991; 40(3):264–267.

13. Turbow MM, Ballon SC, Sikic BI, Koretz MM. Cisplatin, doxorubicin, and cyclophosphamide chemotherapy for advanced endometrial carcinoma. *Cancer Treat Rep* 1985; 69(5):465–467.

14. Dunton CJ, Pfeifer SM, Braitman LE, Morgan MA, Carlson JA, Mikuta JJ. Treatment of advanced and recurrent endometrial cancer with cisplatin, doxorubicin, and cyclophosphamide. *Gynecol Oncol* 1991; 41(2):113–116.

15. Ball HG, Blessing JA, Lentz SS, Mutch DG. A phase II trial of paclitaxel in patients with advanced or recurrent adenocarcinoma of the endometrium: a Gynecologic Oncology Group study. *Gynecol Oncol* 1996; 62(2):278–281.

16. Lissoni A, Zanetta G, Losa G, Gabriele A, Parma G, Mangioni C. Phase II study of paclitaxel as salvage treatment in advanced endometrial cancer. *Ann Oncol* 1996; 7(8):861–863.

17. Markman M, Fowler J. Activity of weekly paclitaxel in patients with advanced endometrial cancer previously treated with both a platinum agent and paclitaxel. *Gynecol Oncol* 2004; in press.

18. Lincoln S, Blessing JA, Lee RB, Rocereto TF. Activity of paclitaxel as second-line chemotherapy in endometrial carcinoma: a Gynecologic Oncology Group study. *Gynecol Oncol* 2003; 88(3):277–281.

19. Woo HL, Swenerton KD, Hoskins PJ. Taxol is active in platinum-resistant endometrial adenocarcinoma. *Am J Clin Oncol* 1996; 19(3):290–291.

20. Dimopoulos MA, Papadimitriou CA, Georgoulias V, Moulopoulos LA, Aravantinos G, Gika D, Karpathios S, Stamatelopoulos S. Paclitaxel and cisplatin in advanced or recurrent carcinoma of the endometrium: long-term results of a phase II multicenter study. *Gynecol Oncol* 2000; 78(1):52–57.

21. Fleming GF, Brunetto V, Bentley R, Rader J, Clarke-Pearson D, Sorosky J, Eaton L, Gallion H, Gibbons W. Randomized trial of doxorubicin (Dox) plus cisplatin (Cis) versus Dox plus paclitaxel (Tax) plus granulocyte colony-stimulating factor (G-CSF) in patients with advanced or recurrent endometrial cancer: a report on Gynecologic Oncology Group (GOG) protocol. *Proc Am Soc Clin Oncol* 2000; 1498.

22. Fleming GF, Brunetto V, Mundt AJ, Burks RT, Look KY, Reid G. Randomized trial of doxorubicin (DOX) plus cisplatin (CIS) versus DOX plus CIS plus paclitaxel (TAX) in patients with advanced or recurrent endometrial carcinoma: a Gynecologic Oncology Group (GOG) study. *Proc Am Soc Clin Oncol* 2002; 807.

23. Long HJ, Pfeifle DM, Wieand HS, Krook JE, Edmonson JH, Buckner JC. Phase II evaluation of carboplatin in advanced endometrial carcinoma. *J Natl Cancer Inst* 1988; 80(4):276–278.

24. Green JB,III, Green S, Alberts DS, O'Toole R, Surwit EA, Noltimier JW. Carboplatin therapy in advanced endometrial cancer. *Obstet Gynecol* 1990; 75(4):696–700.

25. Burke TW, Munkarah A, Kavanagh JJ, Morris M, Levenback C, Tornos C, Gershenson DM. Treatment of advanced or recurrent endometrial carcinoma with single-agent carboplatin. *Gynecol Oncol* 1993; 51(3):397–400.

26. Pinelli DM, Fiorica JV, Roberts WS, Hoffman MS, Nicosia SV, Cavanagh D. Chemotherapy plus sequential hormonal ther-

apy for advanced and recurrent endometrial carcinoma: a phase II study. *Gynecol Oncol* 1996; 60(3):462–467.

27. van Wijk FH, Lhomme C, Bolis G, Scotto di Palumbo V, Tumolo S, Nooij M, de Oliveira CF, Vermorken JB. Phase II study of carboplatin in patients with advanced or recurrent endometrial carcinoma. A trial of the EORTC Gynaecological Cancer Group. *Eur J Cancer* 2003; 39(1):78–85.

28. Hoskins PJ, Swenerton KD, Pike JA, Wong F, Lim P, Acquino-Parsons C, Lee N. Paclitaxel and carboplatin, alone or with irradiation, in advanced or recurrent endometrial cancer: a phase II study. *J Clin Oncol* 2001; 19(20):4048–4053.

29. Miller DS, Blessing JA, Lentz SS, Waggoner SE. A phase II trial of topotecan in patients with advanced, persistent, or recurrent endometrial carcinoma: a gynecologic oncology group study. *Gynecol Oncol* 2002; 87(3):247–251.

30. Wadler S, Levy DE, Lincoln ST, Soori GS, Schink JC, Goldberg G. Topotecan is an active agent in the first-line treatment of metastatic or recurrent endometrial carcinoma: Eastern Cooperative Oncology Group Study E3E93. *J Clin Oncol* 2003; 21(11):2110–2114.

31. Hall J, Higgins R, Naumann R, Groblewski M. Phase II study of topotecan and cisplatinum stages III and IV or for recurrent endometrial cancer. *Proc Am Soc Clin Oncol* 2000; 1622.

32. Escobar PF, Markman M, Zanotti K, Webster K, Belinson J. Phase 2 trial of pegylated liposomal doxorubicin in advanced endometrial cancer. *J Cancer Res Clin Oncol* 2003; 129(11):651–654.

33. Muggia FM, Blessing JA, Sorosky J, Reid GC. Phase II trial of the pegylated liposomal doxorubicin in previously treated metastatic endometrial cancer: a Gynecologic Oncology Group study. *J Clin Oncol* 2002; 20(9):2360–2364.

34. Sutton GP, Blessing JA, DeMars LR, Moore D, Burke TW, Grendys EC. A phase II Gynecologic Oncology Group trial of ifosfamide and mesna in advanced or recurrent adenocarcinoma of the endometrium. *Gynecol Oncol* 1996; 63(1):25–27.

35. Pawinski A, Tumolo S, Hoesel G, Cervantes A, van Oosterom AT, Boes GH, Pecorelli S. Cyclophosphamide or ifosfamide in patients with advanced and/or recurrent endometrial carci-

noma: a randomized phase II study of the EORTC Gynecological Cancer Cooperative Group. *Eur J Obstet Gynecol Reprod Biol* 1999; 86(2):179–183.

36. Carbone PP, Carter SK. Endometrial cancer: approach to development of effective chemotherapy. *Gynecol Oncol* 1974; 2(2–3):348–353.

37. Cohen CJ, Deppe G, Bruckner HW. Treatment of advanced adenocarcinoma of the endometrium with melphalan, 5-fluorouracil, and medroxyprogesterone acetate: a preliminary study. *Obstet Gynecol* 1977; 50(4):415–417.

38. Piver MS, Lele SB, Patsner B, Emrich LJ. Melphalan, 5-fluorouracil, and medroxyprogesterone acetate in metastatic endometrial carcinoma. *Obstet Gynecol* 1986; 67(2):261–264.

39. Cornelison TL, Baker TR, Piver MS, Driscoll DL. Cisplatin, adriamycin, etoposide, megestrol acetate versus melphalan, 5-fluorouracil, medroxyprogesterone acetate in the treatment of endometrial carcinoma. *Gynecol Oncol* 1995; 59(2):243–248.

40. Poplin EA, Liu PY, Delmore JE, Wilczynski S, Moore DF, Jr., Potkul RK, Fine BA, Hannigan EV, Alberts DS. Phase II trial of oral etoposide in recurrent or refractory endometrial adenocarcinoma: a southwest oncology group study. *Gynecol Oncol* 1999; 74(3):432–435.

41. Rose PG, Blessing JA, Lewandowski GS, Creasman WT, Webster KD. A phase II trial of prolonged oral etoposide (VP-16) as second-line therapy for advanced and recurrent endometrial carcinoma: a Gynecologic Oncology Group study. *Gynecol Oncol* 1996; 63(1):101–104.

42. Markman M, Kennedy A, Webster K, Kulp B, Peterson G, Belinson J. Persistent chemosensitivity to platinum and/or paclitaxel in metastatic endometrial cancer. *Gynecol Oncol* 1999; 73(3):422–423.

43. Aalders J, Abeler V, Kolstad P, Onsrud M. Postoperative external irradiation and prognostic parameters in stage I endometrial carcinoma: clinical and histopathologic study of 540 patients. *Obstet Gynecol* 1980; 56(4):419–427.

44. Greven KM, Randall M, Fanning J, Bahktar M, Duray P, Peters A, Curran WJ, Jr. Patterns of failure in patients with

stage I, grade 3 carcinoma of the endometrium. *Int J Radiat Oncol Biol Phys* 1990; 19(3):529–534.

45. Mayr NA, Wen BC, Benda JA, Sorosky JI, Davis CS, Fuller RW, Hussey DH. Postoperative radiation therapy in clinical stage I endometrial cancer: corpus, cervical, and lower uterine segment involvement—patterns of failure. *Radiology* 1995; 196(2):323–328.

46. Lanciano RM, Greven KM. Adjuvant treatment for endometrial cancer: who needs it? *Gynecol Oncol* 1995; 57(2):135–137.

47. Calais G, Descamps P, Vitu L, Reynaud-Bougnoux A, Bougnoux P, Lansac J, Le Floch O. Lymphadenectomy in the management of endometrial carcinoma stage I and II. Retrospective study of 155 cases. *Clin Oncol (R Coll Radiol)* 1990; 2(6):318–323.

48. Grigsby PW, Perez CA, Camel HM, Kao MS, Galakatos AE. Stage II carcinoma of the endometrium: results of therapy and prognostic factors. *Int J Radiat Oncol Biol Phys* 1985; 11(11):1915–1923.

49. Greven KM, Lanciano RM, Corn B, Case D, Randall ME. Pathologic stage III endometrial carcinoma. Prognostic factors and patterns of recurrence. *Cancer* 1993; 71(11):3697–3702.

50. Mackillop WJ, Pringle JF. Stage III endometrial carcinoma. A review of 90 cases. *Cancer* 1985; 56(10):2519–2523.

51. Grigsby PW, Perez CA, Kuske RR, Kao MS, Galakatos AE. Results of therapy, analysis of failures, and prognostic factors for clinical and pathologic stage III adenocarcinoma of the endometrium. *Gynecol Oncol* 1987; 27(1):44–57.

52. Morrow CP, Bundy BN, Homesley HD, Creasman WT, Hornback NB, Kurman R, Thigpen JT. Doxorubicin as an adjuvant following surgery and radiation therapy in patients with high-risk endometrial carcinoma, stage I and occult stage II: a Gynecologic Oncology Group Study. *Gynecol Oncol* 1990; 36(2):166–171.

53. Burke TW, Gershenson DM, Morris M, Stringer CA, Levenback C, Tortolero-Luna G, Baker VV. Postoperative adjuvant cisplatin, doxorubicin, and cyclophosphamide (PAC) chemotherapy in women with high-risk endometrial carcinoma. *Gynecol Oncol* 1994; 55(1):47–50.

54. Reisinger SA, Asbury R, Liao SY, Homesley HD. A phase I study of weekly cisplatin and whole abdominal radiation for the treatment of stage III and IV endometrial carcinoma: a Gynecologic Oncology Group pilot study. *Gynecol Oncol* 1996; 63(3):299–303.

55. Sood BM, Timmins PF, Gorla GR, Garg M, Anderson PS, Vikram B, Goldberg GL. Concomitant cisplatin and extended field radiation therapy in patients with cervical and endometrial cancer. *Int J Gynecol Cancer* 2002; 12(5):459–464.

56. Lewis GC Jr, Slack NH, Mortel R, Bross ID. Adjuvant progestogen therapy in the primary definitive treatment of endometrial cancer. *Gynecol Oncol* 1974; 2(2–3):368–376.

57. Kelley RM, Baker WH. Proges in the treatment of carcinoma of the endometrium. *N Engl J Med* 1961; 216-222

58. Kauppila A. Progestin therapy of endometrial, breast and ovarian carcinoma. A review of clinical observations. *Acta Obstet Gynecol Scand* 1984; 63(5):441–450.

59. Moore TD, Phillips PH, Nerenstone SR, Cheson BD. Systemic treatment of advanced and recurrent endometrial carcinoma: current status and future directions. *J Clin Oncol* 1991; 9(6):1071–1088.

60. Podratz KC, O'Brien PC, Malkasian GD, Jr., Decker DG, Jefferies JA, Edmonson JH. Effects of progestational agents in treatment of endometrial carcinoma. *Obstet Gynecol* 1985; 66(1):106–110.

61. Thigpen JT, Blessing J, DiSaia P. Oral medroxyprogesterone acetate in advanced or recurrent endometrial carcinoma: results of therapy and correlation with estrogen and progesterone levels. The gynecology oncology experience. In: Banlieu EE, Slacobelli S, McGuire WL; eds. *Endocrinology of Malignancy*. Park Ridge, NJ: Parthenon 1986;p.446.

62. Lentz SS, Brady MF, Major FJ, Reid GC, Soper JT. High-dose megestrol acetate in advanced or recurrent endometrial carcinoma: a Gynecologic Oncology Group Study. *J Clin Oncol* 1996; 14(2):357–361.

63. Piver MS, Barlow JJ, Lurain JR, Blumenson LE. Medroxyprogesterone acetate (Depo-Provera) vs. hydroxyprog-

esterone caproate (Delalutin) in women with metastatic endometrial adenocarcinoma. *Cancer* 1980; 45(2):268–272.

64. Muss HB, Case LD, Capizzi RL, Cooper MR, Cruz J, Jackson D, Richards F, II, Powell BL, Spurr CL, White D, et al. High- versus standard-dose megestrol acetate in women with advanced breast cancer: a phase III trial of the Piedmont Oncology *Assoc J Clin Oncol* 1990; 8(11):1797–1805.

65. Thigpen JT, Brady MF, Alvarez RD, Adelson MD, Homesley HD, Manetta A, Soper JT, Given FT. Oral medroxyprogesterone acetate in the treatment of advanced or recurrent endometrial carcinoma: a dose-response study by the Gynecologic Oncology Group. *J Clin Oncol* 1999; 17(6):1736–1744.

66. Quinn MA, Cauchi M, Fortune D. Endometrial carcinoma: steroid receptors and response to medroxyprogesterone acetate. *Gynecol Oncol* 1985; 21(3):314–319.

67. Rendina GM, Donadio C, Fabri M, Mazzoni P, Nazzicone P. Tamoxifen and medroxyprogesterone therapy for advanced endometrial carcinoma. *Eur J Obstet Gynecol Reprod Biol* 1984; 17(4):285–291.

68. Quinn MA, Campbell JJ. Tamoxifen therapy in advanced/recurrent endometrial carcinoma. *Gynecol Oncol* 1989; 32(1):1–3.

69. Thigpen T, Brady MF, Homesley HD, Soper JT, Bell J. Tamoxifen in the treatment of advanced or recurrent endome- trial carcinoma: a Gynecologic Oncology Group study. *J Clin Oncol* 2001; 19(2):364–367.

70. Mortel R, Levy C, Wolff JP, Nicolas JC, Robel P, Baulieu EE. Female sex steroid receptors in postmenopausal endometrial carcinoma and biochemical response to an antiestrogen. *Cancer Res* 1981; 41(3):1140–1147.

71. Carlson JA Jr, Allegra JC, Day TG Jr, Wittliff JL. Tamoxifen and endometrial carcinoma: alterations in estrogen and prog- esterone receptors in untreated patients and combination hor- monal therapy in advanced neoplasia. *Am J Obstet Gynecol* 1984; 149(2):149–153.

72. Fiorica JV, Brunetto V, Hanjani P, Lentz S, Mannel R, Anderson W. A phase II study (GOG 153) of recurrent and advanced endometrial carcinoma treated with alternating

courses of megesterol acetate and tamoxifen citrate. *Proc Am Soc Clin Oncol* 2000; 1499.

73. Whitney CW, Brunetto VL, Zaino RJ, Lentz SS, Sorosky J, Armstrong DK, Lee RB. Phase II study of medroxyprogesterone acetate plus tamoxifen in advanced endometrial carcinoma: a Gynecologic Oncology Group study. *Gynecol Oncol* 2004; in press.

74. Pandya KJ, Yeap BY, Weiner LM, Krook JE, Erban JK, Schinella RA, Davis TE. Megestrol and tamoxifen in patients with advanced endometrial cancer: an Eastern Cooperative Oncology Group Study (E4882). *Am J Clin Oncol* 2001; 24(1):43–46.

75. Sato M, Turner CH, Wang T, Adrian MD, Rowley E, Bryant HU. LY353381.HCl: a novel raloxifene analog with improved SERM potency and efficacy in vivo. *J Pharmacol Exp Ther* 1998; 287(1):1–7.

76. McMeekin DS, Gordon A, Fowler J, Melemed A, Buller R, Burke T, Bloss J, Sabbatini P. A phase II trial of arzoxifene, a selective estrogen response modulator, in patients with recurrent or advanced endometrial cancer. *Gynecol Oncol* 2003; 90(1):64–69.

77. Watanabe K, Sasano H, Harada N, Ozaki M, Niikura H, Sato S, Yajima A. Aromatase in human endometrial carcinoma and hyperplasia. Immunohistochemical, in situ hybridization, and biochemical studies. *Am J Pathol* 1995; 146(2):491–500.

78. Rose PG, Brunetto VL, Van Le L, Bell J, Walker JL, Lee RB. A phase II trial of anastrozole in advanced recurrent or persistent endometrial carcinoma: a Gynecologic Oncology Group study. *Gynecol Oncol* 2000; 78(2):212–216.

79. Soh E, Sato K. Clinical effects of danazol on endometrial hyperplasia in menopausal and postmenopausal women. *Cancer* 1990; 66(5):983–988.

80. Grio R, Piacentino R, Marchino GL, Bocci A, Navone R. Danazol in the treatment of endometrial hyperplasia. *Panminerva Med* 1993; 35(4):231–233.

81. Covens A, Brunetto VL, Markman M, Orr JW, Lentz SS, Benda J. Phase II trial of danazol in advanced, recurrent, or persist-

ent endometrial cancer: a Gynecologic Oncology Group study. *Gynecol Oncol* 2003; 89(3):470–474.

82. Imai A, Ohno T, Iida K, Fuseya T, Furui T, Tamaya T. Presence of gonadotropin-releasing hormone receptor and its messenger ribonucleic acid in endometrial carcinoma and endometrium. *Gynecol Oncol* 1994; 55(1):144–148.

83. Covens A, Thomas G, Shaw P, Ackerman I, Osborne R, Lukka H, Carey M, Franssen E, Roche K. A phase II study of leupro-lide in advanced/recurrent endometrial cancer. *Gynecol Oncol* 1997; 64(1):126–129.

84. Jeyarajah AR, Gallagher CJ, Blake PR, Oram DH, Dowsett M, Fisher C, Oliver RT. Long-term follow-up of gonadotrophin-releasing hormone analog treatment for recurrent endometrial cancer. *Gynecol Oncol* 1996; 63(1):47–52.

85. Markman M, Kennedy A, Webster K, Peterson G, Kulp B, Belinson J. Leuprolide in the treatment of endometrial cancer. *Gynecol Oncol* 1997; 66(3):542.

86. Lhomme C, Vennin P, Callet N, Lesimple T, Achard JL, Chauvergne J, Luporsi E, Chinet-Charrot P, Coudert B, Couette JE, Guastalla JP, Lebrun D, Ispas S, Blumberg J. A multicenter phase II study with triptorelin (sustained-release LHRH agonist) in advanced or recurrent endometrial carci-noma: a French anticancer federation study. *Gynecol Oncol* 1999; 75(2):187–193.

87. Asbury RF, Brunetto VL, Lee RB, Reid G, Rocereto TF. Goserelin acetate as treatment for recurrent endometrial car-cinoma: a Gynecologic Oncology Group study. *Am J Clin Oncol* 2002; 25(6):557–560.

88. Macdonald RR, Thorogood J, Mason MK. A randomized trial of progestogens in the primary treatment of endometrial carci-noma. *Br J Obstet Gynaecol* 1988; 95(2):166–174.

89. Vergote I, Kjorstad K, Abeler V, Kolstad P. A randomized trial of adjuvant progestagen in early endometrial cancer. *Cancer* 1989; 64(5):1011–1016.

90. Burke TW, Wolfson AH. Limited endometrial carcinoma: adju-vant therapy. *Semin Oncol* 1994; 21(1):84–90.

91. Martin-Hirsch PL, Lilford RJ, Jarvis GJ. Adjuvant progesta-gen therapy for the treatment of endometrial cancer: review and meta-analyses of published randomised controlled trials. *Eur J Obstet Gynecol Reprod Biol* 1996; 65(2):201–207.

92. COSA-NZ-UK Endometrial Cancer Study Groups. Adjuvant medroxyprogesterone acetate in high-risk endometrial cancer. *Int J Gynecol Cancer* 1998; 8:387–391.

93. von Minckwitz G, Loibl S, Brunnert K, Kreienberg R, Melchert F, Mosch R, Neises M, Schermann J, Seufert R, Stiglmayer R, Stosiek U, Kaufmann M. Adjuvant endocrine treatment with medroxyprogesterone acetate or tamoxifen in stage I and II endometrial cancer—a multicentre, open, controlled, prospec-tively randomised trial. *Eur J Cancer* 2002; 38(17):2265–2271.

94. Gotlieb WH, Beiner ME, Shalmon B, Korach Y, Segal Y, Zmira N, Koupolovic J, Ben-Baruch G. Outcome of fertility-sparing treatment with progestins in young patients with endometrial cancer. *Obstet Gynecol* 2003; 102(4):718–725.

95. Slomovitz BM, Burke TW, Eifel PJ, Ramondetta LM, Silva EG, Jhingran A, Oh JC, Atkinson EN, Broaddus RR, Gershenson DM, Lu KH. Uterine papillary serous carcinoma (UPSC): a single institution review of 129 cases. *Gynecol Oncol* 2003; 91:463–469.

96. Umpierre SA, Burke TW, Tornos C, Ordonez N, Levenback C, Morris M. Immunocytochemical analysis of uterine papillary serous carcinomas for estrogen and progesterone receptors. *Int J Gynecol Pathol* 1994; 13(2):127–130.

97. Carcangiu ML, Chambers JT, Voynick IM, Pirro M, Schwartz PE. Immunohistochemical evaluation of estrogen and proges-terone receptor content in 183 patients with endometrial car-cinoma. Part I: Clinical and histologic correlations. *Am J Clin Pathol* 1990; 94(3):247–254.

98. Fitzgerald D, Rosenthal S. Uterine papillary serous carci-noma. Complete response to combination chemotherapy. *Cancer* 1985; 56(5):1023–1024.

99. Levenback C, Burke TW, Silva E, Morris M, Gershenson DM, Kavanagh JJ, Wharton JT. Uterine papillary serous carcinoma (UPSC) treated with cisplatin, doxorubicin, and cyclophos-phamide (PAC). *Gynecol Oncol* 1992; 46(3):317–321.

100. Price FV, Chambers SK, Carcangiu ML, Kohorn EI, Schwartz PE, Chambers JT. Intravenous cisplatin, doxorubicin, and cyclophosphamide in the treatment of uterine papillary serous carcinoma (UPSC). *Gynecol Oncol* 1993; 51(3):383–389.

101. Zanotti KM, Belinson JL, Kennedy AW, Webster KD, Markman M. The use of paclitaxel and platinum-based chemotherapy in uterine papillary serous carcinoma. *Gynecol Oncol* 1999; 74(2):272–277.

102. Ramondetta L, Burke TW, Levenback C, Bevers M, Bodurka-Bevers D, Gershenson DM. Treatment of uterine papillary serous carcinoma with paclitaxel. *Gynecol Oncol* 2001; 82(1):156–161.

103. Chambers JT, Rutherford TJ, Schwartz PE, Carcangiu SK. A pilot study of topotecan for the treatment of serous endometrial cancer. *Proc Am Soc Clin Oncol* 2001; 872.

104. Turner BC, Knisely JP, Kacinski BM, Haffty BG, Gumbs AA, Roberts KB, Frank AH, Peschel RE, Rutherford TJ, Edraki B, Kohorn EI, Chambers SK, Schwartz PE, Wilson LD. Effective treatment of stage I uterine papillary serous carcinoma with high dose-rate vaginal apex radiation (192Ir) and chemotherapy. *Int J Radiat Oncol Biol Phys* 1998; 40(1):77–84.

105. Niikura H, Sasano H, Kaga K, Sato S, Yajima A. Expression of epidermal growth factor family proteins and epidermal growth factor receptor in human endometrium. *Hum Pathol* 1996; 27(3):282–289.

106. Khalifa MA, Mannel RS, Haraway SD, Walker J, Min KW. Expression of EGFR, HER-2/neu, P53, and PCNA in endometrioid, serous papillary, and clear cell endometrial adenocarcinomas. *Gynecol Oncol* 1994; 53(1):84–92.

107. Rolitsky CD, Theil KS, McGaughy VR, Copeland LJ, Niemann TH. HER-2/neu amplification and overexpression in endometrial carcinoma. *Int J Gynecol Pathol* 1999; 18(2):138–143.

108. Berchuck A, Rodriguez G, Kinney RB, Soper JT, Dodge RK, Clarke-Pearson DL, Bast RC Jr. Overexpression of HER-2/neu in endometrial cancer is associated with advanced stage disease. *Am J Obstet Gynecol* 1991; 164(1 Pt 1):15–21.

109. Cobleigh MA, Vogel CL, Tripathy D, Robert NJ, Scholl S, Fehrenbacher L, Wolter JM, Paton V, Shak S, Lieberman G, Slamon DJ. Multinational study of the efficacy and safety of humanized anti-HER2 monoclonal antibody in women who have HER2–overexpressing metastatic breast cancer that has progressed after chemotherapy for metastatic disease. *J Clin Oncol* 1999; 17(9):2639–2648.

110. Slomovitz BM, Broaddus RR, Thornton AD, Oh JC, Celestino J, Schmandt R, Burke TW, Gershenson DM, Lu KH. Gleevec (Imatinib Mesylate) targeted kinases are activated in most endometrial cancers. *Gynecol Oncol* 2003; 88:207.

16

Targeted Therapy of Endometrial Cancer

DAVID O. HOLTZ, RONALD BUCKANOVIC,
AND GEORGE COUKOS

Hospital of the University of Pennsylvania,
Philadelphia, Pennsylvania, U.S.A.

INTRODUCTION

Since the discovery of the c-src oncogene it has been clear that molecular changes involving oncogenes and tumor suppressor genes are critical in tumorigenesis. It has been hypothesized that, at a minimum, 3–8 mutational events are needed to disrupt critical cellular pathways and lead to malignant transformation. Steps felt to be critical to oncogenesis include an increase in growth signals, loss of tumor suppressors, disruption of apoptotic pathways, limitless cell divisions from telomerase reactivation, and altered DNA repair mechanisms. Even then, tumor cells can only form 1–2 mm nodules before being limited by diffusion for oxygen, nutrients, growth factors, and elimination of waste. At this point, further growth requires angiogenesis, the ability to stimulate a new vasculature. In addition, metastatic potential requires the ability to penetrate the basement membrane, grow independent of adhesion, and invade host tissues. Molecular alterations detected in each of these steps contribute to various stages of tumor development and thus offer potential molecular therapeutic targets (1).

To date, therapy for endometrial cancer (EC) is primarily surgical with an 80–90% cure rate. Thus, studies of molecular therapeutics have lagged behind other fields. Unfortunately, the median survival for women with advanced or recurrent EC is less than 1 year, indicating the need for new treatments. A variety of important oncogenic pathways have been identified in EC. Clearly, steroid receptor pathways hold a central position in the process of malignant transformation and offer important targets for therapy. These are described in detail in other chapters; in this chapter, we review other important oncogenic pathways identified in EC and summarize potential molecular targets that have been tested to date.

EPIDERMAL GROWTH FACTOR RECEPTORS

Human cells express a variety of growth factors and their receptors that have a role in cell development and growth. Growth factors are critical in stimulating quiescent (G_0 phase) cells into growth (G_1) and past the restriction point into S phase. Tumor cells often overexpress growth factors and receptors, or express mutant receptors that allow for unregulated growth. Signaling through the epidermal growth factor (EGF) family of tyrosine kinases has been implicated as important in endometrial malignant transformation (2). The epidermal growth factor receptor (EGFR) family, also know as ErbB or HER tyrosine kinases (TK), are typical TK receptors comprised of an extracellular binding domain, a lipophilic transmembrane segment, and a cytoplasmic signaling domain. This EGFR family has four homologous receptors: ErbB1 (HER1), ErbB2 (HER2/neu), ErbB3 (HER3), and ErbB4 (HER4). Upon growth factor binding, the EGF family receptors either homodimerize or heterodimerize depending upon ligand and the density of the various receptors (3). Dimerization leads to receptor phosphorylation and increased tyrosine kinase signaling activity. Overexpression of HER2/neu can result in receptor dimerization in the absence of growth signal leading to constitutive signaling and cellular transformation (4).

EGFR family signaling activates multiple cellular pathways. The Ras-Raf-MAP kinase and Akt/PI-3 kinase pathways, responsible for cell proliferation and survival, are both downstream targets of the EGFR receptor. The EGFR family, particularly HER2/neu, has been clearly associated with oncogenesis in solid tumors. Overexpression of EGFR1 and HER2/neu has been observed in many human cancers, including breast, ovarian, and endometrial (5). Modulation of the tyrosine kinase activity of EGF family receptors should have potent antitumor effects.

Growth factor expression plays a role in endometrial response to hormones. EGFR is expressed in normal cycling endometrium, with increased expression in the proliferative phase (6,7). Estrogen stimulates expression of EGFR in the endometrium of hypogonadal women given estrogen replacement (8). In vivo, estradiol (E2) increases Ishikawa cell production of HER2/neu (9). In mice, however, E2 down-regulates HER2/neu and EGFR mRNA (10). In progesterone-responsive EC, there is an inverse relationship between EGFR content and the extent of progesterone suppression (11).

Several large studies have correlated abnormalities in EGFR and poor prognosis (12–14). Hetzel et al. (13) reported on a cohort of 247 ECs where there was a significant difference in 5-year survival between cancers with negative (95%) and intermediate (83%) HER2/neu staining. In another study, EGFR expression was tested on 60 primary human endometrial tumors; of these, 26 were EGFR-positive with 13 expressing high EGFR levels. High EGFR levels correlated well with poor histopathological grade. The disease-free survival rate was significantly shorter in tumors with high EGFR levels than in tumors with low EGFR levels (15). Niikura et al. (16) found 94 of 140 cases positive for EGFR (67.1%). The presence or absence of EGFR correlated with histological grade and patient's age. Furthermore, patients with EGFR-positive endometrial carcinoma had a statistically significant decrease in overall survival than those with EGFR-negative tumors (16). Wang et al. found that expression of EGFR in addition to ErbB2 protein was more frequently observed with advanced stage of disease and was inversely correlated with the grade of differentiation and with the expression of estrogen receptor (ER) or progesterone receptor (PR) of the tumor (17). In addition, there is an inverse relationship between EGFR content and the extent of progesterone suppression in EC (11).

An important endometrial cancer histotype where HER2/neu may be critically implicated is uterine papillary serous carcinoma (UPSC). Eight of ten UPSC's stained heavily for HER2/neu (2+ to 3+). Freshly established primary USPC cell lines were found to express ten-fold more HER2/neu receptor by flow cytometry when compared with HER2/neu-positive primary or established breast or ovarian cancer cell lines. Although these USPC cell lines were resistant to chemotherapy in vivo and to natural killer- and complement-mediated cytotoxicity in vitro, they were found to be highly sensitive to anti-HER2/neu antibody-dependent cellular cytotoxicity (18).

Some studies have questioned the relationship between EGFR and endometrial cancer. Miturski et al. found that clinicopathological features (age, stage, histological type, grade or depth of invasion) and clinical outcome were unrelated to EGF or EGFR immunoreactivity (6). Similarly, in a study of 113 ECs, Yokoyama et al. reported positive immunohistochemistry (IHC) for EGF or EGFR was found in 25.6% or 53.1% of the neoplasms, respectively, while transforming growth factor-alpha (TGF-α) immunoreactivity was found in 67% of endometrial neoplasias. In this study TGF-α expression, but not EGF or EGFR expression, was correlated with poor histological grade and advanced stage (19).

Several strategies have been developed to take advantage of the EGF family involvement in tumor growth dysregulation. Monoclonal antibodies against EGF receptors and small-molecule inhibitors of the EGFR tyrosine kinase have been developed and shown to have activity in several cancers (5,20–22). Many mechanisms for the antitumor effects of monoclonal antibodies against HER2/neu and EGFR have been proposed: direct receptor binding leading to inhibition of HER2 signaling, cell cycle inhibition, increased apoptosis, inhibition of angiogenesis, suppression of invasion, and metastasis. In addition, stimulation of antitumor immune response in the form of antibody-mediated cytotoxicity has been observed (5).

Trastuzumab (Herceptin®, Genentech) is a humanized antibody directed against the external binding domain of the receptor HER2. Trastuzumab, when combined with chemotherapy, improves overall survival in HER2/neu over-expressing breast cancer by up to 25% (23,24). In GOG 160, a phase II trial of trastuzumab in recurrent ovarian and peri-toneal carcinoma, only 95 of 837 patients (11%) overexpressed HER2/neu. The overall response rate was 7%, leading the authors to conclude that single agent trastuzumab is of lim-ited utility in ovarian cancer (25). There are several ongoing phase I/II studies of trastuzumab in recurrent and refractory endometrial carcinoma. Other therapeutic strategies include trastuzumab conjugated to potent cytotoxic drugs and anti-bodies designed to inhibit HER2/neu dimerization (22). Given the degree of HER2/neu overexpression in uterine papillary serous carcinoma (18), trastuzumab may have an important role in this disease.

Cetuximab (Erbitux®, IMC-225; ImClone) is an antibody against the extracellular binding domain of EGFR/ErbB1 (HER1). Several phase II and III studies of cetuximab with cytotoxic chemotherapy have shown safety and efficacy in can-cers of the head and neck, colon, lung, and pancreas. Overall response rates in those cancers ranged from 11–44% (22).

Several small-molecule TK inhibitors of EGFR have been developed and tested against human cancers (20). All function by interfering with ATP or second-messenger binding with the receptor cytoplasmic TK phosphorylation site. The EGFR-TK inhibitors vary in binding specificity: ErbB1 only; dual ErbB1 and ErbB2; and pan-EGFR-TK inhibitors. They also differ in affinity and reversibility of binding.

Gefitinib (Iressa®, ZD-1839; AstraZeneca) is an orally available, reversible inhibitor of ErbB1. Several phase I studies have shown its side effects to be minor: skin rash, nausea, diarrhea, and elevated transaminases at the highest doses (26–29). Phase II studies of gefitinib 250–500 mg per day in colon, non-small cell lung carcinoma (NSCLC), and head-and-neck squamous cell cancers (HNSCC) showed an overall response rate of 20%. In advanced renal cell carcinoma, however, Iressa monotherapy did not affect progression (20). Gefitinib has been approved for third-line treatment of NSCLC in the United States based on symptomatic improvement of patients, however the drug did not have an effect on overall survival. Phase III trials of Iressa in combination with standard chemotherapy in NSCLCs showed no added benefit (30).

Tarceva® (OSI-774; Genentech) is also a well-tolerated selective ErbB1 receptor TK inhibitor. Its side effects are generally mild and similar to Iressa. Dose limiting diarrhea was noted on a 200 mg/day continuous regimen, and phase II/III studies have been conducted with 150 mg/day dosing (31,32). Phase II studies of Tarceva 150 mg/day in ovarian cancer, HNSCC, and NSCLC showed 6–12% partial response rates and 35–41% stable disease rates (33,34). Several phase III studies of Tarceva with combination chemotherapy as first-line therapy for NSCLC have completed patient enrollment. Tarceva and Iressa are the subjects of two phase II trials for recurrent and resistant endometrial cancer (see the NCI website at www.cancer.gov).

TRANSFORMING GROWTH FACTORS

The TGF family includes TGF-α and -β, which are structurally unrelated. TGF-α binds and acts through the EGFR family. Instead, the three isoforms of TGF-β signal through a single common receptor complex that activates a serine/threonine kinase. TGF-β is involved in cell proliferation, tissue repair, hematopoiesis, and embryogenesis. The TGF-β receptor inhibits proliferation and antagonizes the effects of several growth factors, including EGF (35). Activation of TGF-β

receptor causes phosphorylation of signaling proteins (such as Smad), increased expression of cyclin-dependent kinase inhibitors (p21, p27, p15), and G1 cell cycle arrest (2).

TGF-α expression has been correlated to depth of invasion, survival, and stage in endometrial cancer (19, 36). Many human cancer cell lines, including endometrial and breast cancers, develop resistance to the antiproliferative effects of TGF-β. Overexpresssion of TGF-β is also associated with loss of growth inhibition late in carcinogenesis (37). TGF-β mRNA expression is reduced in ECs compared to non-neoplastic tissues, whereas the immunohistochemical expression of TGF- β is enhanced, suggesting that TGF- β acts as a paracrine regulator of endometrial cell proliferation (38).

PTEN–PI3 KINASE

EC is associated with a DNA replication error in 20–25% of cases and is one of the tumor types associated with the hereditary non-polyposis colorectal cancer (HNPCC) familial cancer syndrome. Interestingly, ECs rarely have mutations in the DNA mismatch repair genes hMSH2 and hMLH1 associated with HNPCC, although hMLH1 may be underexpressed in EC due to promoter hypermethylation. EC has been associated with numerous chromosomal abnormalities. Chromosome 17p, which contains the p53 tumor suppressor gene, is frequently involved, and confers a poor prognosis when involved. Chromosome 10q is also frequently affected and contains the tumor suppressor gene PTEN (putative protein tyrosine phosphatase/tensin). Other commonly affected chromosomes include 3p, 8q, 10p, 13q, and 18q, which contains the putative tumor suppressor DCC.

The PTEN tumor suppressor gene encodes a dual-specificity phosphatase that shares homology with the protein tyrosine kinase family as well as the cytoskeletal proteins tensin and auxilin. PTEN mutation or loss of heterozygosity (LOH) has been implicated in several human cancers. Deletions of PTEN are seen in high-grade glioblastoma (39), prostate cancer (40) and hepatocellular carcinoma (41). Loss of heterozygosity for PTEN is seen in breast cancers but germ-line mutations are rare (42–44). Some evidence shows that PTEN mutations may be associated with endometrioid ovarian cancers, but not sporadic serous or mucinous ovarian tumors (45) or BRCA-1 associated ovarian cancers (46).

PTEN function appears to be critical in controlling the cell cycle. Wild-type PTEN products inhibit the phosphatidyl-inositol 3–kinase (PI3–K) and Akt pathways implicated in G1 cell cycle progression (47–51). PTEN dephosphorylates the products of PI3–K, phosphadiylinositol(3,4,5)P_3 and PI(3,4)P_2. Consequently, inactivating PTEN mutations lead to increased levels of PI3–K products, enhanced Akt activity, and cellular transformation (52,53). Part of the transforming effect of mutant PTEN might be mediated through downregulation of the cyclin-dependent kinase inhibitor p27 (52,53). Zhu et al. expressed wild-type or mutant PTEN in EC cell lines. Expression of exogenous PTEN decreased levels of activated Akt in all cell lines and induced a G1 cell cycle arrest specifically in EC cells lacking endogenous wild-type PTEN. PTEN induced a specific reduction of cyclin D3 levels and indirectly regulated p27KIP1 activity (54). Mouse embryonic stem cells with null-mutation of PTEN showed increased growth rates and accelerated transition from G1 to S growth phase (48). In human glioma cell lines, induced overexpression of PTEN blocked progression from G0/1 to S growth phase (55).

In addition to regulation of the cell cycle, PTEN may also play a critical role in apoptosis. In mouse cell lines, PTEN deficient fibroblasts exhibit decreased apoptosis, while expression of exogenous PTEN cells restored apoptosis and Akt phosphorylation (56,57). Similarly, restoration of wild type PTEN in cell lines with mutated PTEN leads to apoptosis (58). Finally, the expression of phosphorylated Bad, a protein involved in cell survival, was greater in PTEN negative tumors (59).

Classic Type I endometrial adenocarcinomas show alterations in the PTEN gene in 34–50% of studied cases. Atypical endometrial hyperplasia, a precursor lesion to endometrial adenocarcinoma, is also associated with PTEN mutations in 20% of cases (60). Both germ-line mutations and LOH at the chromosome 10q23 region are seen. Hypermethylation of the PTEN promoter, another proposed mechanism of tumor suppressor inactivation, has been observed in approximately 20% of ECs and has been associated with metastatic disease (61,62).

The prognostic significance of PTEN expression in EC has not been clear. In other human cancers, PTEN mutation is associated with increased metastatic potential, as indicated by its alternate name: mutated in multiple advanced cancers-1 (MMAC1) (63). In ECs, several studies suggest that PTEN mutation is associated with a less invasive and less metastatic phenotype (64,65). Risinger et al. performed DNA sequencing of mutated PTEN genes in 44 EC, and found that PTEN mutation was associated with early stage, local disease, and more favorable survival (66). In contrast, Kanamori et al. studied 98 pure EC with retroperitoneal lymph node metastasis for PTEN expression by IHC staining. Negative- or mixed-PTEN staining was observed in 64 (65.3%) patients. The survival rate for PTEN-positive patients was significantly higher than that for PTEN-negative or -mixed patients, and the survival rate for PTEN-positive cases was significantly higher than that for PTEN-negative or -mixed cases when patients underwent chemotherapy (62.4% vs. 11.8%). Subsequent multivariate analysis revealed that PTEN staining was an independent prognostic factor for patients undergoing chemotherapy (67).

Inhibitors of the PTEN pathway have been developed as potential chemotherapeutic agents. The mammalian target of rapamycin (mTOR) protein functions downstream of the PI3–K/Akt pathway and is phosphorylated in response to PI3–K/Akt pathway activation (68). Sirolimus (Rapamune®, CCI-779; Wyeth), a soluble ester analog of rapamycin that inhibits mTOR has shown anti-tumor effects and favorable pharmaceutical and toxicological characteristics in preclinical studies (69–71). Phase I studies of sirolimus have shown activity in several tumor types, including uterine papillary serous carcinoma (68).

Several studies have investigated the role of small molecule-inhibitors of PI3–K as potential tumor suppressor agents. For example, the flavonoid derivative, LY294002 (Eli Lilly), a potent PI3–K inhibitor, is a competitive, reversible inhibitor of the kinases ATP binding site (72,73). The agent induces G1 arrest in proliferating cells, leading to inhibition of proliferation in melanoma cells, MG-63 osteosarcoma cells, and OVCAR-3 ovarian cancer cells (73,74). The inhibitor also completely inhibits the retinoblastoma protein (Rb) hyper-phosphorylation that normally occurs during G1 progression and induces up-regulation of the cyclin-dependent kinase inhibitor p27 (74). However, LY294002 is not a pure PI3–K inhibitor, and because of the ubiquity of PI3K distribution, the drug may exhibit unacceptable toxicity.

ANGIOGENESIS

Angiogenesis is the physiologic process of blood vessel growth arising from existing vasculature. This is in contrast to vasculogenesis, the process of de novo vessel generation from stem cells that occurs during embryonic development. Vascular endothelium (VE) in adults is quiescent, but physiologic angiogenesis does occur during wound healing, endometrial cycling, ovulation, and pregnancy. A balance between pro- and anti-angiogenic factors tightly regulates VE growth and regression. Disease can result from either excess (e.g., proliferative retinopathy, cancer) or deficiencies (e.g., coronary artery disease) in angiogenesis (75,76).

Angiogenesis occurs in a complex series of steps with numerous molecular regulators. In response to injury, hypoxia, or genetic changes, cells release proangiogenic growth factors. These growth factors stimulate signaling cascades within the VE cells leading to increased growth, migration, proliferation, and cell survival. In addition, cells upregulate production of enzymes such as matrix metalloproteinases (MMP) that degrade basement membranes and allow VE migration toward the source of growth factors (77,78). VE cells then elongate and migrate forming tubular structures and eventually capillaries (79). Cancer cells are thought to recruit a new vasculature either directly by an overproduction of angiogenic factors, or by recruiting host stromal or immune cells to produce angiogenic factors (80,81).

Numerous observations have suggested that angiogenesis is a critical step in endometrial neoplastic transformation. Abulafia et al. found a significant difference between the microvascular densities of normal endometrium, endometrial hyperplasia (EH), and stage I EC (78). Multiple studies have confirmed that in stage I and II EC, microvascular density is associated with worse grade, depth of myometrial invasion, lymphovascular space invasion, progression-free and overall survival (82–85). The presence of proangiogenic factors such as interleukin 8 (IL-8) has also correlated with disease prognosis and stage (86). Thus, mediators of angiogenesis represent legitimate targets for molecular therapy in EC.

Vascular endothelial growth factor (VEGF) is a potent and specific mitogen of VE cells. It occurs in several isoforms (VEGF-A, VEGF-B, VEGF-C, VEGF-D, VEGF-E, placental growth factor) that are differentially expressed in many human tissues, tumor cells, and peritumoral stroma (81). VEGF activity is limited primarily to arteries, veins, and lymphatics (87,88), although additional targets include leukocytes and tumor cells. Expression is induced by multiple stimuli including hypoxia (81), hypoglycemia (89), pressure of surrounding cells (90), and cytokines. Its expression is critical in embryogenesis as shown by the uniform lethality of VEGF knockout mice (87,91).

The effects of VEGF are mediated by three receptor tyrosine kinases: VEGFR-1 (Flt-1), VEGFR-2 (Flk-1/KDR), and VEGFR-3 (Flt-4). VEGFR-1 is widely expressed in both normal and tumor cells. VEGFR-2 expression is limited to vascular endothelial cells and is the major regulator of angiogenesis (92). VEGFR-3 expression is limited to lymphatic endothelial cells and primarily regulates lymphangiogenesis (93).

Several studies have suggested an important role for VEGF in endometrial cancer. VEGF expression in endometrial carcinoma is associated with poor prognosis. A multivariate analysis of 121 ECs concluded that VEGF and

VEGFR-2/KDR were the only independent negative prognostic variables for patients with stage I endometrioid adenocarcinoma (94). In a study of 81 stage I ECs, hypoxia-inducible factor 1–alpha (HIF-1α) was detected by IHC in 49% of tumors and was associated with increased VEGF expression, microvascular density and poor prognosis (95). In addition, myofibroblasts adjacent to EC cells express VEGF, IGF-1, EGF, and VEGFR-2 by IHC (96). Finally, insulin upregulates VEGF expression in EC cell lines in vitro, thus suggesting a potential mechanism for the link between obesity and diabetes as risk factors for EC (97).

Multiple other factors have been implicated in angiogenesis: thymidine phosphatase (TP), acidic fibroblast growth factor (a-FGF), basic FGF (b-FGF), angiopoietins, IL-8, TGF-β tumor necrosis factor-beta (TNF-β), cyclooxygenase-2 (COX-2) and others (81,98–101). TP induces angiogenesis through catalytic metabolism of thymidine to 2-deoxy-D-ribose, a chemoattractant of endothelial cells (102). In one study on 101 ECs, Tanaka et al. (103) observed expression of TP by IHC in tumor-infiltrating macrophages, where levels of angiogenesis correlated with TP. They concluded that production of TP by tumor-infiltrating macrophages might influence angiogenesis, tumor invasion, and metastasis (103). In a series of 121 endometrial carcinomas, VEGF and stromal TP coexpression was the most potent angiogenic phenotype, suggesting a synergistic function. Survival analysis revealed that VEGF and stromal TP, whether expressed alone or in combination, defined poor prognosis (104).

Cyclooxygenase-1 (COX-1) and COX-2 convert arachidonic acid to prostaglandins (PGE_2, PGD_2, $PGF_{2\alpha}$, PGI_2) and thromboxane A2 (TXA_2). The levels of VEGF and basic FGF increase in response to prostaglandins such as PGE_2, while the link between COX-2 and angiogenesis is multifactoral (105). COX-2 expression is elevated in several human cancers (106), and non-steroidal antiinflammatory agents (NSAIDs) are effective cancer prevention and treatment agents in mice and humans (summarized in Iniguez, 2003). COX-2 is expressed in EC and EH but not normal endometrium. Stromal expression of COX-2 in EC is associated with increased VEGF, TP, and microvascular density. These observations suggest that Cox-2 may play a role in endometrial carcinogenesis and therefore COX-2 inhibitors may be of therapeutic benefit.

In addition to their effects on the vasculature, proangiogenic factors have also been implicated in suppressing antitumor immune response. The presence of tumor infiltrating dendritic cells (antigen presenting cells) has been inversely associated with VEGF levels and directly correlated with survival in breast cancer (107) and ovarian cancer (108). VEGF has also been shown to block dendritic cell maturation. However, tumor infiltrating T-cells and macrophages can express vasculogenic factors, revealing the complexity of tumor-immune interactions (81,109,110).

Unopposed estrogen has long been implicated in the initiation of endometrial hyperplasia and carcinoma. The relative risk of EC in women taking tamoxifen, a mixed estrogen agonist/antagonist, for the prevention or treatment of breast cancer, is increased 2.3 to 7.5-fold (111,112). The proangiogenic effects of estrogens and tamoxifen have been hypothesized to be one potential mechanism for their association with EC. Estrogens have been shown to induce upregulation of endometrial VEGF, (10) b-FGF, and TGF-α expression (113). Hague et al. noted increased expression of a- and b-FGF after treatment with tamoxifen mainly in premenopausal tissue. Vascular density was significantly increased in pre- but not postmenopausal endometrium following tamoxifen treatment (114).

As opposed to estrogens, progestins have long been known to have therapeutic benefit in EC and may exercise a suppressive effect on angiogenesis in EC and EH. Medroxyprogesterone acetate (MPA) inhibits the angiogenic factor plasminogen activator in bovine endothelial cells (115). In the rabbit cornea model, MPA suppresses EC cell b-FGF and TGF-α expression (113) and decreases microvascular density (116). MPA-treated EC also show reductions in tumor angiogenesis factor and FGFs (117). Microvessel counts of uterine specimens from patients with complex endometrial hyperplasia treated with oral MPA were significantly lower than controls (78).

For several reasons, angiogenesis provides an attractive target for cancer therapy. All solid tumors are dependent upon new vessels to support growth more than 2–3 mm in diameter. Suppression of angiogenesis provides a powerful tool to restrain tumor growth. Tumor neovasculature is derived from normal EC cells that respond to normal growth factor regulation. Unlike tumor cells, where genetic heterogeneity can lead to chemoresistant isolates and escape from apoptotic signaling, host vascular endothelial cells do not lose homeostatic control mechanisms and should remain responsive to therapy predictably in a variety of solid tumors (118). Finally, because these therapies may not affect quiescent VE cells, their toxicities should be limited (77,80).

Antiangiogenesis therapies mandate a change in the way we assess antineoplastic treatments. Typically, phase I studies of chemotherapeutics attempt to reach the maximum tolerated dose with the rationale that treatment with MTD maximizes therapeutic efficacy. In contrast, antiangiogenic therapy will likely require lower, physiologic doses administered chronically. Phase II/III studies use objective measurements of complete or partial response to therapy. However, as antiangiogenic therapies are cytostatic and not cytotoxic, time to tumor progression may be a more appropriate endpoint (119). Imaging modalities specific for angiogenesis, such as positron emission tomography or functional magnetic reasonance, are under investigation as means to directly monitor antiangiogenesis therapy.

As discussed in the previous paragraphs, there are several potential molecular targets for the inhibition of angiogenesis. VEGFs and VEGFRs are leading targets for antiangiogenesis therapy. VEGF receptor expression is limited primarily to vascular and lymphatic endothelium (88), and is increased in growing tumors (120). Many strategies have been tested in VEGF pathway inhibition: small molecule VEGFR inhibitors, monoclonal anti-VEGF antibodies, soluble VEGF receptors, and immunotherapy against the VEGFR [summarized in (77)]. All have shown activity alone or in combination with cytotoxic drugs in preclinical trials.

Recombinant humanized monoclonal antibody against VEGF bevacizumab (Avastin®; Genentech) has shown effect in human solid tumors. In a phase II study of standard chemotherapy (5-fluorouracil and leucovorin) with or without bevacizumab (low or high dose) in 104 cases of untreated metastatic colon cancer, the addition of bevacizumab improved the overall response rate (24% to 40% with bevacizumab and chemotherapy versus 17% chemotherapy alone) and median survival (16.1 to 17.3 months versus 13.6 months) (121). Results of a recently concluded phase III trial suggest that bevacizumab, when added to conventional chemotherapy, improves overall survival for metastatic colon cancer patients. Side effects included hypertension and rare instances of bowel perforation (122,123).

VEGFR small molecule tyrosine kinase inhibitors disrupt VEGF-dependent signaling. In murine and xenograft models of solid tumors, these drugs showed promising efficacy leading to human trials (124). In a phase I study, SU5416 (SUGEN, CA) given at the MTD 145 mg/m^2 IV twice weekly was associated with tolerable side effects: nausea, vomiting, diarrhea, and headaches (125). SU5416 has also shown synergistic effects with radiotherapy. Inhibition of vascular endothelial growth factor receptor signaling leads to reversal of tumor resistance to radiotherapy (126).

Unfortunately, the results of phase III trials of SU5416 in combination with chemotherapy of metastatic colon cancer have been disappointing. Addition of the VEGFR-2 inhibitor provided no benefit over standard chemotherapy, despite preclinical evidence of activity. Several reasons have been advanced for the discrepancy between the preclinical and clinical effect of SU5416 (and possibly all antiangiogenesis agents). Xenograft studies in mice involve small (1–2 mm tumors) with immature vasculature. Clinically evaluable tumors are >1 cm with an established vasculature that may respond differently to agents that halt vessel growth. Also, tumors may express multiple redundant angiogenic factors, thus escaping the inhibition provided by a single agent (92). Studies with VEGFR inhibitors for EC are currently in progress. Other VEGFR small-molecule inhibitors, such as PTK787 (Novartis Pharmaceuticals) and ZD6474 (AstraZeneca) are also in phase I/II studies in humans, but none of this class of drugs is under investigation in endometrial carcinoma.

Thalidomide is best known for its teratogenic effects when taken in early pregnancy. Fetal limb defects are a result of its antiangiogenic properties upon the developing extremity (127). Thalidomide downregulates several proangiogenenic factors (TNF-α, VEGF, b-FGF, and IL-6) (128) through unknown mechanisms. As a single agent in phase II studies, thalidomide shows activity in multiple myeloma, Kaposi's sarcoma, renal cell cancer, and glioma. In combination chemotherapy (*n* = 50) with thalidomide, cyclophosphamide, etoposide, and dexamethasone, 4% of patients achieved complete response (CR) and 64% showed a partial response (PR), with an objective response rate of 86.0% (129). Preliminary studies of thalidomide in refractory and resistant epithelial ovarian and peritoneal carcinomas also showed activity (130). The GOG is actively studying thalidomide in recurrent or resistant EC, uterine sarcoma, and ovarian carcinoma (see the NCI website, www.cancer.gov). Although the toxicities of thalidomide can be severe, most side effects are limited to lethargy, constipation, and rashes (128); however, more severe side effects include peripheral neuropathy and thromboembolic events (131,132).

Suramin, a pylsufonated naphtyl urea compound that binds bFGF and VEGF, is in phase II trials for refractory or recurrent EC (133–135). There is also evidence that traditional cytotoxic agents are antiangiogenic under modified dosing regimens. Treatment with chemotherapeutics near the maximum tolerated dose (MTD) requires extended intervals between doses to allow hematopoetic and GI recovery. Angiogenesis can resume during the 3–4 week rest period even in the absence of tumor growth. The terms "antiangiogenic" and "metronomic" have been used to describe frequent (i.e., weekly), low-dose (one-third to one-tenth MTD) regimens designed to reduce the potential for tumor and vascular growth (136,137). Several studies have documented the in

vivo antiangiogenic effects of paclitaxel, etoposide, doxorubicin, and topotecan (136). Clinical responses have been
reported in breast and ovarian cancers refractory to traditional dosing when switched to weekly regimens (138–144).
Havrilesky et al. reported an 83% overall response rate in 29
patients with recurrent ovarian adenocarcinoma treated with
low-dose carboplatin and paclitaxel (138). Because of the
decreased doses utilized, oral agents are also effective and
make outpatient therapy a possibility (145). All studies
reported few serious toxicities. Hopefully, these encouraging
results will be repeated in larger studies. As recurrent EC is
often reponsive to taxanes, this may offer a future avenue for
EC therapy.

INVASION AND METASTASIS

The ability of cancer to invade and metastasize is one of the
most important characteristics clinically. Localized, non-
invasive or superficially invasive tumors are surgically curable and carry a better prognosis than even minimally
invasive disease (146–148). Tumor cells spread using the
same mechanisms of migration as normal cells during
embryogenesis, placentation, wound healing, and immune-
cell trafficking (149).

The understanding of the process of invasion and metastasis has changed since the "seed and soil" hypothesis of
Paget in 1889 (155,156). Cellular migration is a series of
interrelated steps involving the surrounding cells and extracellular matrix (ECM). First, cellular protrusions form owing
to actin polymerization. Along the advancing edge of the cell,
focal adhesion complexes form by the interaction of integrin
family receptors and the ECM. Activation of integrins causes
recruitment and activation of surface proteases (e.g., matrix
metalloprotease, cathepsin) to the attachment site and degradation of ECM. Propulsion forces are generated by actin fila-
ment contraction via the binding and activation of myosin II
by myosin light-chain kinase. Last, the trailing edge of the
cell releases.

Oncogenic Ras can promote tumor metastasis in a variety of cell types (150). The Ras proteins (H-Ras, N-Ras, and K-Ras) are cytoplasmic GTPases that act as intermediary signals from activated receptors to downstream effectors. Change from active GTP-bound Ras to the inactive, GDP-bound state is mediated by variety of guanine exchange factors (GEFs) and GTPase activating proteins (GAPs) (150). *Ras* is constitutively activated owing to mutations in 30% of human cancers and 50–75% of endometrial cancers (151,152). Ras gain-of-function proteins are important in uncontrolled growth and invasion.

In recent years, the number of Ras effectors and the complexity of activated pathways that Ras regulates have grown considerably. The Raf/MEK cascade activates mitogen-activated protein kinases (MAPKs), upregulating transcription factors. Ras also activates Ral GEFs, which phosphorylates the Rho GAP proteins and the fork head transcription factor, providing another pathway to stimulate cell proliferation. The third effector of Ras is the PI3-kinase family. As described above, PI3-K regulates a diverse array of signaling molecules including Akt and focal adhesion kinases (FAK). PI3-K also controls apoptotic pathways and cytoskeleton organization via the Rac GTPase (150). Oncogenic Ras promotes tumor cell motility directly through activation of the Akt/FAK pathways (153,154). It can also increase expression or activity in enzymes necessary for ECM degradation: metalloproteinases (MMPs), cathepsins, and decreased activity in their inhibitors (TIMPs).

Although the process of migration is similar for all cancers, diverse patterns of infiltration can be found. In general, epithelial tumors follow mesenchymal migration patterns: slow migration through elongation, strong focal adhesion formation, and path generation by proteolysis of the ECM (157,158). Groups of cells can invade as strands or sheets, or can detach and invade as clusters. In contrast, leukocytes, lymphomas, and neuroendocrine tumors move through "amoeboid" migration (159). Cells propel themselves through existing ECM gaps, with non-focal binding.

The process is further complicated by the cell's ability to change migration pattern in response to the extracellular environment. The best characterized example of this change is the epithelial-mesenchymal transition (EMT) and its reverse, MET. Epithelial cancer cells can dedifferentiate, detach, and disseminate by weakening of cell–cell adhesion molecules. An example would be tumor invasion of a blood or lymphatic vessel with subsequent invasion and metastasis of single cells. Further cellular changes, in response to inhibition or mutation of ECM proteolytic enzymes or integrins, can lead to mesenchymal-amoeboid transition (MAT) (160).

The contribution of integrins to the metastatic potential of gynecologic cancer is controversial. Beta-1 integrin expression does correlate with invasion and poor survival in ovarian carcinoma (161,162). Ovarian carcinomas have greater expression of $\alpha_v\beta_3$ integrin than low-malignant potential (LMP) tumors (163). In EC, reduced expression of integrins is associated with poor histological grade and nodal metastasis (164,165). The availability of RGD-containing peptides that can inhbit integrin function offers potential therapeutic intervention.

The effect of proteases such as matrix metalloproteinases (MMPs) in gynecologic cancer is also seemingly contradictory. Increased expression of MMPs in vitro correlates with increased ECM invasion and cell motility and in many cancers is correlated with tumor progression and metastasis (166). Overexpression of MMPs is associated with worse stage (167) and poor survival in ovarian carcinoma (168,169), and increased stage and invasion in EC (170). However, MMP expression does not correlate with survival in vulvar cancer (171) or EC in other studies (172,173).

Metalloproteinase inhibitors (MPIs) have been developed as anticancer agents. Preclinical testing of MPIs showed the effectiveness in delaying tumor progression and metastasis (174–176). However, MPI treatment was more effective in early tumors than bulky disease (176).

The results of phase II–III trials with MPIs have been disappointing. Marimastat (BB-2516) testing in patients with advanced ovarian, pancreatic, colorectal, and prostate cancers showed reduction in the rates of rise of tumor-specific markers (177). However, phase III trials in ovarian and other carcinoma have shown no advantage to MPIs alone or in combination with chemotherapeutic agents (178). It has been argued that trials of MPIs in late-stage disease is inappropriate, as metastasis has already occurred. Perhaps MPIs may have a place in secondary prevention regimens aiming at reducing tumor recurrence in patients at high risk for relapse.

CONCLUSIONS

The increased understanding of the molecular pathways involved in carcinogenesis has yielded many potential targets for therapy. The initial hope for drugs with few side effects and highly specific activity has been tempered by experience in phase III trials. In addition, the endpoints for proving efficacy must be re-evaluated for the next generation of targeted therapies. Future trials must classify patients for the expression of specific targets and seek to employ highly targeted therapy in specific subsets of patients. Translational studies must accompany such trials to document whether the targeted pathways have been manipulated adequately. Molecular endpoints and modified clinical response endpoints must be introduced in order to sort through the ever increasing amount of targeted therapeutic tools and understand how best to combine them with conventional chemotherapy.

REFERENCES

1. Hanahan D, Weinberg RA. The hallmarks of cancer. *Cell* 2000; 100(1):57–70.

2. Herbst RS, Onn A, Mendelsohn J. The role of growth factor signaling in malignancy. *Cancer Treat Res* 2003; 115:19–72.

3. Lemmon MA, Schlessinger J. Regulation of signal transduction and signal diversity by receptor oligomerization. *Trends Biochem Sci* 1994; 19(11):459–463.

4. Klapper LN, et al. The ErbB-2/HER2 oncoprotein of human carcinomas may function solely as a shared coreceptor for multiple stroma-derived growth factors. *Proc Natl Acad Sci USA* 1999; 96(9):4995–5000.

5. Mendelsohn J, Baselga J. The EGF receptor family as targets for cancer therapy. *Oncogene* 2000; 19(56):6550–6565.

6. Miturski R, et al. Epidermal growth factor receptor immunostaining and epidermal growth factor receptor-tyrosine kinase activity in proliferative and neoplastic human endometrium. *Tumour Biology* 2000; 21(6):358–366.

7. Konopka B, et al. Changes in the concentrations of receptors of insulin-like growth factor-I, epithelial growth factor, oestrogens and progestagens in adenomyosis foci, endometrium and myometrium of women during menstrual cycle. *Eur J Gyn Oncol* 1998; 19(1):93–97.

8. McBean JH, Brumsted JR, Stirewalt WS. In vivo estrogen regulation of epidermal growth factor receptor in human endometrium. *J Clin Endocrinol Metab* 1997; 82(5):1467–1471.

9. Hata H, et al. Role of estrogen and estrogen-related growth factor in the mechanism of hormone dependency of endometrial carcinoma cells. *Oncology* 1998; 55 Suppl 1:35–44.

10. Dardes RC, et al. Regulation of estrogen target genes and growth by selective estrogen-receptor modulators in endometrial cancer cells. *Gynecol Oncol* 2002; 85(3):498–506.

11. Gershtein ES, et al. Comparative analysis of the sensitivity of endometrial cancer cells to epidermal growth factor and steroid hormones. *Cancer* 1995. 76(12):2524–2529.

12. Berchuck A, et al. Overexpression of HER-2/neu in endometrial cancer is associated with advanced stage disease. *Amer J Obstet & Gynecol* 1991; 164(1 Pt 1):15–21.

13. Hetzel DJ, et al. HER-2/neu expression: a major prognostic factor in endometrial cancer. *Gynecol Oncol* 1992; 47(2):179–185.

14. Pisani AL, et al. HER-2/neu, p53, and DNA analyses as prognosticators for survival in endometrial carcinoma. *Obstet & Gynecol* 1995; 85(5 Pt 1):729–734.

15. Scambia G, et al. Significance of epidermal growth factor receptor expression in primary human endometrial cancer. *In Cancer* 1994; 56(1):26–30.

16. Niikura H, et al. Prognostic value of epidermal growth factor receptor expression in endometrioid endometrial carcinoma. *Human Pathology* 1995; 26(8):892–896.

17. Wang D, et al. Expression of c-erbB-2 protein and epidermal growth receptor in endometrial carcinomas. Correlation with clinicopathologic and sex steroid receptor status. *Cancer* 1993; 72(9):2628–2637.

18. Santin AD, et al. Overexpression of HER-2/neu in uterine serous papillary cancer. *Clin Cancer Res* 2002; 8(5):1271–1279.

19. Yokoyama Y, et al. Immunohistochemical study of estradiol, epidermal growth factor, transforming growth factor alpha and epidermal growth factor receptor in endometrial neoplasia. *Jap J Clin Oncol* 1996; 26(6):411–416.

20. Baselga J, Hammond LA. HER-targeted tyrosine-kinase inhibitors. *Oncology* 2002; 63 (Suppl 1):6–16.

21. Denny WA. Irreversible inhibitors of the erbB family of protein tyrosine kinases. *Pharm Ther* 2002; 93(2–3):253–261.

2.   Ranson M, Sliwkowski MX. Perspectives on anti-HER monoclonal antibodies. *Oncology* 2002; 63 Suppl 1:17–24.

23. Baselga J. Herceptin alone or in combination with chemotherapy in the treatment of HER2–positive metastatic breast cancer: pivotal trials. *Oncology* 2001; 61 Suppl 2:14–21.

24. Slamon D, Pegram M. Rationale for trastuzumab (Herceptin) in adjuvant breast cancer trials. *Seminars in Oncology* 2001; 28(1 Suppl 3):13–19.

25. Bookman MA, et al. Evaluation of monoclonal humanized anti-HER2 antibody, trastuzumab, in patients with recurrent or refractory ovarian or primary peritoneal carcinoma with overexpression of HER2: a phase II trial of the Gynecologic Oncology Group. *J Clin Oncol* 2003; 21(2):283–290.

26. Baselga J, et al. Continuous Administration of ZD1839 (Iressa), a Novel Oral Epidermal Growth Factor Receptor Tyrosine Kinase Inhibitor (EGFR-TKI), in Patients with Five

Selected Tumor Types: Evidence of Activity and Good Tolerability. In *Proceedings of the American Society of Clinical Oncology*, 2000.

27. Ferry D, et al. Intermittent Oral ZD1839 (Iressa), a Novel Epidermal Growth Factor Receptor Tyrosine Kinase Inhibitor (EGFR-TKI), Shows Evidence of Good Tolerability and Activity: Final Results from a Phase I Study. In *Proceedings of the American Society of Clinical Oncology*, 2000.

28. Negoro S, et al. Final Results of a Phase I Intermittent Dose-Escalation Trial of ZD1839 ('Iressa') In Japanese Patients With Various Solid Tumours. In *Proceedings of the American Society of Clinical Oncology*, 2001.

29. Viens P, et al. A phase II trial to evaluate efficacy and safety of gefitinib (ZD1839) in patients with loco-regionally advanced or metastatic squamous-cell carcinoma of the cervix. In *Proceedings of the American Society of Clinical Oncology*, 2003. Abstract No: 1833.

30. Giaccone G, et al. Results of a multivariate analysis of prognostic factors of overall survival of patients with advanced non-small-cell lung cancer (NSCLC) treated with gefitinib (ZD1839) in combination with platinum-based chemotherapy (CT) in two large phase III trials (INTACT 1 and 2). In *Proceedings of the American Society of Clinical Oncology*, 2003. Abstract No: 2522.

31. Hidalgo M, et al. Phase I and pharmacologic study of OSI-774, an epidermal growth factor receptor tyrosine kinase inhibitor, in patients with advanced solid malignancies (comment). *J Clin Oncol* 2001; 19(13):3267–3279.

32. Karp DD, et al. Phase I Dose Escalation Study of Epidermal Growth Factor Receptor (EGFR) Tyrosine Kinase (TK) Inhibitor CP-358,774 in Patients with Advanced Solid Tumors (Meeting abstract). In *Proceedings of the American Society of Clinical Oncology*, 1999.

33. Finkler N, et al. Phase 2 Evaluation of OSI-774, a Potent Oral Antagonist of the EGFR-TK in Patients with Advanced Ovarian Carcinoma. *Proceedings of the American Society of Clinical Oncology*, 2001. Abstract No: 831.

34.   Perez-Soler R, et al. A Phase II Trial of the Epidermal Growth Factor Receptor (EGFR) Tyrosine Kinase Inhibitor OSI-774, Following Platinum-Based Chemotherapy, in Patients (pts) with Advanced, EGFR-Expressing, Non-Small Cell Lung Cancer (NSCLC). In *Proceedings of the American Society of Clinical Oncology*, 2001.

35.   Hunter KE, Sporn MB, Davies AM. Transforming growth factor-betas inhibit mitogen-stimulated proliferation of astrocytes. *GLIA* 1993; 7(3):203–211.

36.   Reinartz JJ, et al. Expression of p53, transforming growth factor alpha, epidermal growth factor receptor, and c-erbB-2 in endometrial carcinoma and correlation with survival and known predictors of survival. *Hum Pathol* 1994; 25(10):1075–1083.

37.   Gold LI, Parekh TV. Loss of growth regulation by transforming growth factor-beta (TGF-beta) in human cancers: studies on endometrial carcinoma. *Semin Reproductive Endocrino* 1999; 17(1):73–92.

38.   Perlino E, et al. Down-regulated expression of transforming growth factor beta 1 mRNA in endometrial carcinoma. *Br J Cancer* 1998; 77(8):1260–1266.

39.   Sano T, et al. Differential expression of MMAC/PTEN in glioblastoma multiforme: relationship to localization and prognosis. *Cancer Research* 1999; 59(8):1820–1824.

40.   Gray IC, et al. Mutation and expression analysis of the putative prostate tumour-suppressor gene PTEN. *Br J Cancer* 1998; 78(10):1296–1300.

41.   Yao YJ, et al. PTEN/MMAC1 mutations in hepatocellular carcinomas. *Oncogene* 1999; 18(20):3181–3185.

42.   Carroll BT, et al. Polymorphisms in PTEN in breast cancer families.[erratum appears in J Med Genet 2000;7(7):559]. *J Med Genet* 1999; 6(2):94–96.

43.   Feilotter HE, et al. Analysis of the 10q23 chromosomal region and the PTEN gene in human sporadic breast carcinoma. *Br J of Cancer* 1999; 79(5–6):718–723.

44.   Freihoff D, et al. Exclusion of a major role for the PTEN tumour-suppressor gene in breast carcinomas. *Br J Cancer* 1999; 79(5–6):754–758.

45. Obata K, et al. Frequent PTEN/MMAC mutations in endometrioid but not serous or mucinous epithelial ovarian tumors. *Cancer Res* 1998; 58(10):2095–2097.

46. Maxwell GL, et al. Mutation of the PTEN tumor suppressor gene is not a feature of ovarian cancers. *Gynecol Oncol* 1998; 70(1):13–16.

47. Ramaswamy S, et al. Regulation of G1 progression by the PTEN tumor suppressor protein is linked to inhibition of the phosphatidylinositol 3–kinase/Akt pathway. *Proc Natl Acad Sci USA* 1999; 96(5):2110–2115.

48. Sun H, et al. PTEN modulates cell cycle progression and cell survival by regulating phosphatidylinositol 3,4,5,-trisphosphate and Akt/protein kinase B signaling pathway. *Proc Natl Acad Sci USA* 1999; 96(11):6199–6204.

49. Gil EB, et al. Regulation of the insulin-like developmental pathway of Caenorhabditis elegans by a homolog of the PTEN tumor suppressor gene. *Proc Natl Acad Sci USA* 1999; 96(6):2925–2930.

50. Dahia PL, et al. PTEN is inversely correlated with the cell survival factor Akt/PKB and is inactivated via multiple mechanisms in haematological malignancies. *Hum Molec Genet* 1999; 8(2):185–193.

51. Wu X, et al. The PTEN/MMAC1 tumor suppressor phosphatase functions as a negative regulator of the phosphoinositide 3-kinase/Akt pathway. *Proc Natl Acad Sci USA* 1998; 95(26):15587–15591.

52. Blume-Jensen, Hunter T. Oncogenic kinase signalling. *Nature* 2001; 411(6835):355–365.

53. Stambolic V, et al. Negative regulation of PKB/Akt-dependent cell survival by the tumor suppressor PTEN. *Cell* 1998; 95(1):29–39.

54. Zhu X, et al. PTEN induces G(1) cell cycle arrest and decreases cyclin D3 levels in endometrial carcinoma cells. *Cancer Res* 2001; 61(11):4569–4575.

55. Cheney IW, et al. Suppression of tumorigenicity of glioblastoma cells by adenovirus-mediated MMAC1/PTEN gene transfer. *Cancer Res* 1998; 58(11):2331–2334.

56. Simpson L, Parsons R. PTEN: life as a tumor suppressor. *Exp Cell Res* 2001; 264(1):29–41.

57. Kandel ES, et al. Activation of Akt/protein kinase B overcomes a G(2)/m cell cycle checkpoint induced by DNA damage. *Molec & Cellular Biolo,* 2002; 22(22):7831–7841.

58. Tian XX, et al. Restoration of wild-type PTEN expression leads to apoptosis, induces differentiation, and reduces telomerase activity in human glioma cells. *J Neuropathol Exp Neurol* 1999; 58(5):472–479.

59. Kanamori Y, et al. Correlation between loss of PTEN expression and Akt phosphorylation in endometrial carcinoma. *Clin Cancer Res* 2001; 7(4):892–895.

60. Levine RL, et al. PTEN mutations and microsatellite instability in complex atypical hyperplasia, a precursor lesion to uterine endometrioid carcinoma. *Cancer Res* 1998; 58(15):3254–3258.

61. Salvesen HB, et al. PTEN methylation is associated with advanced stage and microsatellite instability in endometrial carcinoma. *Int J Cancer* 2001; 91(1):22–26.

62. Bussaglia E, et al. PTEN mutations in endometrial carcinomas: a molecular and clinicopathologic analysis of 38 cases. *Human Pathol* 2000; 31(3):312–317.

63. Steck PA, et al. Identification of a candidate tumour suppressor gene, MMAC1, at chromosome 10q23.3 that is mutated in multiple advanced cancers. *Nature Genetics* 1997; 15(4):356–362.

64. Risinger JI, et al. PTEN/MMAC1 mutations in endometrial cancers. *Cancer Res* 1997; 57(21):4736–4738.

65. Tashiro H, et al. Mutations in PTEN are frequent in endometrial carcinoma but rare in other common gynecological malignancies. *Cancer Res* 1997; 57(18):3935–3940.

66. Risinger JI, et al. PTEN mutation in endometrial cancers is associated with favorable clinical and pathologic characteristics. *Clin Cancer Res* 1998; 4(12):3005–3010.

67. Kanamori Y, et al. PTEN expression is associated with prognosis for patients with advanced endometrial carcinoma

undergoing postoperative chemotherapy. *Int J Cancer* 2002; 100(6):686–689.

68. Hidalgo M, Rowinsky EK. The rapamycin-sensitive signal transduction pathway as a target for cancer therapy. *Oncogene* 2000; 19(56):6680–6686.

69. Grunwald V, et al. Inhibitors of mTOR reverse doxorubicin resistance conferred by PTEN status in prostate cancer cells. *Cancer Res* 2002; 62(21):6141–6145.

70. Neshat MS, et al. Enhanced sensitivity of PTEN-deficient tumors to inhibition of FRAP/mTOR.[comment]. *Proc Natl Acad Sci USA* 2001; 98(18):10314–10319.

71. Podsypanina K, et al. An inhibitor of mTOR reduces neoplasia and normalizes p70/S6 kinase activity in Pten+/- mice [comment]. *Proc Natl Acad Sci USA* 2001; 98(18):10320–10325.

72. Vlahos CJ, et al. A specific inhibitor of phosphatidylinositol 3–kinase, 2–(4–morpholinyl)-8–phenyl-4H-1–benzopyran-4–one (LY294002). *J Biol Chem* 1994; 269(7):5241–52488.

73. Hu L, et al. In vivo and in vitro ovarian carcinoma growth inhibition by a phosphatidylinositol 3–kinase inhibitor (LY294002). *Clin Cancer Res* 2000; 6(3):880–886.

74. Casagrande F, et al. G1 phase arrest by the phosphatidylinositol 3–kinase inhibitor LY 294002 is correlated to up-regulation of p27Kip1 and inhibition of G1 CDKs in choroidal melanoma cells. *FEBS Letters* 1998; 422(3):385–390.

75. Alon T, et al. Vascular endothelial growth factor acts as a survival factor for newly formed retinal vessels and has implications for retinopathy of prematurity. *Nature Medicine* 1995; 1(10):1024–1028.

76. Rosen L. Antiangiogenic strategies and agents in clinical trials. *Oncologist* 2000; 5 Suppl 1:20–27.

77. Rosen LS, Clinical experience with angiogenesis signaling inhibitors: focus on vascular endothelial growth factor (VEGF) blockers. *Cancer Control* 2002; 9(2 Suppl):36–44.

78. Abulafia O, Triest WE, Sherer DM. Angiogenesis in malignancies of the female genital tract. *Gynecol Oncol* 1999; 72(2):220–231.

79. Folkman J, Haudenschild C. Angiogenesis in vitro. *Nature* 1980; 288(5791):551–556.

80. Folkman J. Seminars in Medicine of the Beth Israel Hospital, Boston. Clinical applications of research on angiogenesis [comment]. *New Engl J Med* 1995; 333(26):1757–1763.

81. Li XF, et al. Angiogenic growth factor messenger ribonucleic acids in uterine natural killer cells. *J Clin Endocrinol Metab* 2001; 86(4):1823–1834.

82. Kirschner CV, et al. Angiogenesis factor in endometrial carcinoma: a new prognostic indicator? *Amer J Obstet Gynecol* 1996; 174(6):1879–82; discussion 1882–1884.

83. Giatromanolaki A, et al. Intratumoral angiogenesis: a new prognostic indicator for stage I endometrial adenocarcinomas? *Oncol Res* 1999; 11(4):205–212.

84. Salvesen HB, Iversen OE, Akslen LA. Prognostic significance of angiogenesis and Ki-67, p53, and p21 expression: a population-based endometrial carcinoma study. *J Clin Oncol* 1999; 17(5):1382–1390.

85. Sivridis E. Angiogenesis and endometrial cancer. *Anticancer Res* 2001. 21(6B):4383–4388.

86. Fujimoto J, et al. Clinical implications of expression of interleukin-8 related to myometrial invasion with angiogenesis in uterine endometrial cancers. *Ann Oncol* 2002; 13(3):430–434.

87. Ferrara N, Alitalo K. Clinical applications of angiogenic growth factors and their inhibitors. *Nature Med* 1999; 5(12):1359–1364.

88. Jakeman LB, et al. Binding sites for vascular endothelial growth factor are localized on endothelial cells in adult rat tissues. *J Clin Invest* 1992; 89(1):244–253.

89. Shweiki D, et al. Induction of vascular endothelial growth factor expression by hypoxia and by glucose deficiency in multicell spheroids: implications for tumor angiogenesis. *Proc Natl Acad Sci USA* 1995; 92(3):768–772.

90. Carmeliet P. Mechanisms of angiogenesis and arteriogenesis. *Nature Med* 2000; 6(4):389–395.

91. Carmeliet P, et al. Abnormal blood vessel development and lethality in embryos lacking a single VEGF allele. *Nature* 1996; 380(6573):435–439.

92. McCarty MF, et al. Promises and pitfalls of anti-angiogenic therapy in clinical trials. *Trends in Molecular Medicine* 2003; 9(2):53–58.

93. Korpelainen EI, Alitalo K. Signaling angiogenesis and lymphangiogenesis. *Current Opinion in Cell Biology* 1998; 10(2):159–164.

94. Giatromanolaki A, et al. The angiogenic "vascular endothelial growth factor/flk-1(KDR) receptor" pathway in patients with endometrial carcinoma: prognostic and therapeutic implications. *Cancer* 2001; 92(10):2569–2577.

95. Sivridis E, et al. Association of hypoxia-inducible factors 1-alpha and 2-alpha with activated angiogenic pathways and prognosis in patients with endometrial carcinoma. *Cancer* 2002; 95(5):1055–1063.

96. Orimo, A, et al. Cancer-associated myofibroblasts possess various factors to promote endometrial tumor progression. *Clin Cancer Res* 2001; 7(10):3097–3105.

97. Bermont L, et al. Insulin up-regulates vascular endothelial growth factor and stabilizes its messengers in endometrial adenocarcinoma cells. *J Clin Endocrinol Metab* 2001; 86(1):363–368.

98. Folkman J, Klagsbrun M. Angiogenic factors. *Science* 1987; 235(4787):442–447.

99. Davis S, et al. Isolation of angiopoietin-1, a ligand for the TIE2 receptor, by secretion-trap expression cloning [comment]. *Cell* 1996; 87(7):1161–1169.

100. Maisonpierre PC, et al. Angiopoietin-2, a natural antagonist for Tie2 that disrupts in vivo angiogenesis [comment]. *Science* 1997; 277(5322):55–60.

101. Frater-Schroder M, et al. Tumor necrosis factor type alpha, a potent inhibitor of endothelial cell growth in vitro, is angiogenic in vivo. *Proc Natl Acad Sci USA* 1987; 84(15):5277–5281.

102. Haraguchi M, et al. Angiogenic activity of enzymes. *Nature* 1994; 368(6468):198.

103.   Tanaka Y, et al. Thymidine phosphorylase expression in tumor-infiltrating macrophages may be correlated with poor prognosis in uterine endometrial cancer. *Hum Pathol* 2002; 33(11):1105–1113.

104.   Sivridis E, et al. Angiogenic co-operation of VEGF and stromal cell TP in endometrial carcinomas. *J Pathol* 2002; 196(4):416–422.

105.   Gupta RA, Dubois RN. Colorectal cancer prevention and treatment by inhibition of cyclooxygenase-2. Nature Reviews. *Cancer* 2001; 1(1):11–21.

106.   Soslow RA, et al. COX-2 is expressed in human pulmonary, colonic, and mammary tumors. *Cancer* 2000; 89(12):2637–2645.

107.   Iwamoto M, et al. Prognostic value of tumor-infiltrating dendritic cells expressing CD83 in human breast carcinomas. *Int J Cancer* 2003; 104(1):92–97.

108.   Zhang L, et al. Intratumoral T cells, recurrence, and survival in epithelial ovarian cancer [comment]. *New Engl J Med* 2003; 348(3):203–213.

109.   Freeman MR, et al. Peripheral blood T lymphocytes and lymphocytes infiltrating human cancers express vascular endothelial growth factor: a potential role for T cells in angiogenesis. *Cancer Res* 1995; 55(18):4140–4145.

110.   Barbera-Guillem E, et al. Vascular endothelial growth factor secretion by tumor-infiltrating macrophages essentially supports tumor angiogenesis, and IgG immune complexes potentiate the process. *Cancer Res* 2002; 62(23):7042–7049.

111.   Bokhman JV. Two pathogenetic types of endometrial carcinoma. *Gynecol Oncol* 1983; 15(1):10–17.

112.   Fisher B, et al. Endometrial cancer in tamoxifen-treated breast cancer patients: findings from the National Surgical Adjuvant Breast and Bowel Project (NSABP) B-14 [comment]. *J National Cancer Instit* 1994; 86(7):527–537.

113.   Yamamoto T, et al. Angiostatic activities of medroxyprogesterone acetate and its analogues. *Int J Cancer* 1994; 56(3):393–399.

114.   Hague S, et al. Tamoxifen induction of angiogenic factor expression in endometrium. *Br J Cancer* 2002; 86(5):761–767.

115. Ashino-Fuse H, et al. Medroxyprogesterone acetate, an anti-cancer and anti-angiogenic steroid, inhibits the plasminogen activator in bovine endothelial cells. *Int J Cancer* 1989; 44(5):859–864.

116. Jikihara H, et al. Inhibitory effect of medroxyprogesterone acetate on angiogenesis induced by human endometrial cancer. *Amer J Obstet Gynecol* 1992; 167(1):207–211.

117. Fujimoto J, et al. Inhibition of tumor angiogenesis activity by medroxyprogesterone acetate in gynecologic malignant tumors. *Invasion & Metastasis* 1989; 9(5):269–277.

118. Boehm T, et al. Antiangiogenic therapy of experimental cancer does not induce acquired drug resistance [comment]. *Nature* 1997; 390(6658):404–407.

119. Eatock MM, Schatzlein A, Kaye SB. Tumour vasculature as a target for anticancer therapy. *Cancer Treatment Reviews* 2000; 26(3):191–204.

120. Cherrington JM, Strawn LM, Shawver LK. New paradigms for the treatment of cancer: the role of anti-angiogenesis agents. *Adv Cancer Res* 2000; 79:1–38.

121. Bergsland E, et al. A Randomized Phase II Trial Comparing rhuMAb VEGF (Recombinant Humanized Monoclonal Antibody to Vascular Endothelial Cell Growth Factor) Plus 5–Fluorouracil/Leucovorin (FU/LV) to FU/LV Alone in Patients with Metastatic Colorectal Cancer. In *Proceedings of the American Society of Clinical Oncology*, 2000; Abstract No: 939.

122. Gray R, et al. The safety of adding angiogenesis inhibition into treatment for colorectal, breast, and lung cancer: The Eastern Cooperative Oncology Group's (ECOG) experience with bevacizumab (anti-VEGF). In *Proceedings of the American Society of Clinical Oncology* 2003; Abstract No: 825.

123. Benson AB, et al. Bevacizumab (anti-VEGF) plus FOLFOX4 in previously treated advanced colorectal cancer (advCRC): An interim toxicity analysis of the Eastern Cooperative Oncology Group (ECOG) study E3200. In *Proceedings of the American Society of Clinical Oncology* 2003; Abstract No: 975.

124. Fong TAT, et al. SU5416 Is a Potent and Selective Inhibitor of the Vascular Endothelial Growth Factor Receptor (Flk-

1/KDR) That Inhibits Tyrosine Kinase Catalysis, Tumor Vascularization, and Growth of Multiple Tumor Types. *Cancer Res* 1999; 59(1):99–106.

125.   Rosen P, et al. A Phase I/II Study of SU5416 in Combination with 5–FU/Leucovorin in Patients with Metastatic Colorectal Cancer. Abstract No. 5D. In *Proceedings of the American Society of Clinical Onocology* 2000.

126.   Geng L, et al. Inhibition of vascular endothelial growth factor receptor signaling leads to reversal of tumor resistance to radiotherapy. *Cancer Res* 2001 61(6):2413–2419.

127.   D'Amato RJ, et al. Thalidomide is an inhibitor of angiogenesis. *Proc Natl Acad Sci USA* 1994; 91(9):4082–4085.

128.   Eisen T. Thalidomide in solid malignancies [comment]. *J Clin Oncol* 2002; 20(11):2607–2609.

129.   Moehler TM, et al. Salvage therapy for multiple myeloma with thalidomide and CED chemotherapy. *Blood*   2001; 98(13):3846–3848.

130.   Abramson N, et al. Ovarian and papillary-serous peritoneal carcinoma: pilot study with thalidomide. *J Clin Oncol* 2002; 20(4):1147–149.

131.   Govindarajan R. Irinotecan and thalidomide in metastatic colorectal cancer. *Oncology* (Huntington) 2000; 14(12 Suppl 13):29–32.

132.   Desai AA, et al. A high rate of venous thromboembolism in a multi-institutional phase II trial of weekly intravenous gemcitabine with continuous infusion fluorouracil and daily thalidomide in patients with metastatic renal cell carcinoma. *Cancer* 2002; 95(8):1629–1636.

133.   Takano S, et al. Suramin, an anticancer and angiosuppressive agent, inhibits endothelial cell binding of basic fibroblast growth factor, migration, proliferation, and induction of urokinase-type plasminogen activator. *Cancer Res* 1994; 54(10):2654–2660.

134.   Pesenti E, et al. Suramin prevents neovascularisation and tumour growth through blocking of basic fibroblast growth factor activity. *Br J Cancer* 1992; 66(2):367–372.

135. Lozano RM, et al. Solution structure of acidic fibroblast growth factor bound to 1,3, 6–naphthalenetrisulfonate: a minimal model for the anti-tumoral action of suramins and suradistas. *J Mol Biol* 1998; 281(5):899–915.

136. Browder T, et al. Antiangiogenic scheduling of chemotherapy improves efficacy against experimental drug-resistant cancer. *Cancer Res* 2000; 60(7):1878–1886.

137. Hanahan D, Bergers G, Bergsland E. Less is more, regularly: metronomic dosing of cytotoxic drugs can target tumor angiogenesis in mice [comment]. *J Clin Invest* 2000; 105(8):1045–1047.

138. Havrilesky LJ, et al. Weekly Low-Dose Carboplatin and Paclitaxel in the Treatment of Recurrent Ovarian and Peritoneal Cancer. *Gynecol Oncol* 2003; 88(1):51–57.

139. Abu-Rustum NR, et al. Salvage weekly paclitaxel in recurrent ovarian cancer. *Seminars in Oncology* 1997; 24(5 Suppl 15):S15–62–S15–67.

140. Burstein HJ, et al. Docetaxel administered on a weekly basis for metastatic breast cancer. *J Clin Oncol* 2000; 18(6):1212–1219.

141. Fennelly D, et al. Phase I and pharmacologic study of paclitaxel administered weekly in patients with relapsed ovarian cancer. *J Clin Oncol* 1997; 15(1):187–192.

142. Greco FA. Oral etoposide in lymphoma. *Drugs* 1999; 58 Suppl 3:35–41.

143. Bolis G, et al. Response to second-line weekly cisplatin chemotherapy in ovarian cancer previously treated with a cisplatin- or carboplatin-based regimen [comment]. *European J Cancer* 1994; 30A(12):1764–1768.

144. Cocconi G, et al. Mature results of a prospective randomized trial comparing a three- weekly with an accelerated weekly schedule of cisplatin in advanced ovarian carcinoma. *Am J Clin Oncol: Cancer Clinical Trials* 1999; 22(6):559–567.

145. Colleoni M, et al. Low-dose oral methotrexate and cyclophosphamide in metastatic breast cancer: antitumor activity and correlation with vascular endothelial growth factor levels [comment]. *Ann Oncol* 2002; 13(1):73–80.

146. Mariani A, et al. Surgical stage I endometrial cancer: predictors of distant failure and death. *Gynecol Oncol* 2002; 87(3):274–280.

147. Phelan C, et al. Outcome and management of pathological stage I endometrial carcinoma patients with involvement of the lower uterine segment. *Gynecol Oncol* 2001; 83(3):513–517.

148. Rotman M, et al. Endometrial carcinoma. Influence of prognostic factors on radiation management. *Cancer* 1993; 71(4 Suppl):1471–1479.

149. Friedl, Wolf K, Tumour-cell invasion and migration: diversity and escape mechanisms. Nature Reviews. *Cancer* 2003; 3(5):362–374.

150. Ulku AS, Der CJ Ras signaling, deregulation of gene expression and oncogenesis. *Cancer Treatment & Res* 2003; 115:189–208.

151. Semczuk A, et al. Ras p21 immunohistochemical detection in human endometrial carcinomas. *Gynecol Obstet Investig* 1997; 44(2):132–135.

152. Esteller M, Xercavins J, Reventos J Advances in the molecular genetics of endometrial cancer (review). *Oncology Reports* 1999; 6(6):1377–1382.

153. Kumar R, Vadlamudi RK. Emerging functions of p21–activated kinases in human cancer cells. *J Cellular Physiol* 2002; 193(2):133–144.

154. Chubb JR, et al. Pseudopodium dynamics and rapid cell movement in Dictyostelium Ras pathway mutants. *Cell Motility & Cytoskeleton* 2002; 53(2):150–162.

155. Paget S. The distribution of secondary growths in cancer of the breast. *Lancet* 1889; 1:571–573.

156. Fidler IJ. The pathogenesis of cancer metastasis: the "seed and soil" hypothesis revisited. Nature Reviews. *Cancer* 2003; 3(6):453–458.

157. Tester AM, et al. MMP-9 secretion and MMP-2 activation distinguish invasive and metastatic sublines of a mouse mammary carcinoma system showing epithelial-mesenchymal

transition traits. *Clin Experimental Metastasis* 2000; 18(7):553–560.

158. Putz E, et al. Phenotypic characteristics of cell lines derived from disseminated cancer cells in bone marrow of patients with solid epithelial tumors: establishment of working models for human micrometastases. *Cancer Res*, 1999. 59(1):241–248.

159. Farina, K.L., et al. Cell motility of tumor cells visualized in living intact primary tumors using green fluorescent protein. *Cancer Res* 1998; 58(12):2528–2532.

160. Thiery JP. Epithelial-mesenchymal transitions in tumour progression. Nature Reviews. *Cancer* 2002; 2(6):442–454.

161. Muller-Klingspor V, et al. Prognostic value of beta1–integrin (=CD29) in serous adenocarcinomas of the ovary. *Anticancer Res* 2001; 21(3C):2185–2188.

162. Strobel T, Cannistra SA. Beta1–integrins partly mediate binding of ovarian cancer cells to peritoneal mesothelium in vitro. *Gynecol Oncol* 1999; 73(3):362–367.

163. Liapis H, et al. Expression of alpha(v)beta3 integrin is less frequent in ovarian epithelial tumors of low malignant potential in contrast to ovarian carcinomas. *Human Pathol* 1997; 28(4):443–449.

164. Miyamoto S, et al. Loss of motility-related protein 1 (MRP1/CD9) and integrin alpha3 expression in endometrial cancers. *Cancer* 2001; 92(3):542–548.

165. Lessey BA, et al. Distribution of integrin cell adhesion molecules in endometrial cancer. *Am J Pathol* 1995; 146(3):717–726.

166. Koblinski JE, Ahram M, Sloane BF. Unraveling the role of proteases in cancer. *Clinica Chimica Acta* 2000; 291(2):113–135.

167. Herrera CA, et al. Expression of metastasis-related genes in human epithelial ovarian tumors. *Intl J Oncol* 2002; 20(1):5–13.

168. Davidson B, et al. EMMPRIN (extracellular matrix metalloproteinase inducer) is a novel marker of poor outcome in serous ovarian carcinoma. *Clin Experimental Metastasis*, 2003. 20(2):161–169.

169. Westerlund A, et al. Gelatinase A-immunoreactive protein in ovarian lesions- prognostic value in epithelial ovarian cancer. *Gynecol Oncol* 1999; 75(1):91–98.

170. Di Nezza LA, et al. Presence of active gelatinases in endometrial carcinoma and correlation of matrix metalloproteinase expression with increasing tumor grade and invasion. *Cancer* 2002; 94(5):1466–1475.

171. Kerkela E, et al. Metalloelastase (MMP-12) expression by tumour cells in squamous cell carcinoma of the vulva correlates with invasiveness, while that by macrophages predicts better outcome. *J Pathol* 2002; 198(2):258–269.

172. Moser PL, et al. Immunohistochemical detection of matrix metalloproteinases (MMP) 1 and 2, and tissue inhibitor of metalloproteinase 2 (TIMP 2) in stage I and II endometrial cancer. *Anticancer Res* 1999; 19(3B):2365–2367.

173. Inoue Y, et al. Immunohistochemical studies on matrix metalloproteinase-9 (MMP-9) and type-IV collagen in endometrial carcinoma. *J Obstet Gynaecol Res* 1997; 23(2):139–145.

174. Sledge GW, Jr., et al. Effect of matrix metalloproteinase inhibitor batimastat on breast cancer regrowth and metastasis in athymic mice. *J Natl Cancer Inst* 1995; 87(20):1546–1550.

175. Eccles SA, et al. Control of lymphatic and hematogenous metastasis of a rat mammary carcinoma by the matrix metalloproteinase inhibitor batimastat (BB-94). *Cancer Res* 1996; 56(12):2815–2822.

176. Bergers G., et al. Effects of angiogenesis inhibitors on multistage carcinogenesis in mice. *Science* 1999; 284(5415):808–812.

177. Rasmussen HS. In Antiangiogenic Agents in Cancer Therapy, Teicher BA ed. 1999, Humana Press: Totowa, N.J., pp. 399–405.

178. Coussens LM, Fingleton B, Matrisian LM. Matrix metalloproteinase inhibitors and cancer: trials and tribulations. *Science* 2002; 295(564):2387-2392.

17

Management of Uterine Sarcomas

GREGORY SUTTON

St. Vincent Hospitals and Health Services,
Indianapolis, Indiana, U.S.A.

HEIDI J. GRAY

University of Pennsylvania Medical Center,
Philadelphia, Pennsylvania, U.S.A.

EPIDEMIOLOGY AND INCIDENCE

The epidemiology of uterine sarcomas has been difficult to clarify given their relative rarity. An excess of carcinosarcomas of the uterus following pelvic radiotherapy was recognized early on and may account for as many as 14% of such tumors in some series (1).

It appears that patients with carcinosarcomas are on the average older (mean 65, and 67 years) (1,2) than those with endometrial adenocarcinomas (mean, 59.1 years) (3), müllerian adenosarcomas (mean, 57.4 and 58 years) (4,5), leiomyosarcomas (mean, 53.5, 55, and 56.2 years)-(6–8), and endometrial stromal tumors (mean, 41, 46, 48 years) (9–11).

Silverberg et al. (12) champion the idea that carcinosarcomas are metaplastic variants of endometrial adenocarcinomas, arguing that the carcinomatous element of mixed tumors usually dictates prognosis and that the clinical behavior of carcinosarcomas closely resembles that of poorly differentiated endometrial adenocarcinomas with regard to lymph node metastases and survival. They also draw a parallel between carcinosarcomas of the uterus and "metaplastic" carcinomas of the breast.

Supporting Silverberg's contention is the work of Zelmanowicz et al. (3), which demonstrates similar risk-factor profiles between patients with carcinosarcomas and endometrial adenocarcinomas. Both populations share the risk factors of obesity, exogenous estrogen use, nulliparity, are protected by oral contraceptive use, and are currently smoking.

Zelmanowicz et al. are among recent authors to note that women with carcinosarcomas are much more likely to be of African-American descent (28% vs. 4%; $p = .001$) than those with endometrial adenocarcinomas.

The overall and relative incidences of the three main uterine sarcomas—carcinosarcoma, leiomyosarcoma, and endometrial stromal tumors—have been reported by a number of authors. Bartsich et al. (6) noted in 1968 that 125 of 1562 (8%) uterine malignancies encountered at Columbia Presbyterian Medical Center in New York City between 1917 and 1966 were sarcomas and that 56 of 125 (44.8%) were leiomyosarcomas, 57 (45.6%) were carcinosarcomas, and 12 (9.6%) were endometrial stromal tumors. Knocke et al. (13) evaluated 72 patients with sarcomas in referral during a 12-year period during which 1782 women with uterine adenocarcinomas were seen, for a relative incidence of 3.9%. Distribution by histology was similar to Bartsich et al. (6); 30 of 72 (41.7%) were leiomyosarcomas, 28 (38.9%) were carcinosarcomas, and 11 (15.3%) endometrial stromal tumors.

Endometrial stromal lesions are usually subclassified in accordance with the seminal work of Norris and Taylor (14) into two broad groups of tumors with invasive (stromal sarcomas) and noninvasive (stromal nodules) characteristics; the former is further stratified into low- or high-grade sarcomas based upon mitotic indices (<10 and >10 mitoses/10 high power fields, respectively).

Although some authors include müllerian adenosarcomas in the category of carcinosarcomas or mixed müllerian tumors, most have identified them separately since their description in 1974 by Clement and Scully (4). They are distinctly rare, fewer than 200 cases having been reported as of 1990. Of note is the report in 1996 of Clement et al. (5) of six patients who developed müllerian adenosarcomas of the uterine corpus after taking tamoxifen for periods of 6 months to 4 years. An additional such case was reported by Bocklage et al. (15).

PROGNOSTIC FACTORS

Carcinosarcomas

Silverberg et al.'s (12) review of Gynecologic Oncology Group (GOG) materials demonstrated that features of the stromal component of these lesions had little bearing on the presence of metastases; however, high-risk epithelial constituents such as clear-cell and papillary serous malignancies influenced the frequency of metastases and, conversely, overall outcome. Other adverse prognostic indicators included deep myometrial invasion, lymphatic or vascular space involvement, or uterine isthmus or cervical spread.

Patients with extrauterine disease have a poor outlook regardless of adjuvant therapy, as do those with large tumors, uterine serosal spread, and lesions which are composed predominantly of an epithelial as opposed to stromal component.

Leiomyosarcomas

A number of investigators have explored prognostic factors in uterine leiomyosarcomas. Since Kempson and Bari (16) first described vascular invasion, necrosis, and mitotic count as indicators of aggressiveness, few other meaningful features have been identified. Markers that probably are of limited prognostic importance include Epstein-Barr nuclear antigen (17), cytokeratin and epithelial membrane antigen (18), Mdm-2 protein, HER-2/neu, and K- or H-ras (19,20). Potentially useful markers include AgNORS, PCNA, and p53 expression (21). Other potential markers include Glut1, CD44s, bcl2 (22), and Ki-67 (23). Other correlates which may warrant evaluation are angiolymphatic invasion, tumor size, patient age, pushing versus infiltrative tumor/myometrium interface, and mitotic count. As the role of Epstein-Barr virus in leiomyosarcomas among immunosuppressed patients is elucidated, additional intermediate regulatory factors may be identified as well.

Endometrial Stromal Sarcomas

In their review of 117 patients with primary endometrial stromal neoplasms, Chang et al. (24) found that neither mitotic index nor cytologic atypia were predictive of recurrence in patients with stage I tumors.

Müllerian Adenosarcomas

Kaku et al. (25) indicated that müllerian adenosarcoma usually were locally invasive; only 30% of the 31 cases in their review suffered recurrences. Factors associated with poor outcome were extrauterine spread, deep myometrial invasion, sarcomatous overgrowth, and rhabdomyosarcomatous differentiation.

SURGICAL STAGING OF UTERINE SARCOMAS

In agreement with other authors, Yamada et al. (26) noted that uterine sarcomas are excluded from the staging systems of the International Federation of Obstetricians and Gynecologists (FIGO). By default, and in conformity with the opinions of other authors, the FIGO staging system for corpus cancer is utilized (Table 1). This staging system presuppposes that all patients undergo not only hysterectomy and bilateral salpingo-oophorectomy but also at least sampling of the pelvic and para-aortic lymph nodes and peritoneal washings for cytology.

Table 1 FIGO Staging of Corpus Cancer (1988)

Stage I	Carcinoma confined to corpus
	IA Tumor limited to endometrium
	IB < 1/2 myometrial invasion
	IC > 1/2 myometrial invasion
Stage II	Involvement of corpus and cervix
	IIA Endocervical glandular involvement only
	IIB Cervical stromal invasion
Stage III	Extension outside uterus, but not outside true pelvis
	IIIA Tumor invades serosa, or adnexa, or + cytology
	IIIB Vaginal metastasis
	IIIC Positive pelvic and/or para-aortic nodes
Stage IV	Extension outside true pelvis or obvious involvement of bladder or rectal mucosa
	IVA Tumor invasion of bladder and/or bowel mucosa
	IVB Distant metastasis, including intrabdominal (omentum) or inguinal lymph nodes

Exhaustive surgical staging is advocated by most authors in uterine sarcomas where feasible. The relative merit of this approach in carcinosarcomas has been highlighted in Yamada et al.'s study (26). Extrauterine spread was identified in 61% of patients undergoing surgery for carcinosarcomas whose disease was clinically confined to the uterus. Although this figure is somewhat higher than observed by others (27), it does demonstrate that exclusion of patients with occult stage II–IV lesions is associated with the extremely favorable 5-year survival figure (74%) for stage I disease reported in the study. This figure is even more remarkable given the fact that only 32% of patients received adjuvant radiotherapy.

Although nodal extrauterine spread is common in carcinosarcomas and endometrial stromal tumors, this is a relative rarity in leiomyosarcomas (3.5% lymph node or adnexal metastases and 5.3% malignant cytology) (27). The diagnosis of carcinosarcoma is usually made by endometrial biopsy or curettage; appropriate preoperative referral to a gynecologic oncologist is made and lymph node sampling is accomplished at the time of hysterectomy. Conversely, most leiomyosarcomas are diagnosed after hysterectomy at the time of histologic review of the surgical specimen. More often than not, lymph node sampling is omitted from the procedure. This dichotomy in presentation of the two main uterine sarcomas was highlighted in a staging study published by the GOG (27). Fewer patients with leiomyosarcomas were enrolled in the study than those with the diagnosis of carcinosarcoma. Re-staging after primary surgery was an obstacle to enrollment in patients with leiomyosarcoma. Major et al. (27) therefore concluded that given the small number of positive lymph nodes in leiomyosarcomas, re-exploration for the sole purpose of staging is not recommended in patients with leiomyosarcomas. This approach was supported by Giuntoli (28) in an exhaustive review of patients with uterine leiomyosarcomas seen at the Mayo Clinic in Minnesota.

Kaku et al. (25) recommended staging laparotomy with lymph node sampling and peritoneal cytology based upon their review of 31 patients with adenosarcomas of the uterus accrued to a GOG staging study. Extrauterine spread was observed to the vagina, pelvic lymph nodes, peritoneal washings, parametria, and ovary in their study.

Extended Staging of Uterine Sarcomas

Since the most common sites of metastases for non-leiomyosarcoma uterine sarcomas are pelvic and para-aortic lymph nodes, studies such as computerized tomography (CT) of the abdomen and pelvis are probably not justified in patients with clinical stage I and II disease. On the other hand, if an extensive uterine mass is present, these evaluations may suggest a palliative rather than curative approach to the patient. Radionuclide bone scans and imaging of the brain are of little value in the absence of pulmonary metastases. Preoperative radiographs are helpful in excluding pulmonary metastases and are often indicated preoperatively in patients of advanced age.

The utility of chest tomography in uterine sarcomas has not been formally addressed, but should be considered in patients with high-grade lesions, especially if palliation rather than curative therapy seems appropriate based upon advanced age and/or poor performance status. Porter et al. (29) reviewed

600 patients with nonthoracic T2 soft-tissue sarcomas and concluded that routine chest CT identified metastases in 19.2% of patients but at a cost of $27,594 per patient with metastases. If scanning was limited to patients with high-grade histologies only, the cost per patient with metastases was reduced to $418 per patient with metastases. Since no specific data are in place for uterine sarcomas, CT scanning seems indicated in the triage of patients with high-grade sarcomas to differentiate between those with surgically-resectable and thus curable lesions and those with more extensive pelvic lesions, in whom the focus is control of symptoms.

ADJUVANT CHEMOTHERAPY IN EARLY UTERINE SARCOMAS

Carcinosarcomas

Although hysterectomy may be curative in a small proportion of patients with early carcinosarcomas of the uterus, therapy of these sarcomas has been largely unsuccessful. Reported 5-year survival rates in stage I disease seldom exceed 50%. Several drugs with phase II activity in the 20–30% range suggest a role for adjuvant chemotherapy in these malignancies. However, although the role of adjuvant chemotherapy has been established for treatment of rhabdomyosarcomas, osteosarcomas, and Ewing's sarcomas, Antman contends that it "remains controversial" in the setting of gynecologic sarcomas (30).

Several pilot studies have evaluated the use of adjuvant chemotherapy in early carcinosarcomas of the uterus. Hannigan et al. (31) treated 17 patients with adjuvant vincristine, actinomycin D, and cyclophosphamide (VAC) and compared them to 67 patients who received no adjuvant treatment. Nearly all patients with carcinosarcoma received pelvic radiotherapy postoperatively. Five-year survival for all patients in this study (including the 30% with non-carcinosarcomatous sarcomas) was 46.8% for those receiving chemotherapy versus 50.7% for those who did not. Interestingly, a similar study from the University of Kentucky (32) demonstrated a favorable outcome in four of five patients with early carcinosarcomas treated with postoperative VAC chemotherapy without radiation. In a study conducted by the GOG (33), patients with stage I disease treated with doxorubicin postoperatively had no better survival than controls undergoing surgery alone. In patients with early stage carcinosarcomas, 24 of 44 were progression-free and 23 were alive after adjuvant doxorubicin compared with 25 of 49 progression-free and 27 alive after surgery. Nearly 39% of the patients on this study received pelvic radiotherapy. In a different GOG study of adjuvant ifosfamide and cisplatin without pelvic radiotherapy (34), progression-free and overall survival were slightly better than those of the previous GOG doxorubicin adjuvant trial. Perhaps the greatest concern of the study was the large fraction of patients who developed pelvic (10/23, or 43.5%) or abdominal (15/23, or 65%) failures; presumably these were potentially preventable with postoperative radiotherapy to the pelvis or whole abdomen.

The GOG is presently engaged in an evaluation of adjuvant cisplatin/ifosfamide chemotherapy versus whole abdominal radiotherapy in patients with completely resected carcinosarcomas of the uterus (GOG protocol 150). Depending upon the results of this study, a trial of sequential, concomitant, or "sandwiched" chemo- and radiotherapy in such patients would be of interest.

Leiomyosarcomas

Pelvic radiotherapy did not improve outcome in patients with leiomyosarcomas treated as part of GOG protocol 20 (35); additionally, adjuvant doxorubicin failed to improve survival in the same study. To date, the use of adjuvant chemotherapy in sarcomas has been considered appropriate only in Ewing's, primitive neuroectodermal tumors, and rhabdomyosarcomas (36). Although individual trials fail to demonstrate a survival advantage for adjuvant chemotherapy in other soft tissue sarcomas, a recent meta-analysis does suggest a highly-significant improvement in overall and disease-free survival for adjuvant chemotherapy (37). Additionally, a cooperative Italian study utilizing 5'-epidoxorubicin and ifosfamide was strongly positive (38). Since GOG protocol 87F demonstrated superior activity of doxorubicin and ifosfamide in advanced or recurrent leiomyosarcomas of the uterus, a trial of 5'-epidox-orubicin and ifosfamide in the adjuvant would be highly interesting. In this uncommon tumor, it would be necessary to compare disease-free and overall survival to controls from previous trials. Since the risk of nodal metastases in early leiomyosarcomas of the uterus is low, formal staging should not be required in a study of adjuvant chemotherapy if CT evaluation is negative. If necessary, subjects could be strati-fied into "clinical" and "surgically-staged" stage I and II groups. This would improve accrual considerably since many of these patients are diagnosed postoperatively.

ADJUVANT RADIOTHERAPY IN UTERINE SARCOMAS

Carcinosarcomas

As noted previously, surgical therapy alone of early carci-nosarcomas has proven ineffective for long-term disease con-trol in at least half of patients with stage I and II disease. Adjuvant pelvic radiotherapy has been utilized for many years in these patients and effectively reduces pelvic and vaginal recurrences, but has not been convincingly shown to decrease disease-related mortality. Salazar et al. (39) recom-mended postoperative pelvic radiotherapy in early disease, noting a reduction in pelvic recurrences from 100% with sur-gery alone to 59% with postoperative pelvic radiotherapy. Similarly, DiSaia and Pecorelli (40) found that 8 of 10 patients treated with surgery alone had local recurrences. Perez et al. (41) reported a 44% local recurrence rate for sim-ilar patients. In a study by Spanos et al. (42), patients with carcinosarcoma limited to the uterus had a 5-year survival of 52% after surgery and radiotherapy; at a median 24 months, approximately 50% of patients were living.

Gerszten et al. (43) also advocated postoperative radio-therapy, noting a reduction of postoperative pelvic recur-rences from 35% in 31 patients treated with surgery alone to 3% (1 patient) among 29 who received radiation. Median sur-vival times for the two groups were 12 and 77 months, respec-tively. Sartori et al. (44) reported a 42% recurrence rate in patients with stage I and II carcinosarcomas; patients had a 2-year actuarial survival of 27%. In those receiving postoperative radiotherapy, 34.3% had recurrences compared with 45.5% treated with surgery alone.

Podczaski et al. (45) treated 27 patients with stage I or II carcinosarcomas and noted a 2-year survival rate of 52%. Three of 21 patients (14%) developed local recurrences after radiotherapy in comparison with five of ten patients treated with adjuvant chemotherapy with cisplatin or doxorubicin. Molpus et al. (46) found a survival advantage for postoperative pelvic radiotherapy, but only 12 patients with early stage cancers were analyzed. Pelvic recurrences were reduced from 87.5% to less than 10% with radiotherapy. In a review by Chi et al. (47), a similar reduction in pelvic recurrences was seen when radiotherapy was given postoperatively (6/28 or 21% in those treated with radiotherapy versus 5/10 or 50% treated with surgery alone), and 2-year survival for the radiotherapy group trended toward improvement (79% vs. 60%).

Leiomyosarcomas

As previously noted, pelvic radiotherapy did not improve outcome in patients with leiomyosarcomas treated as part of Gynecologic Oncology Group protocol 20, which randomized patients to adjuvant doxorubicin or no chemotherapy, but allowed pelvic radiation therapy at the discretion of the individual clinician (35). In this study, 19 of 23 patients (83%) who developed recurrences had the first evidence of disease occur outside the pelvis.

PALLIATIVE CHEMOTHERAPY IN UTERINE SARCOMAS

Carcinosarcomas

Hysterectomy with or without radiotherapy may be curative in a number of patients with carcinosarcoma limited to the uterus at the time of diagnosis, yet reported 5-year survival rates are typically in the 50% range. Thus, many patients will present with either advanced or recurrent carcinosarcomas for which chemotherapy represents perhaps the best option for palliation. Unfortunately, chemotherapy-induced responses are usually partial and of brief duration. Evaluation of chemotherapeutic agents in carcinosarcomas of the uterus has been hampered because many studies in the past failed to differentiate these cancers from other uterine or soft tissue sarcomas. The GOG first demonstrated the differential sensitivity of uterine sarcomas to drug therapy in a report wherein 25% of patients with metastatic leiomyosarcomas responded to doxorubicin, but only 15% of those with carcinosarcomas responded to the same therapy (50).

Conversely, cisplatin has definite activity in treatment of refractory carcinosarcomas, but has very limited effectiveness in leiomyosarcomas of the uterus. Thigpen et al. (51) reported a 19% response rate in chemotherapy-naive patients with carcinomsarcomas given cisplatin at dose of 50 mg/m^2 intravenously every 3 weeks.

Combination therapy may produce results more favorable than those obtained with single agent therapy. Baker et al. (52) reported a 23% response rate with 12% complete responses to a combination of cyclophosphamide, vincristine, doxorubicin, and dacarbazine. Hannigan et al. (53) also reported a 29% response rate (13.3% complete response) in patients with uterine sarcomas treated with cyclophosphamide, actinomycin-D, and vincristine.

Ifosfamide-based combination regimens showed promise in the management of soft tissue sarcomas. Response rates of 36% and 41% were reported by Schutte et al. (55) and Sledge et al. (56), respectively, in patients treated with combination ifosfamide and doxorubicin. Elias et al. (57) added dacarbazine to these drugs and observed responses in 45% of patients with advanced sarcomas. Ifosfamide therapy for advanced and metastatic carcinosarcomas of the uterus was associated with an unusually high response rate (34.8%) in a GOG trial (54).

In carcinosarcomas of the uterus, other combinations have yielded results no better than those obtained with cisplatin, doxorubicin, or ifosfamide as single agents. Muss et al. (58) reported a negative study of the GOG comparing doxorubicin to doxorubicin plus cyclophosphamide in uterine sarcomas. Omura et al. (59) reported the experience of the GOG in a group of patients with uterine sarcomas treated with doxorubicin with or without DTIC. Best response rate was 24% with no statistical difference between the two treatment arms. In a later GOG study, Currie et al. (60) reported a 15% rate of response in 32 patients treated with etoposide, hydroxyurea, and DTIC.

Combination therapy of soft tissue sarcomas has generally resulted in greater rates of response at the expense of myelotoxicity; no striking survival advantage has been reported. In three randomized trials, ifosfamide combinations have been compared with doxorubicin alone. In an Intergroup phase III trial of 170 patients reported by Antman et al. (61), MAID (doxorubicin, DTIC, and ifosfamide) was associated with significantly higher rates of both response and myelosuppression than doxorubicin and ifosfamide. Survival was significantly shorter in the three-drug arm and deaths were limited to patients over age 50. Similarly, an ECOG study (62) of doxorubicin alone versus doxorubicin plus ifosfamide showed greater response and myelosuppression in the combination arm with no overall survival difference. Finally, in a three-arm prospective study of the EORTC (63), there was no difference in response rates, remission duration, or survival among patients treated with doxorubicin alone, in combination with ifosfamide, or in combination with cyclophosphamide, vincristine, and DTIC. An increase in myelotoxicity and cardiotoxicity was observed in patients receiving doxorubicin in combination with ifosfamide.

In carcinosarcomas of the uterus, a randomized, phase III trial of ifosfamide versus ifosfamide plus cisplatin was conducted by the GOG. The response rate to the combination therapy was superior (54% vs. 36%), but neuro- and myelotoxicity was great enough in the combination arm to dampen enthusiasm for these drugs in this population. In addition, median survivals were 9.4 and 7.6 months with no identifiable advantage for the combination (64).

Future directions in the treatment of recurrent or metastatic carcinosarcomas of the uterus remain unclear.

Although Balcerzak et al. (65) found that only 12% of 48 patients with soft tissue sarcomas responded to paclitaxel 250 mg/m^2, a study of paclitaxel by Curtin et al. (66) demonstrated an 18.2% response rate in previously treated patients with carcinosarcomas. Furthermore, half of the responses were complete. Docetaxel therapy was associated with a response rate of 17% in a study of 29 patients with soft tissue sarcomas reported by van Hoesel (67). The GOG is presently engaged in a randomized trial of ifosfamide versus ifosfamide plus paclitaxel in patients with advanced or metastatic carcinosarcomas of the uterus.

Leiomyosarcomas

As noted above, few early chemotherapeutic trials distinguished between leiomyosarcomas and carcinosarcomas of the uterus. Omura et al. (50) compared doxorubicin alone or in combination with dacarbazine in uterine sarcomas. Twenty-five percent of patients with leiomyosarcomas responded to treatment whereas responses were observed in only 9.8% of those bearing carcinosarcomas. Similarly, when dacarbazine was added, the response rates for patients with the two tumors were 30% and 22.6%, respectively. In a later GOG trial (49), cisplatin administration was associated with a response rate of 18% in patients with doxorubicin-refractory carcinosarcomas but only 5.3% of patients with similarly treated leiomyosarcomas. Of 33 chemotherapy-naive patients with recurrent or metastatic leiomyosarcoma, only one partial response (3%) was observed with cisplatin administration in a GOG study (51). The differential sensitivity to chemotherapy in these two types of sarcomas resulted in segregation of leiomyosarcomas from carcinosarcomas in all subsequent GOG phase II drug studies.

Ifosfamide has proven to be an active drug in leiomyosarcomas in GOG trials. Among untreated patients, 17.2% responded to single-agent therapy (65), which compares with other drugs studied by the group. Etoposide administration was associated with a response rate of only 10.7% in patients previously exposed to other chemotherapy agents (66). In a study combining doxorubicin and ifosfamide, 30.3% of patients responded to therapy, but response duration was only 4 months and toxicity was of concern (67).

A phase II trial of paclitaxel in women with advanced or recurrent leiomyosarcomas of the uterus who had not received other chemotherapy was conducted by the GOG (68). The starting dose of paclitaxel was 175 mg/m^2/3 hours for 3 weeks. The starting dose of paclitaxel was reduced to 135 mg/m^2/3 hours in patients who had previously received radiotherapy. Of 33 patients evaluable for toxicity and response, there were only two complete responses of short duration. Toxicity was not noteworthy, suggesting that a higher dose of paclitaxel might deserve evaluation in these patients.

Endometrial Stromal Tumors

There is a paucity of literature regarding the chemotherapy of metastatic endometrial stromal sarcomas. As few as 150 cases occur annually in the United States. In a review from the Memorial Sloan-Kettering Cancer Center, Berchuck et al. (9) reported a 50% response rate to doxorubicin either alone or in combination with other drugs, in 10 patients with recurrent endometrial stromal sarcomas. Two partial responses were also recorded in women treated with vincristine, actinomycin, and cyclophosphamide or mitomycin and velban. Mansi et al. (69) from the Royal Marsden Hospital reported a partial response to cholorambucil therapy and one of three responses to cyclophosphamide, vincristine, adriamycin, and dacarbazine. In Omura et al.'s GOG study (50), doxorubicin alone or with dacarbazine was associated with a 20% response rate in "other" sarcomas, about half of which were endometrial stromal sarcomas. Similarly, when doxorubicin was given alone or with cyclophosphamide, 2 of 9 patients with "other" sarcomas had responses (58). In Piver et al.'s survey (70) of patients treated for recurrent endolymphatic stromal myosis, one complete response of 19-months duration was reported in a patient who received doxorubicin, cyclophosphamide, methotrexate, and megestrol acetate. Ten

other patients failed to respond to a variety of chemotherapeutic agents and combinations. Other reports are scattered
through the literature. Hoovis (71) reported a response to
cyclophosphamide in a single patient with recurrent endometrial stromal sarcoma, whereas 5-fluorouracil failed to induce
a response in two patients. Lehner et al. (72) reported a complete response following treatment with doxorubicin, vincristine, and cyclophosphamide. Goff et al. also reported a
favorable response with doxorubicin combination chemotherapy (8). While the best cytotoxic treatment for metastatic
endometrial stromal sarcoma may never be entirely clarified,
it appears that a combination containing doxorubicin would
be preferred. The observed activity of ifosfamide (73) in this
group of patients suggests that a combination of doxorubicin
and ifosfamide may be highly active as well.

Müllerian Adenosarcomas

There are few reports of chemotherapy treatments of recurrent or metastatic müllerian adenosarcoma. Verschraegen et
al. (74) reviewed the M.D. Anderson Cancer Center experience with these tumors and reported a very high rate of
response to cisplatin chemotherapy and cisplatin-chemora-
diotherapy.

HORMONAL THERAPY IN UTERINE SARCOMAS

Although the role of hormone therapy is clear in breast and
endometrial cancers, few uterine sarcomas contain sufficient
estrogen- or progesterone-receptor protein to influence therapy, the only exception being low-grade endometrial stromal
sarcomas or stromal nodules. Sutton et al. (75) found that a
large proportion of uterine sarcomas possessed estrogen and
progesterone receptors, but that the median concentrations
were substantially lower than those observed in breast or
endometrial cancers. Uniquely, low-grade endometrial stromal sarcomas are hormonally-responsive in roughly two-
thirds of cases.

Lantta et al. (76) published two cases of extensive intraperitoneal low-grade endometrial stromal sarcomas in complete remission with hormone therapy and associated with high concentrations of progesterone receptor. Three additional patients reported by Baker et al. (77) had partial responses or stabilization of disease on oral megestrol; all had progesterone receptor concentrations exceeding 674 fmol/mg. Piver et al. (70), in a collaborative survey of endolymphatic stromal myosis, recorded complete or partial responses to hormonal therapy in 6 of 13 patients (46%) treated with progestational agents.

MULTIMODALITY ADJUVANT THERAPY

Well-controlled, prospective treatment trials of consistent combination adjuvant therapy with radiation and modern chemotherapy are few. Since pelvic radiotherapy does not prevent distant metastases and adjuvant chemotherapy is associated with pelvic failures, such an approach is highly desirable. In a recent study from Sidney, Australia, Manolitsas et al. (78) piloted sequential postoperative tailored radiotherapy followed by cisplatin and epirubicin in 38 patients with stage I and II carcinosarcomas. Patients with surgically negative pelvic lymph nodes received vaginal vault radiotherapy and others received customized external beam therapy. Cisplatin and epirubicin were given at doses of 75 mg/m^2 each "sandwiched" around the radiotherapy administration. Four cycles of therapy were administered to patients with stage I and six cycles to those with more advanced disease. Twenty-seven of the 38 patients had stages IA–IC. Overall survival was 74% for the group with 95% of the patients who completed therapy alive and 90% disease-free at 26 months. Patients not completing protocol therapy had an overall survival of 47%. Such results hold promise for women with early carcinosarcomas. The toxicity of combination therapy in women of advanced age must be taken into consideration, however, and confirmatory trials are essential.

REFERENCES

1. Meredith RJ, Eisert DR, Kaka Z, Hodgson SE, Johnston GA Jr, Boutselis JG. An excess of uterine sarcomas after pelvic irradiation. *Cancer* 1986; 58:2003–2007.

2. Nielsen SN, Podratz KC, Scheithauer BW, O'Brien PC. Clinical-pathologic analysis of uterine malignant mixed müllerian tumors. *Gynecol Oncol* 1988; 34:372–378.

3. Zelmanowicz A, Hildesheim A, Sherman MA, Sturgeon SR, Kurman RJ, Barrett RJ, Berman ML, Mortel R, Twiggs LB, Wilbanks GD, Brinton LA. Evidence for a common etiology for endometrial carcinomas and malignant mixed müllerian tumors. *Gynecol Oncol* 1998; 69:253–257.

4. Clement PB, Scully. Müllerian adenosarcoma of the uterus: clinicopathologic analysis of ten cases of distinctive type of müllerian mixed tumor. *Cancer* 1974 34:1138–1149.

5. Clement PB, Oliva E, Young RH. Müllerian adenosarcoma of the uterine corpus associated with tamoxifen therapy: report of six cases and review of tamoxifen-associated endometrial lesions. *Int J Gynecol Pathol* 1996; 15:222–229.

6. Bartsich EG, Bowe ET, Moore JG. Leiomyosarcoma of the uterus. *Obstet Gynecol* 1968; 32:101–106.

7. Christopherson WM, Williamson FO, Gray LA. Leiomyosarcoma of the uterus. *Cancer* 1972; 29:1512–1517.

8. Goff BA, Rice LW, Fleischhacker D, Muntz HG, Falkenberry SS, Nikrui N, Fuller AF. Uterine leiomyosarcoma and endometrial stromal sarcoma: lymph node metastases and sites of recurrence. *Gynecol Oncol* 1993; 50:105.

9. Berchuck A, Rubin SC, Hoskins WJ, Saigo PE, Pierce VK, Lewis JL Jr. Treatment of endometrial stromal tumors. *Gynecol Oncol* 1990; 36:60–65.

10. Mansi JL, Ramachandra S, Wiltshaw E, Fisher C. Endometrial stromal sarcomas. *Gynecol Oncol* 1990; 36:113–118.

11. Lehner LM, Miles PA, Enck RE. A complete remission of widely metastatic endometrial stromal sarcoma following combination chemotherapy. *Cancer* 1979; 433:1189.

12. Silverberg SG, Major FJ Blessing JA, Fetter B, Askin FB, Liao S-Y, and Miller A. Carcinosarcoma (malignant mixed mesodermal tumor of the uterus). *Int J Gynecol Pathol* 1990; 9:1–19.

13. Knocke TH, Kucera H, Dorfler D, Pokrajac B, Potter R. Results of postoperative radiotherapy in the treatment of sarcoma of the corpus uteri. *Cancer* 1998; 83:1972–1979.

14. Norris HJ, Taylor HB. Mesenchymal tumors of the uterus. I. A clinical and pathological study of 53 endometrial stromal tumors. *Cancer* 1966; 19:755–766.

15. Bocklage T, Lee KR, Belinson JL Uterine müllerian adenosarcoma following adenomyoma in a woman on tamoxifen therapy. *Gynecol Oncol* 1993; 44:104–109.

16. Kempson RL, Bari W. Uterine sarcomas: Classification, diagnosis, and prognosis. *Human Pathol* 1970; 1:331–349.

17. Hill MA, Araya JC, Eckert MW, Gillespie AT, Hunt JD, Levine EA. Tumor specific Epstein-Barr virus infection is not associated with leiomyosarcoma in human immunodeficiency virus negative individuals. *Cancer* 1997; 80:204–210.

18. Iwata J, Fletcher CD. Immunohistochemical detection of cytokeratin and epithelial membrane antigen in leiomyosarcoma: a systematic study of 100 cases. *Pathol Internat* 2000; 50:7–14.

19. Layfield LJ, Liu K, Dodge R, Barsky SH. Uterine smooth muscle tumors: utility of classification by proliferation, ploidy, and prognostic markers versus traditional histopathology. *Arch Pathol Lab Med* 2000; 124:221–227.

20. Yoo J, Robinson RA, Lee JY. H-ras and K-ras gene mutations in primary human soft tissue sarcoma: concomitant mutations of the ras genes. *Modern Pathol* 1999; 12:775–80.

21. Zhai Y, Kobayashi Y, Mori A, Orii A, Nikaido T, Konishi I, Fuji S. Expression of steroid receptors, Ki-67, and p53 in uterine leiomyosarcomas. *Int J Gynecol Pathol* 1999; 18:20–28.

22. Blom R, Guerrieri C, Stal O, Malmstrom H, Simonsen E. Leiomyosarcoma of the uterus: clinicopathologic, DNA flow cytometric, p53, and mdm-2 analysis of 49 cases. *Gynecol Oncol* 1998; 68:54–61.

23. Konomoto T, Fukuda T, Hayashi K, Kumazawa J, Tsuneyoshi M. Leiomyosarcoma in soft tissue: examination of p53 status and cell proliferating factors in different locations. *Human Pathol* 1998; 29:74–81.

24. Chang KL, Crabtree GS, Lim-Tan SK, Kempson RL, Hendrickson MR. Primary uterine endometrial stromal neoplasms; a clinicopathologic study of 117 cases. *Am J Surg Pathol* 1990; 1415:415–438.

25. Kaku T, Silverberg SG, Major FJ, Miller A, Fetter B, Brady MF. Adenosarcoma of the uterus: Gynecologic Oncology Group clinicopathologic study of 31 cases. *Int J Gynecol Pathol* 1992; 11:75–88.

26. Yamada DS, Burger RA, Brewster WR, Anton D, Kohler MF, Monk BJ. Pathologic variables and survival for patients with surgically evaluated carcinosarcoma of the uterus. *Cancer* 2000; 88:2782–2786.

27. Major FJ, Blessing JA, Silverberg SG, Morrow CP, Creasman WT, Currie JL, Yordan E, Brady MF. Prognostic factors in early-stage uterine sarcoma. *Cancer* 1993; 71:1702–1709.

28. Giuntoli R Jr. Personal communication.

29. Porter GA, Cantor SB, Ahmad SA, Lenert JT, Ballo MT, Hunt KK, Feig BW, Pater SR, Benjamin RS, Pollock RE, Pisters PW. Cost-effectiveness of staging computed tomography of the chest in patients with T2 soft tissue sarcomas. *Cancer* 2002; 94:197–204.

30. Antman K. Adjuvant therapy of sarcomas of soft tissue. *Sem Oncol* 1997; 24:556–60.

31. Hannigan EV, Freedmans RS, Rutledge FN. Adjuvant chemotherapy in early uterine sarcoma. *Gynecol Oncol* 1983; 15:56–64.

32. van Nagell JR, Hanson MB, Donaldson ES, Gallion HH. Adjuvant vincristine, dactinomycin, and cyclophosphamide therapy in stage I uterine sarcomas. *Cancer* 1986; 57:1451–54.

33. Omura GA, Blessing JA, Major F, Lifschitz S, Ehrlich CE, Mangan C, Beecham J, Park R, Silverberg S. A randomized clinical trial of adjuvant adriamycin in uterine sarcomas:

Gynecologic Oncology Group study. *J Clin Oncol* 1985; 3:1240–1245.

34. Sutton GP, Blessing JA, Carson LF, Lentz SS, Whitney CW, Gallion HH. Adjuvant ifosfamide, mesna, and cisplatin in patients with completely resected stage I or II carcinosarcomas of the uterus: a study of the Gynecologic Oncology Group. *J Clin Oncol* 1997; 16:47–54.

35. Hornback N, Omura GA, Major FJ. Observations on the use of adjuvant radiation therapy in patients with stage I and II uterine sarcoma. *Int J Rad Oncol Biol Phys* 1986; 12:2127–2130.

36. Mazanet R, Antman KH. Adjuvant therapy for sarcomas. *Sem Oncol* 1991; 18:603–612.

37. Tierny J. Meta-analysis of adjuvant sarcoma trials. *Lancet* 1997; 350:1647–1650.

38. Frustaci S, Gherlinzoni F, De Paoli A, Bonetti M, Azzarelli A, Comandone A, Olmi P, Buonadonna A, Pignatti G, Barbieri E, Apice G, Zmerly H, Serraino D, Picci P. Adjuvant chemotherapy for adult soft tissue sarcomas of the extremities and girdles: results of the Italian randomized cooperative trial. *J Clin Oncol* 2001; 19:1238–1247.

39. Salazar OM, Bonfiglio TA, Patten SF, Keller BE, Feldstein, Dunne ME, Rudolph JH. Uterine sarcomas. An analysis of failures with special emphasis on the use of adjuvant radiation therapy. *Cancer* 1978; 42:1161–1170.

40. DiSaia PJ, Pecorelli S. Gynecologic sarcomas. *Sem Surg Oncol.* 1994; 10:369–73.

41. Perez CA, Askin F, Baglan RJ, Kao M-S, Kraus FT, Perez BM, Williams CF, Weiss D. Effects of irradiation on mixed müllerian tumors of the uterus. *Cancer* 1979; 43:1274–1284.

42. Spanos WJ, Peters LJ, Oswald MJ. Patterns of recurrence in malignant mixed müllerian tumor of the uterus. *Cancer* 1986; 57:155–159.

43. Gerszten K, Faul C, Kounelis S, Huang Q, Kelley J, Jones MW. The impact of aduvant radiotherapy on carcinosarcoma of the uterus. *Gynecol Oncol* 1998; 68:8–13.

44. Sartori E, Bazzurini L, Gadducci A, Landoni F, Lissoni A, Maggin T, Zola P, La Face B. Carcinosarcoma of the uterus: clinicopathologic multicenter CTF study. *Gynecol Oncol* 1997; 67:70–75.

45. Podczaski ES, Woomert CA, Stevens Jr CW, Manetta A, Larson JE, Zaino RJ, Mortel R. Management of malignant mixed mesodermal tumors of the uterus. *Gynecol Oncol* 1989; 32:240–244.

46. Molpus KL, Redlin-Frazier S, Reed G, Burnett LS, Jones HW III. Postoperative pelvic irradiation in early stage uterine mixed müllerian tumors. *EuropJ Gynecol Oncol* 1999; 19:541–546.

47. Chi DS, Mychalczak B, Saigo PE, Rescigno J, Brown CL. The role of whole-pelvic irradiation in the treatment of early-stage uterine carcinosarcoma. *Gynecol Oncol* 1997; 65:493–498

48. Badib AO, Vongtama V, Kurohara SS, et al. Radiotherapy in the treatment of sarcomas of the corpus uteri. *Cancer* 1969; 24:724–729.

49. Thigpen JT, Blessing JA, Wilbanks GD. Cisplatin as second-line chemotherapy in the treatment of advanced or recurrent leiomyosarcomas of the uterus: phase II trial of the Gynecologic Oncology Group. *Am J Clin Oncol* 1986; 9:18–20.

50. Omura GA, Major FJ, Blessing JA, Sedlacek T, Thigpen JT, Creasman WT, Zaino RT. A randomized study of adriamycin with and without dimethyl triazenoimidazole carboxamide in advanced uterine sarcomas. *Cancer* 1983; 62:626–632.

51. Thigpen JT, Blessing JA, Beecham J, Homesley H, Yordan E. Phase II trial of cisplatin as first-line chemotherapy in patients with advanced or recurrent uterine sarcomas: Gynecologic Group Study. *J Clin Oncol* 1991; 9:1962–1966.

52. Baker TR, Piver MS, Caglar H, Piedmonte M. Prospective trial of cisplatin, adriamycin, and dacarbazine in metastatic mixed mesodermal sarcomas of the uterus and ovary. *Am J Clin Oncol* 1991; 14:246–250.

53. Hannigan EV, Freedman RS, Elder KW, Rutledge FN. Treatment of advanced uterine sarcoma with vincristine, actinomycin D, and cyclophosphamide. *Gynecol Oncol* 1983; 15:224–229.

54. Sutton GP, Blessing JA, Rosenshein N, Photopulos G, DiSaia PJ. Phase II trial of ifosfamide and mesna in mixed mesodermal tumors of the uterus (a Gynecologic Oncology Group study). *Am J Obstet Gynecol*, 1989; 161:309–312.

55. Schutte J, Dombernowsky P, Santoro A. Adriamycin and ifosfamide, a new effective combination in advanced soft tissue sarcoma; preliminary report of a phase II study of the EORTC soft tissue and bone sarcoma group [abstr]. *Proc Am Soc Clin Oncol* 1986; 5:145.

56. Sledge G, Loehrer P, Brenner D, Hainsworth J, Martello O. Treatment of adanced soft tissue sarcomas with ifosfamide and adriamycin [abstr]. *Proc Am Soc Clin Oncol* 1988; 7:273.

57. Elias AD, Ryan L, Sulkes A, Collins J, Aisner J, Antman KH. Response to mesna doxorubicin, ifosfamide and dacarbazine in 108 patients with metastatic or unresectable sarcoma and no prior chemotherapy. *J Clin Oncol* 1989; 7:1208–1216.

58. Muss HB, Bundy B, DiSaia PJ, Homesley HD, Fowler WC, Creasman W, Yordan E. Treatment of recurrent or advanced uterine sarcoma: A randomized trial of doxorubicin versus doxorubicin and cyclophosphamide (phase III trial of the Gynecologic Oncology Group). *Cancer* 1985; 55:1648–1653.

59. Omura GA, Major FJ, Blessing JA, Sedlacek TV, Thigpen JT, Creasman WT, Zaino RJ. A randomized study of adriamycin with and without dimethyl triazenoimidazole carboxamide in advanced uterine sarcomas. *Cancer* 1983; 52:626–632.

60. Currie JL, Blessing JA, McGehee R, Soper JT, Berman M. Phase II trial of hydroxyurea, dacarbazine (DTIC), and etoposide (VP-16) in mixed mesodermal tumors of the uterus: a Gynecol Oncol Group study. *Gynecologic Oncology* 1996; 61:94–96.

61. Antman KH, Blum RH, Wilson RE, Corson JM, Greenberger JS, Amato DA, Canellos GP, Frei E. Survival of patients with localized high-grade soft tissue sarcoma with multimodality therapy. A matched control study. *Cancer* 1983; 51:396–401.

62. Blum RH, Edmonson J, Ryan L, Pelletier L. Efficacy of ifosfamide in combination with doxorubicin for the treatment of metastatic soft-tissue sarcoma. The Eastern Cooperative Oncology Group. *Cancer Chemo Pharmacol* 1993; 31(supp):s238–240.

63. Santoro A, Tursz T, Mouridsen H, Verweij J, Steward W, Somers R, Buesa J, Casali P, Spooner D, Rankin E. Doxorubicin versus CYVADIC versus doxorubicin plus ifosfamide in first-line treatment of advanced soft tissue sarcomas: a randomized study of the European Organization for Research and Treatment of Cancer Soft Tissue and Bone Sarcoma Group. *J Clin Oncol* 1995; 13:1537–1545.

64. Sutton GP, BrunettoVL, Kilgore L, Soper JT, McGehee R, Olt G, Lentz SS, Sarosky J, and Hsiu JG. A phase III trial of ifosfamide with or without cisplatin in carcinosarcoma of the uterus: A Gynecologic Oncology Group study. *Gynecol Oncol* 2000; 79:147–153.

65. Balcerzak SP, Benedetti, Weiss GR, Natale RB. A phase II trial of paclitaxel in patients with advanced soft tissue sarcomas. A Southwest Oncology Group study. *Cancer* 1995; 76:2248–2252.

66. Curtin JP, Blessing JA, Soper JT, DeGeest K. Paclitaxel in the treatment of carcinosarcoma of the uterus: A Gynecologic Oncology Group Study. *Gynecol Oncol* 2001; 83:268–270.

67. van Hoesel QG, Verweij J, Catimel G, Clavel M, Kerbrat P van Ooterom AT, Kerger J, Tursz T, van Glabbeke M, van Pottelberghe C. Phase II study with docetaxel (Taxotere) in advanced soft tissue sarcomas of the adult. EORTC Soft Tissue and Bone Sarcoma Group. *Ann Oncol* 1994; 5:539–542.

68. Sutton GP, Blessing JA, Barrett RJ, McGehee R. Phase II trial of ifosfamide and mesna in leiomyosarcoma of the uterus: a Gynecologic Oncology Group study. *Am J Obstet Gynecol* 1992; 166; 556–559.

69. Slayton RE, Blessing JA, Angel C, Berman M. A phase II clinical trial of etoposide in the management of advanced or recurrent leiomyosarcoma of the uterus: A Gynecologic Oncology Group trial. *Cancer Treat Rep* 1987; 71:1303–1304.

70. Sutton GP, Blesing JA, Malfetano JH. Ifosfamide and doxorubicin in the treatment of advanced leiomyosarcomas of the uterus: A Gynecologic Oncology Group study. *Gynecologic Oncology* 1996; 62:226–229.

71. Sutton GP, Blessing JA, Ball HG. A phase II study of paclitaxel in leiomyosarcoma of the uterus: A Gynecologic Oncology Group study. *Gynecol Oncol* 1999; 74:346–349.

72. Mansi JL, Ramachandra S, Wiltshaw E, Fisher C. Case report: endometrial stromal sarcomas. *Gynecol Oncol* 1990; 36:113–118.

73. Piver MS, Rutledge FN, Copeland L, Webster K, Blumenson L, Suh O. Uterine endolymphatic stromal myosis. *Obstet Gynecol* 1984; 63:725–745.

74. Hoovis ML. Response of endometrial stromal sarcoma to cyclophophamide. *Am J Obstet Gynecol* 1970; 108:1072–1088.

75. Lehner LM, Miles PA, Enck RE. Complete remission of widely metastatic endometrial stromal sarcoma following combination chemotherapy. *Cancer* 1979; 433:1189–1194.

76. Sutton GP, Blessing JA, DiSaia PJ, Rosenshein N. Ifosfamide treatment of recurrent or metastatic endometrial stromal sarcomas previously unexposed to chemotherapy: a study of the Gynecologic Oncology Group. *Obstet Gynecol* 1996; 87:747–750.

77. Verschraegen CF, Vasuratna A, Edwards CL, Kudelka AP, Wharton JT, Freedman RS, Silva EG, Benjapibal M, Torns C, Kavanagh JJ. Clinicopathologic analysis of müllerian adenosarcomas. *Proc Am Soc Clin Oncol* 1998; 17:1452.

78. Sutton GP, Stehman FB, Michael H, Young PCM, Ehrlich CE. Estrogen and progesterone receptors in uterine sarcomas. *Obstet Gynecol* 1986; 68:709–714.

79. Lantta M, Kahanpaa K, Karkkainen J, Lehtovirta P, Wahlstrom T, Widholm O. Estradiol and progesterone receptors in two cases of endometrial stromal sarcoma. *Gynecol Oncol* 1984; 18:233–239.

80. Baker TR, Piver MS, Lele SB, Tsukada Y. Stage I uterine adenosarcoma: a report of six cases. *J Surg Oncol* 1988; 37:128–132.

81. Manolitsas T, Wain GV, Williams KE, Hacker NF. Multimodality therapy for patients with clinical stage I and II malignant mixed müllerian tumors of the uterus. *Cancer* 2001; 91:1437–1443.

18

Hormone Replacement in the Patient with Uterine Cancer

KATHLEEN LIN
New York Presbyterian Hospital/New York Weill
Cornell Center, New York, New York, U.S.A.

CAROLYN D. RUNOWICZ
St. Luke's-Roosevelt Hospital Center and
Women's Health Service Line of Continuum
Health Partners, Inc., New York, New York, U.S.A.

Although endometrial cancer (EC) is the most common gynecologic cancer in women, the majority of the cancers are early stage. Since the overall 5-year survival rate for patients with stage I disease is 86%, the number of women who have survived EC represents an enlarging and ever-increasing population of cancer survivors (1). The question of estrogen replacement therapy (ERT) for the relief of menopausal symptoms, prevention of osteoporosis, and colon cancer becomes evermore relevant for this group of women. Because of shared epidemiologic and genetic risk factors, woman with EC may also be at increased risk for breast cancer, thus further complicating considerations for ERT or hormone replacement theraphy (HRT) in these patients.

Osteoporosis affects more than 22 million U.S. women, resulting in approximately 1.5 million fractures a year, including 250,000 hip fractures which carries great morbidity and mortality. As many as 20% of women are affected by postmenopausal osteoporosis within 15 to 20 years of menopause, and at least 75% of bone loss during this period is attributable to lack of estrogen, not to aging (2). A quarter of patients over the age of 50 die within a year after hip fracture. Estrogen has an antiresorptive effect on bone by inhibiting osteoclast activity and ERT may reduce fractures by 50% (4). As shown in the Postmenopausal Estrogen/Progestin Interventions (PEPI) trial, which included 875 postmenopausal women randomized to ERT (conjugated equine estrogen, 0.625 mg/day) or combination estrogen and progesterone replacement therapy (HRT), those taking hormones actually had increases in the bone mineral density of vertebrae from 3.5% to 5% and in the hip of 1.7%. In contrast, the placebo group lost an average of 1.7% in vertebrae and 1.8% in hip bone mineral density (5). 17β-estradiol (at least 1.0 mg/day) administered cyclically for 23 of 28 days for 18 months also showed a significant increase in spinal trabecular bone density of 1.8–2.5% in a dose-dependent fashion. The addition of calcium to ERT/HRT further enhances the positive effect on bone mineral density (6).

ERT/HRT clearly has a beneficial role not only in the preservation of bone, but also in reversing the worsening progression of osteoporosis. However, other pharmacologic agents are available which are comparable or better at preventing and treating osteoporosis. Bisphosphonates resemble estrogen in inhibiting osteoclast activity and preventing further bone breakdown. Alendronate has been approved by the FDA for the prevention and treatment of osteoporosis. Studies reveal an increase in bone mineral density of 6% at the hip and 8.8% at the spine after 3 years of treatment.

Furthermore, there was a 48% reduction in vertebral fractures. Risedronate has been shown to reduce the risk of nonvertebral fractures in several clinical trials (7). Raloxifene, a nonsteroidal benzothiophene, is a selective estrogen-receptor modulator that has been shown to increase bone mineral density. Studies have demonstrated a 2.4% increase for the lumbar spine, 2.4% for the total hip, and 2.0% for the total body when used at doses of 60 mg/day. In contrast, the placebo group lost an average of 0.8% in bone mineral density, both at the lumbar spine and hip over the 24 months of study (9–11). Furthermore, a 75% reduction in the risk of breast cancer has been reported at 4 years. Calcitonin can also be considered a second-line treatment for osteoporosis in a patient who is not a candidate for the aforementioned therapies (7). Lastly, exercise and a diet supplemented by 1500 mg/day of elemental calcium and 400 IU/day of vitamin D can be adjuncts to other medications for osteoporosis or as sole therapy in elderly women (7).

Colorectal cancers are the third leading cause of cancer deaths in woman (1). In the Women's Health Initiative study, colorectal cancers were reduced by 37% (19). Although there are biologically plausible mechanisms to explain this protective effect, there are other lifestyle and pharmacologic intervention strategies to prevent colon cancer. Approximately 90% of all colorectal cancers are thought to be preventable, based on temporal and international variations and existing approaches to prevention and early detection (1).

Cardiovascular disease, including coronary heart disease (CHD) and stroke, accounts for more deaths among women each year than any other disease, including cancer (12). Based on observational studies, ERT/HRT use, particularly long-term use, has been associated with a decreased overall mortality (RR, 0.27; 95% CI, 0.1, 0.71), which has been attributed to its reversal of harmful postmenopausal cardiovascular pathophysiology (13,14). As estrogen and progesterone levels decrease with menopause, lipid profiles worsen with an increase in low-density lipoproteins (LDL) and a reduction of high-density lipoproteins (HDL). Both conjugated equine estrogens, as used in the PEPI trial, and newer synthetic estrogens, such as 17β-estradiol alone or in combination with different progesterones, result in an increase in HDL, a decrease in LDL, a decrease in total cholesterol, and an increase in triglycerides (14,16). Observational studies have found lower rates of coronary heart disease in post-menopausal woman who take estrogen than in women who did not. However, this potential benefit was not confirmed in recent clinical trials.

The Heart and Estrogen/Progestin Replacement Group Study (HERS) was the first large prospective, randomized placebo-controlled clinical trial of HRT for the secondary prevention of coronary heart disease (17). Conjugated equine estrogens and medroxy-progesterone acetate (0.625 mg/2.5 mg daily) were used to prevent secondary coronary outcomes, i.e., myocardial infarction or CHD death, in postmenopausal women with established coronary artery disease. No significant difference in nonfatal myocardial infarction or coronary heart disease death was found among the treatment and control groups (RR, 0.99; 95% CI, 0.8–1.22). An unexpected finding was an increased rate of coronary heart disease events in the first year of HRT use, despite a more favorable cholesterol profile in the HRT users. By years 4 and 5, however, CHD events were found to be lower for the HRT group than the placebo group. Furthermore, a higher incidence of venous thromboembolism (RR, 2.89; 95% CI, 1.50–5.58) and gallbladder disease (RR, 1.38; 95% CI, 1.00–1.92) were found in the treatment groups. Based on a median follow-up of 4 years, the study concluded that HRT did not reduce the overall rate of coronary heart disease events in postmenopausal women with established coronary disease.

The Estrogen Replacement and Atherosclerosis (ERA) trial also examined the effect of ERT/HRT on patients with existing coronary atherosclerosis by angiography (18). Women with >30% stenosis in one or more coronary arteries were randomized to conjugated equine estrogens alone, conjugated equine estrogens/medroxyprogesterone acetate, or placebo. Despite a significant improvement in cholesterol profiles, no difference was found in the progression of atherosclerosis or clinical coronary events. The authors concluded that such women should not use estrogen replacement with an expectation of cardiovascular benefit

The third study refuting the once universally believed benefical effect of ERT/HRT on cardiovascular disease is the large, randomized prospective Women's Health Initiative that recently reported a higher rate of coronary heart disease, stroke, and thromboembolic events in HRT users without pre-existing CHD (19).

At the present time, ERT alone or in combination with progesterone (i.e., HRT) is considered by many to be contraindicated in survivors of EC because of the fear that estrogens may accelerate the growth of occult disease. Only a handful of studies have investigated the important issue of ERT/HRT after primary treatment for EC (Table 1). Although in aggregate, no increase in rates of recurrence or death have been reported in these studies, these reports are limited by small sample size, short follow-up, and retrospective trial design (20–23). In 1986, Creasman et al. were the first to address this issue when they published retrospective data on 221 patients treated surgically for stage I EC (20). 47 patients received estrogen postsurgery, with the remaining 174 patients serving as controls. 75% of the estrogen users received either vaginal estrogen alone or combined vaginal and oral estrogen, while only 7 of the 47 patients received only oral estrogen. The interval to starting estrogen was 0 to 81 months (median, 15 months) after primary cancer therapy and the length of HRT use varied from 3 to 84 months (median, 26 months). The median follow up period was approximately 3 years after initiating therapy in the estrogen users.

The study retrospectively matched the stage, grade, depth of invasion, nodal metastasis, peritoneal cytology, and hormone receptor status between the estrogen and non-estrogen users. In detail, 64% of estrogen users and 67% of non-estrogen users were stage IA, while the remainder were stage IB. 39% of estrogen users and 50% of non-estrogen users had moderate or poor grade tumors. 2% of estrogen users and 7% of nonestrogen users had pelvic or para-aortic nodal metastases, while 20% of users and 14% of non-users showed posi-

Table 1 Effect of Hormone Replacement Therapy on Endometrial Cancer Recurrence

Study	No. of Subjects	Stage					Interval to Treatment Postsurgery (mo)	Treatment Duration (mo)	Duration of Follow-up (mo)	Recurrences
		IA	IB	IC	II	III				
Creasman et al. (20)	47	30	17	—	—	—	0–81	3–84	6–84	1 (22 mo)
Lee et al. (21)	44	24	20	—	—	—	1–>60	>2	25–150	0
Chapman et al. (22)	62	—	60	—	2	—	0–108	>3	3–107	2 (24 mo, 32 mo)
Suriano et al. (23)	75[a] / 228[a] (198)[b]	14	44	6	7	4	0–>12	Not stated	18–245	2

[a]Contains 30 patients from Chapman's study.
[b]Excludes double counting of 30 patients.

tive peritoneal cytology. The majority of patients had superficial invasion of the myometrium (not defined). None of these factors was significantly different between the two groups. However, the number of patients in this study was very small for such a subset analysis.

Their result showed a 2.1% (1 patient) recurrence rate in the estrogen-treated group compared to 14.9% (26 patients) in the estrogen-untreated group, suggesting that the groups were not evenly matched. Of the 26 patients with recurrence in non-estrogen users, 16 died from their disease. Furthermore, in this group, 10 other patients died of intercurrent diseases. Based on small sample size and short follow-up, the authors concluded that estrogen provided a protective effect as noted by a significantly longer disease-free survival in the treated group. However, the methodologic limitations of this study limit the significance of these results.

A second study addressing the issue of ERT in survivors of stage I EC found no recurrences or deaths in the group using ERT (44/144 patients) after complete surgical resection (21). On the other hand, an 8% recurrence rate was reported among non-estrogen users, but there were no deaths from recurrent disease. In fact, the 8 deaths reported in the study were due to intercurrent diseases, the leading cause being myocardial infarctions (5) followed by a second primary cancer (3). They concluded that estrogen use was safe in low-risk, early stage EC survivors. They reinforced the cardioprotective effects of estrogen by highlighting that none of the estrogen users died of myocardial infarctions.

The groups were not evenly matched, as all estrogen users had disease ≥ stage IB grade 2, and of the non-estrogen users, only 12/99 had grade 3 tumors. Another methodologic limitation of this study was the great variability in the interval between surgery and initiation of ERT. While the majority (57%) started within 12 months of surgery, 13% did not initiate therapy until 5 years after surgery, when recurrence risk can be considered equivalent to the general population. One advantage of this study over the previous study was that all the estrogen replacement users took oral estrogen rather than an assortment of oral and/or vaginal preparations. Also, the dosages of estrogen were clearly reported to be 0.625 or 1.25 mg every day for 25 days each month.

In 1996, Chapman et al. reported a retrospective, case-control study that included 62 patients who received ERT, the majority (60%) starting less than 12 months from initial surgical treatment for EC (22). Oral estrogens were used predominantly (92%) and half opted for simultaneous progesterone therapy. These cases were matched to 61 patients with EC who did not receive ERT. The great majority of patients from both groups were stage IA or 1B (87% of ERT users and 71% of controls); however, estrogen users tended to have earlier-stage disease with only 3% stage II and 10% grade 3, while the controls had 15% stage II and 16% grade 3. Furthermore, the estrogen users had a statistically significant less depth of myometrial invasion than the controls, had longer follow-up periods (57 vs. 39 months), and were generally healthier with less co-morbidities. These discrepancies demonstrate the patient and investigator bias introduced into retrospective observational studies.

3.2% of patients (2/62) in the ERT group as compared to 9.8% of controls (6/61) had recurrent disease. In the ERT group, one patient had stage IA group 2 disease, while the other had stage IB grade 1 disease. In the controls, one patient with recurrence had stage IIB grade 1, while the others had less advanced disease. Recurrence occurred within an average of 28 months after initial treatment. In comparing deaths, one patient in the ERT group versus two patients in the control group died due to recurrent disease. There was one death in the ERT group and two deaths in the control group from co-morbid illness(es). Overall, the authors concluded that the ERT group had a better disease-free survival than the controls, but this result was not significant given the small numbers in the study. As noted, this study suffers from the same methodologic limitations as those previously discussed (20,21).

A retrospective case-control study by Suriano et al. reported the long-term followup of a cohort of patients (23). They expanded the cohort of patients by including patients with stage III disease. 30 of these patients were included in the Chapman et al. report (22). It is unclear what criteria the authors used in selecting these 30 patients from their prior report. 75 treatment-control pairs were compared to 130 women with stage I, II, or III EC who received estrogen with or without progesterone. Nearly 60% of the patients were stage IB and the great majority (>90%) had endometrioid adenocarcinomas. Approximately 73% of the patients started hormone replacement ≤12 months from surgery.

Over a mean interval of 83 months, 2 recurrences were detected in the treatment group, one of whom died of disease, while the other was alive and without evidence of disease. In the control group, 11 recurrences were reported over a 69-month mean interval of follow-up, of which 1 resulted in death due to a distant recurrence, 5 were alive and without evidence of disease, and 3 were alive with disease. The authors concluded that ERT with or without progesterone does not increase the rate of recurrence and/or death among survivors of EC. However, this study has methodologic limitations due to its small sample size, retrospective design, and investigator bias.

The American College of Obstetricians and Gynecologists issued a Committee Opinion in 2000 that stated that the effect of HRT on the recurrence risk of EC is unknown. It further stated that in the absence of well-designed studies, the selection of appropriate candidates for estrogen replacement should be based on prognostic indicators, including depth of invasion, degree of differentiation, and cell type. These predictors can assist the physician in describing the risks of recurrent tumors to the patient in determining the amount of risk she is willing to assume. The Committee Opinion concludes that the decision to prescribe HRT for a patient with a history of EC should be based on the patient's perceived benefits and risks after careful counseling (24).

CONCLUSION

Routine use of ERT/HRT (either estrogen alone or estrogen with progesterone) is not recommended for women who have had EC. Randomized controlled trials are required to guide recommendations for this group of women. The Gynecologic Oncology Group has a study underway which is addressing this issue. Women who have had EC are at risk of recurrence. Since women with EC also share epidemiologic risk factors with women with breast cancer, they are at increased risk for breast cancer. The potential effect of ERT/HRT on these outcomes in women with EC has not been determined in methodologically sound studies. Postmenopausal women with EC should be encouraged to consider alternatives to ERT/HRT for the control of symptoms or prevention of osteoporosis (25–27). Only in women with symptoms not controlled by non-hormonal treatment strategies should ERT be considered.

REFERENCES

1. Cancer Facts & Figures 2002. American Cancer Society. Atlanta, Georgia.

2. Riggs BL, Melton LJ III. Involutional osteoporosis. *N Engl J Med* 1986; 314:1676–1686.

3. http://www.nof.org/osteoporosis/stats.htm.

4. Ettinger B, Genant HK, Cann CE. Long-term estrogen replacement therapy prevents bone loss and fractures. *Ann Intern Med* 1985; 2:319–324.

5. Effects of hormone therapy on bone mineral density: results from the postmenopausal estrogen/progestin intervention (PEPI) trial. The Writing Group for the PEPI. *JAMA* 1996; 276:1389–1396.

6. Ettinger B, Genant HK, Steiger P, Madvig P. Low-dosage micronized 17 beta-estradiol prevents bone loss in postmenopausal women. *Am J Obstet Gynecol* 1992; 166:479–488.

7. Bolognese M. Effective pharmacotherapeutic interventions for the prevention of hip fractures. *The Endocrinologist* 2002; 12:29–37.

8. Liberman UA, Weiss SR, Broll J, Knickerbocker RK, Nicelsen T, Genant HK, Christiansen C, Delmas PD, Zanchetta JR, Stakkestad J, Gluer CC, Krueger K, Cohen FJ, Eckhert S, Ensrud KE, Avioli LV Lips P, Cummings SR. Effect of oral

alendronate on bone mineral density and the incidence of fractures in postmenopausal osteoporosis. The Alendronate Phase III Osteoporosis Treatment Study Group. *N Engl J Med* 1995; 333:1437–1443.

9. Ettinger B, Black DM, Mitlak BH, Helmut MW, Quan H, Bell NH, Portales JR, Downs RW Jr, Dequeker J, Fagvus M, Seeman E, Recker RR, Capizi T, Santora AC 2nd, Lombardi A, Shah RV, Hirsch LJ, Karpf DBl. Reduction of vertebral fracture risk in postmenopausal women with osteoporosis treated with raloxifene: results from a 3-year randomized clinical trial. Multiple Outcomes of Raloxifene Evaluation. (MORE) Investigators. *JAMA* 1999; 282:637–645.

10. Delmas PD, Bjarnason NH, Mitlak BH, Ravvoux AC, Shah AS, Huster WJ, Draper M, Christiansen C. Effects of raloxifene on bone mineral density, serum cholesterol concentrations, and uterine endometrium in postmenopausal women. *N Engl J Med* 1997; 337:1641–1647.

11. Johnston CC Jr, Bjarnason NH, Cohen FJ, Shah A, Lindsay R, Mitlak BH, Huster W, Draper MW, Harper KD, Heath H III, Gennari C, Arnaud CD, Delmas PD. Long-term effects of raloxifene on bone mineral density, bone turnover, and serum lipid levels in early postmenopausal women: three-year data from two double-blind, randomized, placebo-controlled trials. Arch Intern Med 2000; 160:3444–3450.

12. 2002 Heart and Stroke Statistical Update, Dallas Texas: American Heart Association; 2001.

13. Ettinger B, Friedman G, Bush T, Quesenberry CP Jr. Reduced mortality associated with long-term postmenopausal estrogen therapy. *Obstet Gynecol* 1996; 87:6–12.

14. Effects of estrogen or estrogen/progestin regimens on heart disease risk factors in postmenopausal women. The Postmenopausal Estrogen/Progestin Interventions (PEPI) Trial. The Writing Group for the PEPI Trial. *JAMA* 1995; 273:199–208.

15. Stampfer MH, Colditz GA. Estrogen replacement therapy and coronary heart disease: a quantitative assessment of the epidemiologic evidence. *Preventive Medicine* 1991; 20:47–63.

16. Lobo RA, Zacur HZ, Caubel P, Lane R. A novel intermittent regimen of norgestimate to preserve the beneficial effects of

17β-estradiol on lipid and lipoprotein profiles. *Am J Obstet Gynecol* 2000; 182:41–49.

17.   Hulley S, Grady D, Bush T, Furberg C, Herrington D, Riggs B, Vittinghoff E. Randomized trial of estrogen plus progestin for secondary prevention of coronary heart disease in postmenopausal women. Heart and Estrogen/Progestin Replacement Study (HERS) Research Group. *JAMA* 1998; 280:605–613.

18.   Herrington DM, Reboussin DM, Brosnihan KB, Sharp PC, Shumaker SA, Snyder TE, Furberg CD, Kowalchuk GJ, Stuckey TD, Rogers WJ, Givens DH, Waters D. Effects of estrogen replacement on the progression of coronary-artery atherosclerosis. *N Engl J Med* 2000; 343:522–529.

19.   Writing Group for the Women's Health Initiative Investigators. Risks and benefits of estrogen plus progestin in healthy postmenopausal women. *JAMA* 2002; 288:321–333.

20.   Creasman WT, Henderson D, Hinshaw W, Clarke-Pearson DL. Estrogen replacement therapy in the patient treated for endometrial cancer. *Obstet Gynecol* 1986; 67:326–330.

21.   Lee RB, Burke TW, Park RC. Estrogen replacement therapy following treatment for stage I endometrial carcinoma. *Gynecol Oncol* 1990; 36:189–191.

22.   Chapman JA, DiSaia PJ, Osann K, Roth PD, Gilotte DL, Berman ML. Estrogen replacement in surgical stage I and II endometrial cancer survivors. *Am J Obstet Gynecol* 1996; 175:1195–2000.

23.   Suriano KA, McHale M, McLean CE, Li KT, Re A, DiSaia PJ. Estrogen replacement therapy in endometrial cancer patients: a matched control study. *Obstet Gynecol* 2001; 97:555–560.

24.   Hormone replacement therapy in women treated for endometrial cancer. ACOG committee opinion: Committee on Gynecologic Practice, No. 235. May 2000. The American College of Obstetricians and Gynecologists, Washington, DC.

25.   Gass MLS, Taylor MB. Alternatives for women through menopause. *Am J Obstet Gynecol* 2001; 185:547–556.

26.   Cass I, Runowicz CD. Non-hormonal alternatives to treating menopausal symptoms. *Am J Managed Care* 1998; 4:732–739.

27.   Loprinzi CL, Barton DL, Rhodes D. Management of hot flashes in breast-cancer survivors. *Lancet Oncol* 2001; 2:199–204.

Index

Abnormal uterine bleeding. *See* AUB.

Adencanthoma, prognosis of, 253

Adencarcinoma
clinical disease I–III, 172–173
criteria for, 99–100
medroxyprogesterone acetate, 231
squamous epithelium, 100
TP53 gene mutation, 12

Adenosarcoma, 170–174, 171
clinical features, 170
clinicopathologic correlation, 172
differential diagnoses, 172
pathology, 170–172

Adenosquamous tumors, prognosis of, 253

Adjuvant chemotherapy
early stage EEC, 412–413
early uterine sarcomas, 475–477

Adjuvant hormonal therapy, EEC and, 416–417

Adjuvant radiotherapy, in uterine sarcomas, 477–478

Adnexal metastasis
endometrial cancer, 308–309
prognostic factors, 256–257
surgery for, 309
survival rates, 308

Age, as prognostic factor, 253

Akt serine/theronine kinase, PIP-3 and, 13

Akt/PI3 kinase pathway, 13, 437

Alendronate vs. ERT/HRT, for osteoporosis, 494

Amsterdam I/II, clinical diagnosis of HNPCC, 40

Anastrozole, 415

Androgen receptors, 52, 53

Aneuploidy, as prognostic factor, 259

Angiogenesis suppression
  as cancer therapy, 448–449
  VEGF/VEGFRs, 448
  definition of, 436, 444–451
  endometrial neoplastic
    transformation, 445
  TP (thymedine phosphatase),
    446
Antiangiogenesis, therapies for,
  448
APC/beta-catenin (CTNNB1),
  14–15
Apoptosis, and PTEN, 442
Arzoxifene, 415
Atypical hyperplasia, 94
  vs. adenocarcinoma, 102–103
  work-up for, 238
AUB (abnormal uterine
    bleeding), 193
  benign lesions, 197
  diagnosis, 220
  diet and stress, effects of, 204
  foreign bodies in vagina, 201
  herbal medicines, 203
  imaging technique, 204
  medications for, 202
  pregnancy and, 195
  systemic causes, 195
  tamoxifen, 202–203
  transvaginal sonography
    (TVS), 204
Avastin (VEGF bevacizumab),
  449

Bad, phosphorylated and
    PTEN, 442
BAX mutations
  colon cancers, 13
  MSI-positive endometrial
    cancers, 13
  TP53 gene mutation, 12

bcl-2, molecular genetics in
    endometrioid carcinoma,
    137
Benign lesions, 197
Beta-1 integrin expression,
  453
Bethesda criteria, for HNPCC,
  40
Bisphosphonates vs. ERT/HRT,
  for osteoporosis, 494
Bowel herniation, as
    complication of
    laparoscopy, 293
Brachytherapy
  high-dose rate, for inoperable
    patients, 394–396
  for vaginal recurrence, 389
Bulky residual disease,
    pathologic stage III,
    380–381

CA-125
  extrauterine disease and, 236
  as indicator of treatment
    failure, 236
Calcitonin vs. ERT/HRT, for
    osteoporosis, 495
Carbon dioxide retention, as
    complication of
    laparoscopy, 292
Carboplatin
  in chemotherapy, 409
  for ovarian adenocarcinoma,
    451
Carboplatin/paclitaxel,
    combination
    chemotherapy, 444
Carcinoma
  undifferentiated, 134
  well-differentiated, work-up
    for, 238

Carcinosarcoma, 174–178, 176,
  471
  adjuvant chemotherapy,
    475–476
  adjuvant radiotherapy,
    477–478
  clinical features, 175
  differential diagnoses,
    177–178
  gross pathology, 175
  microscopic pathology,
    175–177
  müllerian carcinoma, 175
  palliative chemotherapy,
    478–481
  uterine sarcomas, 354, 470
Cardiovascular disease,
  ERT/HRT, 495
Cellular atypia, endometrial
  hyperplasia and, 54
Cellular matrix, in cellular
  migration, 451
Cellular migration
  cellular matrix, 451
  integrin family receptors,
    451
  process of, 451
Cervical cancer, 200–201
Cervical involvement, in
  endometrioid carcinoma,
  110–111
Cetuximab (Erbitux), 439
c-fos, 52
CHD (coronary heart disease),
  495
Chemotherapy
  5–fluorouracil (5–FU), 444
  for advanced and recurrent
    EEC, 408–412
  carboplatin, 409
  cisplatin, 408, 479
  doxorubicin, 408, 479

etoposide, 444
isofamide, 444
paclitaxel, 409
radiation and, 413
topotecan, 444
Chromosome 10 deletions, 15
Chromosome 10q, 441
Chromosome 17p, 441
Cisplatin, 408, 479
Clear cell carcinoma, 129–130,
  131
  prognosis of, 253
ClinD-4 vs. ESS, 149
Clinical outcomes of surgical
  therapy (COST) study
  group, quality-of-life
  outcomes, 276
c-myc, 52
Colon cancer
  laparoscopy and, 295
  BAX mutations, 13
Colorectal cancer
  ERT/HRT, 495
  HNPCC, 37
    vs. familial adenomatous
      polyposis (FAP), 38
Combination chemotherapy
Carboplatin and paclitaxel, 444
  for uterine sarcomas, 479
Complex atypical hyperplasia
  vs. adenocarcinoma,
  98–99
COX-2, angiogenesis and, 446
Cross-talk, endometrial glands
  and stroma, 59–60
CTNNB1
  APC/beta-catenin and, 14–15
  MSI and, 15
Cytologic atypia, endometrial
  hyperplasia, 94, 234
Cytologic sampling,
  endometrial, 210

Cytoreductive surgery
  definition of, 306
  endometrial cancer and,
    313–315
  ovarian cancer, 307
  stage III, endometrial cancer,
    307–308
  theoretical basis, 306–307
  UPSC, 318–319
  various cancers and, 306
Cytosolic receptors, 65

Danazol, 416
DBD (DNA binding domain), 61
Dendritic cells and VEGF, 447
Dimethisterone, in endometrial
    hyperplasia, 233
DNA analysis, prognostic
    factor, 259–260
DNA binding domain (DBD), 61
DNA mismatch repair genes,
    441
  and cancer risk, 7
  defects in, 9–12
  endometrial cancer, 9
  frequency in endometrial
    cancer, 10
  gene mutation, cancer
    risk, 6
  HNPCC, 5, 39
  in uterine cancer, 3–4, 9
DNA replication error,
    endometrial cancer and,
    441
Doxorubicin, 408, 479
  vs. doxorubicin plus
    cyclophosphamide, 480
Dysfunctional uterine bleeding
    (DUB), 199–200
Dysmenorrhea, definition of,
    194

Edema, as complication of
    laparoscopy, 293
EEC (endometrioid endometrial
    carcinoma), 408–421
  chemotherapy for advanced
    and recurrent, 408–412
  hormonal therapy, 413–417
  molecular therapies, 420–421
  radiation, chemotherapy, 413
EGE, tumor growth
    dysregulation and,
    438–439
EGF, epidermal growth factor,
    52, 436
EGFR, 52
  endometrial cancer and, 438
  prognosis and, 437
EGFR families, oncogenesis
    and, 437
EGFR levels, survival and, 437
EMB (endometrial biopsy),
    210–212
  hysteroscopy and, 216
EMT (epithelial-mesenchymal
    transition), 453
EMX2 mutation, in endometrial
    cancer, 15–16
Endometrial carcinoma,
    radiation treatment for,
    343–345
Endometrial adenocarcinoma,
    and projestins, 55
Endometrial biopsy (EMB),
    210–212
Endometrial cancer, 200,
    435–454
  adnexal metastasis, 308–309
  advanced/recurrent, radiation
    treatment, 367–396
  classification of, 93
  clinical characteristics, 228,
    229–230

conservative treatment of, 227–454

cure rate, 436

cytoreductive surgery, 313–315

DNA mismatch repair, 9, 441

EMX2 mutation, 15–16

ERT/HRT, 497–498

endometrioid subtype, 92

gene defects in type I and II, 18

hereditary, incidence of, 35

HNPCC, 5, 36–37

hormone use, 92

hyperestrogenic states, 54–55

KRAS2 and MSI mutation in, 17

lymph node metastasis, 309–312

mixed types, 131–132

molecular genetics of, 134–139

MSI, HNPCC-related, 39

MSI, MLH1, 11

nonpolyposis colorectal cancer syndrome, 35–47

obesity and, 92

pathogenetic forms, 92

pathologic, stage III, 368–379

precursors of, 94

progesterone receptors in, 230

progestin, 231

prognostic factors, 248

radiation treatment and, 345–353

recurrence, effect of hormone replacement therapy, 498–501

serous carcinoma, 92

stage(s) I and II
  irradiation and, 345–346, 351–352

postoperative management, 345–353

risk of recurrence, 345–346

treatment regimen for, 240, 345–346

stage I and II, treatment recommendations, 352–348

stage III, 307–312

stage IV, 312–316

survival rates, 312–313

stage(s) I and II
  irradiation and, 345–346, 351–352

  postoperative management, 345–353

  risk of recurrence, 345–346

suramin, 450

surgical management of, 245–264

surgical studies, 316

systemic therapies, 407–421

taxmoifen and, 78–80

thalidomide, 450

Type I vs. Type II, 2–3

Type I, 2, 92

Type II, 2, 92

Endometrial cytologic sampling, 210

Endometrial glands, cross-talk with stroma, 59–60

Endometrial hyperplasia, 2, 436
  atypical, *98*

  causes of, 95

  cellular atypia and, 54

  complex, 97

  conservative treatment of, 227–454

  cytologic atypia, 94, 234

  definition of, 228

  diagnosis of, 95–97

  dimethisterone and, 233

Endometrial hyperplasia (*contd.*)
  medroxyprogesterone acetate
    and, 233
  megestrol acetate and, 233
  nuclear atypia, 96–97
  oxyprogesterone caproate
    (OPC), 232
  progestin therapy, 230–235
  progression of, 103
  rate of, 54
  simple vs. complex, 94
  simple, 96
  treatment failure, indicators
    of, 235
  treatment regimens, 238
Endometrial intraepithelial
    carcinoma (EIC),
    104–105
Endometrial sampling, 209–210
  tamoxifen screening, 86–87
Endometrial sarcoma,
    undifferentiated, 153
Endometrial stromal invasion,
    99
Endometrial stromal lesions,
    470
Endometrial stromal nodule
    (ESN), clinical features,
    148
Endometrial stromal sarcoma.
    See ESS.
Endometrial stromal tumors
  palliative chemotherapy and,
    482–483
  uterine sarcomas, 470
Endometrial tumorigenesis,
    and MSI, 11
Endometrioid adenocarcinoma
  DNA mismatch repair, 9
  KRAS2 mutation, 17
  squamous differentiation,
    118

villoglandular type, 114, 115
  well-differentiated, 100, 101
Endometrioid carcinoma,
    106–122
  cervical involvement, 110–111
  CTNNB1 and, 15
  differential diagnosis,
    107–108
  extrauterine factors, 108
  grading, 108–109
  gross findings, 106
  hormone receptor expression,
    112
  microscopic findings, 106–107
  molecular genetics of,
    134–138
  bcl-2, 137
  HER-2/neu, 138
  K-ras proto-oncogene, 137
  microsatellite instability,
    137–137
  oncogenes, 137
  patterns of spread, 113
  peritoneal cytology,
    prognostic factors,
    111
  positive aortic lymph nodes,
    112
  prognostic factors, 108–113
  PTEN tumor suppressor gene
    in, 135–136
  squamous dfferentiation,
    116–120
  behavior, 120
  differential diagnosis,
    119
  gross and microscopic
    findings, 117–119
  tumor grading, 106–107
  two-tiered vs. FIGO, 109
  Type I tumors, MSI, 11
  uterine factors, 108

vascular invasion, prognostic factors, 111

Endometrioid endometrial carcinoma. *See* EEC.

Endometrioid subtype, of endometrial carcinoma, 92

Endometrium, estrogen receptors and, 52–54

Endrometrial sampling, complications with, 213–214

EORTC study, uterine sarcoma, 355

Epidermal growth factor (EGF) in endometrial malignant transformation, 436

Epidermal growth factor receptors (EGFR), 436–440

Epithelial elements, classification of, 158–159

Epithelial neoplasms, 147–148
  epithelial/mesenchymal neoplasm, 147–148
  uterine sarcomas, classification of, 147–148, 149

Epithelial/mesenchymal neoplasm, 147–148

Epithelial-mesenchymal transition (EMT), 453

Epithelioid leiomyosarcomas, 164

ER, 52–54
  endometrium and, 52

ER level, tumor phenotype and, 56–57

ERA (estrogen replacement and atherosclerosis) trial, 496

Erbitux (cetuximab), 439

ERT (estrogen replacement therapy), 493–502
  vs. alendronate, for osteoporosis, 494
  vs. bisphosphonates, for osteoporosis, 494
  vs. calcitonin, for osteoporosis, 495
  for cardiovascular disease, 495
  for colorectal cancer, 495
  for coronary heart disease (CHD), 495
  for endometrical cancer, 497–498
  heart and estrogen/progestin replacement group study (HERS), 496
  vs. raloxifene, for osteoporosis, 495
  vs. risedronate, for osteoporosis, 495
  stroke and, 495
  women's health initiative, 497

ESN (endometrial stromal nodule), clinical features, 148

ESS (endometrial stromal sarcoma), 148–156, 358–360, 472
  antibody CD, 10, 152
  vs. clinical disease I—IV conditions, 154–156
  clinical features, 148–150
  clinicopathologic correlation, 153–154
  differential diagnosis, 154–156
  endometrial stromal sarcoma, 148–156
  gross pathology, 150

ESS (endometrial stromal
sarcoma) (*contd.*)
microscopic pathology,
150–152
prognosis of, 153
radiation and, 358–360
stages I and II, radiation
treatment alone, 359
with sex cord-like areas, *157*
undifferentiated, 168
uterine sarcoma, 354–355
Estrogen receptor level, as
prognostic factor, 258
Estrogen receptors. *See* ER.
Estrogen replacement and
atherosclerosis (ERA)
trial, 496
Estrogen replacement therapy.
See ERT.
Estrogen stimulaton,
endometrial cancer and,
54
Etoposide, chemotherapy, 444
Exenteration, pelvic recurrence,
treatment of, 384–390
External irradiation, technique
of, 360–361
Extrauterine spread, 473

5-Fluorouracil (5–FU), in
chemotherapy, 444
Familial adenomatous
polyposis (FAP)
vs. colorectal cancer, HNPCC
and, 38
manifestations of, 38
Fertility preservation,
hormonal therapy for
EEC, 417
FIGO (International Federation
of Obstetrics and

Gynecology) staging, 107,
247, 248, 251, 278, 367,
473
Focal adhesion kinases (FAK),
452

GEF (guanine exchange
factors), 452
Gefitinib (Iressa), 440
Genetics
changes in sporadic cancers,
9–17
DNA mismatch repair genes,
3–4
oncogenes, 3–4
tumor suppressor genes, 3–4
of uterine malignancies, 1–18
Genotypic progression in
cancer, 4
Germ line testing, HNPCC and,
41
GOG experience, laparoscopy,
297
GOG Phase III study, radiation
therapy, 346
GOG surgical staging study,
349
GOG-99 study, radiation
therapy, 346–347
GRA vs. GRB, 64–65
Guanine exchange factors
(GEF), 452

HDR brachytherapy, techniques
for, 361–362
Heart and estrogen/progestin
replacement group study
(HERS), 496
HER-2/neu
breast cancer and, 16

endometrioid carcinoma,
  molecular genetics of,
  138
oncogeneses and, 437
UPSC and, 438
Herbal medicines, 203
Herceptin (trastuzumab), 439
Hereditary nonpolyposis
  colorectal cancer. *See*
  HNPPC.
Histologic grade, and prognosis,
  249
HNPCC (hereditary
  nonpolyposis colorectal
  cancer), 5–7, 35
  chemoprevention, 46
  clinical criteria for diagnosis,
  40, 42
    Amsterdam I and II
    criteria, 40
    Bethesda criteria, 40
  colon cancer screening, 6
  colorectal cancer surgery, 37,
  47
  diagnosis of, 6–7
  DNA mismatch repair, 5
  endometrial cancer and,
  36–37
  fecal screening, 41
  gene mutation, MLH1 and
  MSH2, 3
  genetic basis of, 39–40
  germ line testing, 41
  gynecologic cancer surgery,
  46–47
  lifestyle effects, 46
  mismatch repair (MMR)
  genes, 36
  MSI screening, 41
  ovarian cancer, 37
  prophylactic surgery, 46–47

screening for, 44–45
testing recommendations,
  41–44
HNPCC-associated inherited
  endometrial cancer, 7
HNPCC-related cancers,
  clinical and pathologic
  features, 36–39
HNPCC-related endometrial
  cancer, 39
  genetic testing for, 41
HNPCC syndrome
  Lynch syndrome II, 36
  other malignancies, 38–39
Holbert study group. 205
Hormone receptor expression,
  prognostic factors in
  endometrioid carcinoma,
  112
Hormone receptor status,
  prognostic factor, 258
Hormone receptors, 54–56
Hormone replacement therapy
  (HRT), 493–502
  in EEC, 492, 47–45
HRT (hormone replacement
  therapy), 493–502.
HSG (hysterosalpingogram),
  208
Hyperplasia, atypical, 94
Hypomenorrhea, definition of,
  194
Hysterectomy
  alternatives to traditional
  abdominal, 261
  endometrial hyperplasia,
  234
  vs. progestin therapy, 234
  prognosis, with, 260
Hysterosalpingogram (HSG),
  208

Hysteroscopy, 214
  complications with, 216–217
  EMB, 216
  tumor cells, 220

Ifosfamide, 444, 481
  combinations, uterine
    sarcomas, 479, 480
  plus cisplatin, 480
IHC
  ER levels and, *57,* 57–58
  PR levels and, *58*
  steroid receptor status and,
    56–59
Immunohistochemistry. *See*
  IHC.
Infralevator, pelvic
  exenteration, 333
Inherited risk, of uterine
  cancer, 4–8
Inoperable patients, radiation
  therapy and, 390–396
Integrin family receptors, in
  cellular migration, 451
Intermenstrual bleeding,
  definition of, 194
International Federation of
  Obstetrics and
  Gynecology (FIGO)
  surgical staging system,
  246
Iressa (gefitinib), 440
Irradiation, technique of
  external, 360–361
Isofamide, 444
Isoforms, receptor, 61–65
  ERα vs. ERβ, 63–64
  GRA vs. GRB, 64–65
  PRA vs. PRB, 61–63
Isolated adnexal invasion
  pathologic stage III, 372–373

K-ras, serous carcinoma,
    molecular genetics of,
    139
K-ras proto-oncogene,
    molecular genetics of,
    137
K-ras2 and MSI mutation
  in colon cancer, 17
  in endometrial cancers, 17

Laparoscopic equipment,
    development of, 279
Laparoscopically assisted
    vaginal hysterectomy,
    bilateral salpingo-
    oophorectomy
    (LAVH/BSO), 280
Laparoscopy
  age as contraindication, 286
  bowel herniation, 293
  carbon dioxide retention, 292
  colon cancer, 295
  complications of, 291–297
  development of, 277
  edema, 293
  GOG experience, 297
  vs. laparotomy, 276
  obesity as contraindication,
    285
  positive peritoneal cytology,
    294
  potential benefits, 289–290
  pros and cons, 276
  public demand for, 275–279
  quality of life, 290
  recurrence and survival risk,
    294–297
  surgical candidate selection,
    284–288
  surgical techniques, 280
  training for, 288

treatment algorithms, 284
vascular lacerations, 291
Laparotomy vs. laparoscopy, 276
LAVH/BSO (laparoscopically assisted vaginal hysterectomy, bilateral salpingo-oophorectomy), 280
 clinical disease I, 166
 clinical disease II, 166
 clinical disease III, 167–168
 clinical disease IV, 168
Leiomyosarcoma, 471
 adjuvant chemotherapy, 476–477
 adjuvant radiotherapy, 478
 vs. clinical disease(s) I-IV, 166–168
 clinical features, 161
 clinicopathologic correlation, 165–166
 definition of, 160
 diagnostic criteria, 166–167
 gross pathology, 161–162
 microscopic appearance, 162–164
 palliative chemotherapy, 481–482
 prognosis, 165
 uterine sarcoma, 354, 357–358, 470
Ligand binding assays, steroid receptor status and, 56–59
Loss of heterozygosity (LOH), 15
PTEN, 441–442
LVSI (lymph-vascular space invasion), prognostic factor, 257–258
LY260022, as PI3–K inhibitor, 444

Lymph node metastasis, lymphadenectomy, 309–310
 clinical stage I vs. II (occult) disease, 251
 prognostic factors, 250
 survival rates, 311–312
 tri-modality therapy, 311
Lymph node pathologic stage III, 374–378
Lymphadenectomy
 determination of, 261
 safety of, 262
Lymph-vascular space invasion (LVSI), prognostic factor, 257–258
Lynch syndrome II (HNPCC syndrome), 5, 36

Magnetic resonance imaging (MRI), 209
Malignancies, molecular genetics of, 1–18
Malignant mesodermal mixed tumor (MMMT)/ carcinosarcoma, 132–134
Malignant mixed müllerian tumor (MMMT). *See* carcinosarcoma.
Matrix metallo-proteinases (MMP), 444
 in gynecologic cancer, 453
Medroxyprogesterone acetate (MPA)
 adencarcinoma, 231
 endometrial cancer and, 447
 endometrial hyperplasia, 233, 238
Megace regimen, atypical hyperplasia, 239

Megestrol acetate, endometrial hyperplasia, 230, 233, 238

Menomemorrhagia, definition of, 194

Menopause, definition of, 194

Mesenchymal epithelial neoplasms, 147–148

Mesenchymal-epithelial transition (MET), 453

Metabolite E, tamoxifen and, 80

Metalloptroteinase inhibitors (MPIs) as anticancer agents, 453

Microsatellite instability (MSI), 5, 39
  endometrioid carcinoma, molecular genetics of, 136–137
  phenotype, endometrial cancer, 9

Mismatch repair (MMR) genes, HNPCC and, 36

Mixed mesenchymal elements, classification of, 158–159

Mixed mesodermal tumors, uterine sarcoma, 354, 356–357

MLH1
  analysis, clinical implications of, 11
  endometrial cancer MSI, 11
  HNPCC gene mutation, 39

MLH1 promoter, methylatin of, 11

MMMT (malignant mixed müllerian tumor). *See* Carcinosarcoma.

MMMT/carcinosarcoma, malignant mesodermal mixed tumor, 132–134

MMP (matrix metallo-proteinases), 444

MMR (mismatch repair) genes, 36

Molecular markers, indicator of treatment failure, 236

Molecular therapies, in EEC, 420–421

MRI (magnetic resonance imaging), 209
  as indicator of treatment failure, 237

MSH2, HNPCC gene mutation, 39

MSH6 mutation and cancer risk, 7

MSI (microsatellite instability)
  endometrial tumorigenesis, 11
  endometrioid endometrial carcinoma, 10–11
  HNPCC-related endometrial cancer, 39
  Hyperplasia and, 11
  K-ras2 mutation and, 17
  levels and cancer risk, 7
  microsatellite instability, 5, 9, 39
  screening, HNPCC, 41

MSI-positive endometrial cancers
  BAX mutations, 13
  somatic mutations, 11

Mucinous adenocarcinoma, 120–122, *121*

Müllerian adenosarcomas, 472
  palliative chemotherapy, 483

Müllerian neoplasms, mixed, 169–170

Multimodality adjuvant therapy, 484

Myometrial invasion, and
    prognosis, 109, 248, 250
Myxoid leiomyosarcoma, 164

National Cancer Institute of
    Canada—Clinical Trials
    Group (NCIC) study on
    radiation, 347
Neo-vagina, pelvic
    exenteration, 336
Nonpolyposis colorectal cancer
    syndrome, endometrial
    cancer, 35–47
Nordic Society for Gynecologic
    Oncology (NSG 9501)
    study on radiation,
    348–349
Nuclear atypia, endometrial
    hyperplasia, 96–97

Obesity
    and endometrial carcinoma,
        92
    in surgical candidate
        selection for laparoscopy,
        285
Oligomenorrhea, definition of,
    194
Oncogenes, 16–17
    endometrioid carcinoma,
        molecular genetics of, 137
    tumorigenesis and, 435–436
    in uterine cancer, 3–4
Oncogenic Ras, in tumor
    metastasis, 451–452
OPC (oxyprogesterone
    caproate), 232
Optimally debulked stage III,
    pathologic stage III,
    373–374

Osteoporosis, ERT/HRT, 494
Ovarian adenocarcinoma
    carboplatin in, 451
    paclitaxel in, 451
Ovarian cancer
    cytoreductive surgery, 307
    HNPCC, 36
Oxyprogesterone caproate
    (OPC), and endometrial
    hyperplasia, 232

p53 expression, indicator of
    treatment failure, 236
Pathologic stage III, clinical
    stage IV, 381–382
Paclitaxel
    in chemotherapy, 409
    for ovarian adenocarcinoma,
        451
Palliative chemotherapy in
    uterine sarcomas,
    337–338, 478–483
Papillary serous carcinomas,
    prognosis of, 253
Para-aortic lymphadenectomy,
    281–283
    lymph node matastasis,
        lymphadenectomy, 310
Para-aortic node metastases,
    incidence of, 252
Pathologic stage III, 368–379
    bulky residual disease after
        surgery, 380–381
    clinical stage III/IV, 379–380
    debulked stage III,
        373–374
    hormonal therapy, 371
    isolated adnexal invasion,
        372–373
    lymph node positive stage
        IIIC, 374–378

Pathologic stage III (*contd.*)
  positive peritoneal cytology,
    368–372
  prognosis, 370
  radiation, 370–371
Pelvic exenteration
  anterior infralevator, with
    vulvectomy, 335
  classification of, 333
  definition of, 333
  indications for/preoperative
    evaluation, 330–331
  for recurrent EC, 329–337
  resection of pelvic organs,
    332–334
  surgical exploration
    331–332
  surgical reconstruction,
    334–335
  types of, 334
Pelvic lymphadenectomy,
  280–281
Pelvic node metastases,
  incidence of, 252
Pelvic radiation, PORTEC
  randomized trial,
  383–384
Pelvic recurrence, incidence of,
  382–384
  radiation therapy for,
    382–390
  treatment of, 384–390
    exenteration, 384–390
    radical radiation,
      384–389
    vaginal recurrence,
      386–390
Peritoneal cytology
  in early stage endometrial
    cancer, 255
  prognostic factor, 111,
    254–255

Phase III studies,
  advanced/recurrent
  endometrial cancer, 411
Phenotypic progression, in EC,
  4
Phosphatidylinositol (3,4,5)
  triphosphate (PIP-3), 13
Phosphorylated band, PTEN
  and, 442
PI3–K (p-13 kinase) family, 452
  inhibitor, LY260022, 444
PIP-3 and Akt serine/theronine
  kinase, 13
Polycystic ovarian syndrome
  (PCOS), 228
Polymenorrhea, definition of,
  194
PORTEC randomized trial,
  pelvic radiation,
  383–384
Positive aortic lymph nodes,
  prognostic factors, 112
Positive peritoneal cytology,
  pathologic stage III,
  368–372
Positive peritoneal washings,
  in, stage IIIA
  endometrial carcinoma,
  370
Postmenopausal bleeding,
  definition of, 194
Postmenopausal
  estrogen/progestin
  interventions (PEPI)
  trial, 494
Progesterone receptor (PR),
  52–54
  concentration, indicator of
    treatment failure, 235
  in endometrial cancers, 230
  level, as prognostic factor,
    258

expression, 55–56
tumor phenotype and, 56–57
PRA and PRB, 52–53, 53,
    61–63
Pregnancy, AUB, 195
Proangiogenic growth factors,
    444
Progesterone, endometrial
    cancer and, 54–55
Progestin, and endometrial
    cancer, 54, 231
Progestin therapy
  in advanced recurrent EEC,
    413–417
  endometrial adenocarcinoma
    and, 55
  in endometrial carcinoma,
    231, 447
  in endometrial hyperplasia,
    230–235, 238
  vs. hysterectomy, 234
  metestrol, 230
  side effects of, 239, 413
Prognositic factors
  adnexal metastases, 256–257
  age as, 253
  cervical involvement, in
    endometriod carcinoma,
    110–111
  DNA analysis, 259–260
  for endometriod carcinoma,
    111
  FIGO grade, 248
  hormone receptor expression,
    112
  lymph node metastases, 250
  myometrial invasion, 109,
    248
  peritoneal cytology, 254–255
  positive aortic lymph nodes,
    112
  tumor histology, 252

tumor size, 258
Proteases, effect of, 453
Protooncogenes, 52
PTEN (putative protein tyrosine
    phospatase/tensin), 441
  apoptosis and, 442
  phosphorylated Bad and, 442
PTEN mutation
  cancer and 441–442
  loss of heterozygosity (LOH)
    cancer and, 441–442
  metastatic potential, 443
  PI3–K products and, 442
  serous carcinoma, molecular
    genetics of, 139
  type I and II cancers, 14, 442
  uterine sarcoma, 16
  wild-type, 442
PTEN pathway inhibitors,
    443–444
PTEN tumor suppressor gene,
    8, 13–14
PTEN-P13 kinase, 441–444
Putative protein tyrosine
    phosphatase/tenisin. *See*
    PTEN.

Rac GTPase, 452
Radiation therapy
  for advanced recurrent
    endometrial cancer,
    367–396
  vs. chemotherapy, EEC, 413
  for clinical stage III/IV
    disease, pathologic stage
    III, 379–380
  for clinical stage IV, pathologic
    stage III, 381–382
  endometrial cancer
    (PORTEC) study group,
    350–351

Radiation therapy *(contd.)*
  for endometrial cancer,
      345–353
  for endometrial stromal
      sarcoma, 358–360
  GOG phase III/GOG-99
      study, 346–347
  inoperable EC patients,
      390–396
  National Cancer Institute of
      Canada–Clinical Trials
      Group (NCIC) study,
      347
  operable vs. inoperable
      patients, 392–394
  pelvic recurrence and, 382–390
  treatment sequelae,
      inoperable patients,
      396–397
  uterine sarcoma, 354–358
Radical hysterectomy, 261
Radical radiation, pelvic
      recurrence, treatment of,
      384–389
Ral GEFs, 452
Raloxifene, 415
  vs. ERT/HRT, for
      osteoporosis, 495
Rapamycin (mTOR) protein, 443
Ras effectors, 452
Ras genes, 16–17
Ras proteins, 451
Ras-Raf-MAP kinase pathway,
      437
Receptor isoforms, 61–65
  ERa vs. ERb, 63–64
  GRA vs. GRB, 64–65
  PRA vs. PRB, 61–63
Receptor tyrosine kinases,
      VEGF and, 445
Recurrent EC
  definition of, 328

pelvic exenteration and,
      329–337
  treatment for, 328
  surgical management of,
      327–337
Retroperitoneal left-sided para-
      aortic lymphadectomy,
      283
Right para-aortic
      lymphadenectomy,
      281
Risedronate vs. ERT/HRT, for
      osteoporosis, 495
RTOG 99–05 trial, radiation,
      347–348

Salvage therapy for vaginal
      recurrence, survival
      rates, 387
Sarcoma
  TP53 gene mutation in, 12
  miscellaneous pure, 169
Selective estrogen receptor
      modulators (SERMs),
      414–415
Serous carcinoma, 122–129,
      124, 125, 126, 127
  behavior, 128
  differential diagnosis,
      127–128
  endometrial carcinoma, 92
  gross findings, 122
  microscopic findings,
      123–126
  molecular genetics of,
      138–140
  k-ras, 139
  PTEN, 139
  vs. villoglandular carcinoma,
      127
Sirolimus mTOR and, 443

Smooth muscle neoplasm, predictor of malignancy, 160–161

Society of Gynecologic Oncologists (SGO), conservative therapy survey, 234

Somatic mutations, MSI-positive endometrial cancers, 11

Sonographic staging, of endometrial cancer, 237

Sonohysterography (SIS), 207–208

S-phase function, prognostic factor, 259
  genetic changes, 9–17
  and PTEN tumor suppressor gene, 8

"Sporadic" disease, uterine cancer, 4, 9–12

Squamous epithelium. and adencarcinoma, 100

SR suppression, genomic effects of, 60–61

Stage(s) of disease, 246
  at diagnosis, distribution by, 246
  stage(s) I and II, irradiation alone, 359
  stage III endometrial cancer, 307–312, 368–379
  stage IIIA, positive peritoneal washings only, results, 370
  stage IIIC patients with positive pelvic or para-aortic lymph nodes, radiation, 376
  stage III-IV, radiation, 368–382

stage IV, 312–316

Steroid hormone, non-genomic effects of, 65–66

Steriod hormone receptors, 51–66
  endometrial cancer, 54–56
  IHC and, 56–59
  ligand binding assays and, 56–59
  normal endometrium, 52–54

Stroke, ERT/HRT, 495

Stroma, cross-talk with endometrial glands, 59–60

Supralevator pelvic exenteration, 333

Suramin, endometrial cancer and, 450

Surgery
  approaches, 260–263
  contraindications for, 390

Survival curves, 319

Susceptibility genes, familial breast cancer, 8

Systemic therapies, endometrial carcinoma, 407–421

Tamoxifen, 202–203, 415
  breast cancer and, 81–82
  effects on endometrium, 77–87
  endometrial cancer and, 78–80, 447
  histology in uterine cancer, 80–84
  incidence of endometrial cancer and, 84
  metabolite E and, 80
  screening, 84–87

Tamoxifen (*contd.*)
    transvaginal sonography
        (TVS), 84–86
    studies relating to, 78–80
    uterine cancer and, recent
        series, 83
Tarceva, 440
TGF-a expression, 441
TGF-b expression, 441
TGF, transforming growth
    factors, 440–441
Thalidomide, endometrial
    carcinoma and, 450,
Thymedine phosphatase (TP),
    in angiogenesis, 446
TK receptors, 436
Topotecan, in chemotherapy,
    410
TP (thymedine phosphatase), in
    angiogenesis, 446
TP53 gene mutation, 12–16
    adenocarcinomas, 12
    BAX, 12
    sarcoma, 12
    type I and II cancers, 12
Transforming growth factors
    (TGF), 440–441
Transvaginal sonography
    (TVS), 84–86
Trastuzumab (herceptin), 439
Tri-modality lymph node
    matastasis,
    lymphadenectomy, 311
Triphosphate PIP-3,
    phosphatidylinositol(3,4,
    5), 13
Tumor histology, prognostic
    factor, 252
Tumor phenotype, high PR/ER
    level and, 56–57
Tumor size, prognostic factor, 258
Tumor suppressor genes

defects, 12–16
tumorigeneisis, 3–4, 435–436
uterine cancer, 3
Tumorigenesis, uterine cancer
    and, 3–4
TVS (transvaginal sonography),
    204
Type I endometrial carcinoma,
    2, 14, 18, 92
Type II carcinomas, 2, 92,
    104–105

Undifferentiated ESS, 168
UPSC, 438, 417–420
    adjuvant therapy for, 419–420
    chemotherapy for, 417–418
    cytoreductive surgery, 318–319
    features of, 317
    incidence of, 318
    survival rates, 317
Uterine mesenchymal elements,
    classification of, 158–159
Uterine neoplasms, with sex
    cord-like elements,
    156–159
Uterine papillary serous
    carcinoma. *See* UPSC.
Uterine sarcoma, 147–178
    adjuvant chemotherapy in,
        475–477
    adjuvant radiotherapy in,
        477–478
    carcinosarcomas, 354
    combination therapy, 479
    DNA mismatch repair, 9
    endometrial stromal sarcoma,
        354–355
    EORTC study, 355
    epidemiology and incidence,
        469–471
    extended staging of, 474–475

familial inherited
    susceptibility, 7
hormonal therapy in,
    483–484
ifosfamide-based combination
    regimens, 479
leiomyosarcomas, 354,
    357–358
management of, 469–484
mixed mesodermal tumors,
    354, 356–357
palliative chemotherapy in,
    478–483
prognostic factors, 354,
    471–472
radiation treatment for,
    354–358
stages I and II, postoperative
    management, 354–358
surgical staging of, 472–475
types of, 354

Vaginal hysterectomy, 261
Vaginal recurrence
brachytherapy for, 389
pelvic recurrence, treatment
    of, 386–390
results of treatment of, 388
Vascular endothelial growth
    factor (VEGF), 445
isoforms of, 445
Vascular endothelium (VE), 444

Vascular invasion, prognostic
    factors, 111
Vascular lacerations,
    complications of
    laparoscopy, 291
Vascular space invasion,
    indicator of treatment
    failure, 236
VE (vascular endothelium), 444
VEGF
activity, 445
receptor tyrosine kinases,
    445
bevacizumab (Avastin), 448
dendritic cells and, 447
expression, in endometrial
    carcinoma, 445
vascular endothelial growth
    factor, 445
Villoglandular adenocarcinoma,
    113–116, *114, 115*
vs. serous carcinoma, 127
von Willebrand's disease, 200

WHO classification of
    endometrial carcinoma,
    93, 107
WHO histopathologic
    classification, 107
Wild-type, PTEN, 442
Women's health initiative,
    ERT/HRT, 497